Clear Skin For Everyone

Clear Skin For Everyone

A practical lifestyle guide
to clear, healthy skin
for good, for real.

Kimberly Yap Tan

Clear Skin For Everyone
A practical lifestyle guide to clear, healthy skin for good, for real.

ISBN 978-1-7364772-0-5

Copyright © 2023 by Kimberly Yap Tan

All rights reserved. No part of this publication may be reproduced, stored in a retrieval system, or transmitted in any form or by any means - electronic, mechanical, photocopying, recording, or any other - except for brief quotations in printed reviews, without prior permission of the copyright holder.

www.withandwithin.com

Cover design, interior design and illustrations: Hester van Toorenburg
www.naiabookdesign.com

Liberation for all, with & within.

Clear Skin for Everyone

Contents

Clear Skin for Good, for Real 10
San Francisco's First Holistic Adult Acne Clinic 12
How to Use This Book 14
What to Expect... 20

Section 1 - Start with the Obvious - Your Skincare Face Regimen 22

Plan Overview 24
Understand Skin Types and Conditions 26
Understand Products 34
How to Start the Clearing Process 50
What to Expect During the Clearing Process 65
How to Wash Your Face and Use Your Products 70
Body and Hair Care in the Shower 90
Makeup 94
Hairstyling Products 100
Picking 102

Section 2 - Acne 101 110

Genetics and Acne 112
Acne Types 115
Inspiring (and Real) Acne Case Studies 132
Other Acne Approaches 139

Section 3 - The 5 Types of Hormone Stress Responsible for Acne 148

Understanding "Stress" 150

Contents

The Five Types of Stress 152

Section 4 - Lifestyle 160
Practical Daily Life 163
Travel 185
With & Within Acne Face Map 197

Section 5 - The Digestive System, Diet and Acne 202
How to Eat 204
Eating Acne-safe 216
Medications and Nutritional Supplements 231

Section 6 - Candida 236
What is Candida? 238
Other Candida Approaches 240
How to Get it Under Control 241
The Acne-safe Candida Cleanse 244
What to Do with Your Face 252

Section 7 - Working With a Professional Esthetician 254
How to Find One 256
What to Look for & What to Ask 257
The Treatment 260
Give It Time 262

Section 8 - The With & Within Standard of Treatment 264

Our Therapists 266
Our Acne Treatments 267

Section 9 - Feeling Stuck? Let's Reassess 276

Let's Check-in 278
Strengthen Your Program 280
Professional Help: an Esthetician 284

Section 10 - Maintaining Your Clear Skin 286

What Does My Maintenance Regimen Look Like? 288
Regimen Adjustment Ideas 289
Reintroducing Questionable Variables 291
When Do I Need Treatments? 292
Importance of Maintaining an Acne-safe Lifestyle and Diet 292
Scarring 292

Section 11 - Additional Resources 296

With & Within Lifestyle Library Blog 298
Books on Skin 299
Comedogenic Ingredients 299
With & Within Products and Shop 300
Body-Focused Repetitive Behaviors (BFRB) 302
Food 305
General Wellness 306

Contents

Communication and Relational Skills 307
Self-care and Meditation 308

Section 12 - Finale 310
Finale 312
Gratitude 312
About Kim and With & Within's Story 315

Section 13 - Glossary 318
Glossary 320

Section 14 - Index 326
Index 328

Clear Skin for Good, for Real

You've got acne, and you've probably had it for a while now. Maybe you grew up with it as a teen. Or maybe it came out of nowhere (the adult onset kind). Or acne didn't run in your family at all. You're an adult who just shouldn't be breaking out anymore. You're over it. Done with caking on the makeup, hiding behind your hair or caps pulled low, the physical pain of the zits themselves (let alone the emotional hit on your self-esteem). You're overusing all the filters and photo editing tricks. Aunties at family parties giving you unsolicited advice on how to fix your face, feeling like you're not confident enough to date. Not being taken seriously when you're up to get that promotion you deserve. Taking forever to get ready and leave the house. Or maybe you just avoid going out altogether. You're over it. All of it.

And so, being the empowered adult you are, you've taken the initiative to do some research to figure out what on earth is going on with your skin and what to do about it. Why does your face make you look like a teen when you're a fully grown adult? You're constantly internet-searching for what to do about those damn zits, trying all the things and spending all the time and resources to try and get your skin under control. You've bought all the miracle skin products on your Instagram feed, gotten countless skin treatments, tried all kinds of extreme diets, did some 26-step face routine some beauty blogger *swore* would get rid of your acne in three days. And when that didn't work, you took all the supplements and prescription drugs that sensitize your skin, incite yeast infections or digestive troubles, that maybe worked just okay for a while or didn't do anything.

By the time you were done doing everything you could to get rid of your acne, you hit rock bottom, completely giving up and resigning yourself to a life with zits. It may feel like you've reached a dead end on the road to decent, if not clear, skin. Thankfully, a detour is available, and you're holding it in your very hands.

I'm Here to Help!

This book is your detailed roadmap to long-term clear skin, tested and proven thousands of times over nearly two decades of my career as a holistically acne-focused esthetician. We'll actually get to the root source of the skin problems in order to correct them instead of using temporary bandages for a temporary fix.

Running With & Within (then called skinSALVATION), San Francisco's first holistic adult acne skincare clinic, taught me and my thousands of clients so many things about solving the acne problems many people face, and in this book, I share them all with you. Everything I've learned, observed, and researched in our brick-and-mortar clinic since we first opened in 2008 is distilled into this book to help save you time, resources, and disappointment and gain more confidence, fulfillment, and joy. To make all these clear skin "secrets" accessible for everyone everywhere to achieve their best health, lives, and world through clear skin and a more intentional, thoughtful, and informed lifestyle. By using the techniques inside these pages, not only will your skin look better, you'll gain more awareness and thus control over what's happening on your face and in your body. You'll soon be feeling and living better *in your own skin*, every inch of it.

I'm not a skincare guru, fanatic, or any kind of skin fairy miracle worker. I like to think of myself more as a guide or facilitator because it's *you* who's going to have to do the work day in and day out. Healthy, clear skin comes down to a good and consistent routine that includes skincare, dietary and lifestyle changes to optimize your body functions and genetics (which is something one can't completely or easily control). Everything else, though, to some degree, you *can* influence. And I will show you exactly how.

By gaining self-awareness and learning to use the tools that'll more positively influence the things in your life affecting your skin, you (likely) won't need to pay anyone to fix your skincare problems. And you won't need to rely on others—or monthly facials for life—to keep your skin healthy and clear. With this book, you *will* learn to identify and fix these acne-causing imbalances yourself. We'll take a deep dive into what we're dealing with and then plunge deeper into skin, body, and lifestyle best practices so you can get to the true root source of your skin problems.

Time + money + emotional stress + physical stress + negative effects from all the products or diets you may be trying can all equal more acne. With so much information to sort through, it can be very confusing and overwhelming, and the lackluster results may make you want to give up altogether. But have no fear; I'll give you very specific and actionable directions to guide you.

One Last Thing...

Be easy on yourself. Life is hard enough, and dealing with acne can certainly be devastating on so many levels. None of this acne is your fault, so let go of that. Things you will learn in this book, you didn't know until you knew! And it's only once you know that you can have the agency to make changes as you see fit.

I hope this book helps you stop obsessing over your skin so that you can be your best and fullest self. That your newfound freedom and confidence will open up whole new meaningful worlds for you to explore and grow into, contributing positively to your loved ones, community, and society. The world needs a happy and healthy you now more than ever. Self-care is not selfish; it is, in fact, the foundation for all positive change to happen. The compounding beneficial effects of self-care reverberate through your actions, touching your community and the world. I am so glad to put everything I know into this book to get you feeling healthy in your body, peaceful in your mind, and happy in your own skin!

If the injustices that are happening in the world bother you, the first radical step to changing the world truly is self-care.

> "Caring for myself is not self-indulgence. It is self-preservation, and that is an act of political warfare." – Audre Lorde, *A Burst of Light and Other Essays*.

San Francisco's First Holistic Adult Acne Clinic

After working all around the San Francisco Bay Area as an esthetician, I started working with Laura Cooksey of Face Reality Skincare in San Leandro, California and studying in-person with Dr. James E. Fulton Jr. (pioneer researcher of acne, co-creator of Retin-A, stabilizer of benzoyl peroxide for acne, among many other achievements, from Miami, Florida). Drawing from these pioneers, I combined my work and study experience with my own journey and learning in holistic healing to start With & Within (then called skinSALVATION), San Francisco's first holistic adult acne skincare clinic, in 2008. Since then, my team and I have helped thousands of adults naturally clear and successfully manage their acne in an average of three months through skin treatments, acne-safe skin products, and lifestyle education—no prescription medications needed.

In all my years of treating skin, I found that only treating the skin topically offered short-term results; the real secret to long-term clear skin is living an acne-safe lifestyle. Attacking acne on all three fronts with effective skincare products, lifestyle education, and treatments cleared people up the fastest, for the longest. Repeating this process with thousands of clients with consistently good results over the years has proven our approach effective, safe, and reliable.

And although it's just one significant part of our lifestyle, using good, effective skin products consistently in the right way twice daily makes a big impact in getting and keeping skin its clearest—much like brushing your teeth in-between dentist visits. Meeting the needs of our clients shaped our product philosophy and best practices sourcing (and eventually formulating) them to ensure we only sell products that are acne-safe.

For my clinic, I carefully shopped for products with acne-safe ingredient listings. After finding products that looked good on paper, I would test them in-house for several months on my clear-skinned team and clients before selling them in the shop. These folks were perfect test subjects, because since they were already living an acne-safe lifestyle, any new breakouts could be isolated to that one variable–the product they were testing. As you can imagine, finding these products is a very painstaking and time-consuming process because the vast majority available on the market are comedogenic. A very special thanks to employees and clients over the years who have willingly tested products for us, helping to ensure what we offer is safe for all to use.

I soon realized that all the things we taught our clients to help clear their skin were generally good practices for *everyone* to embody, not just those acne-affected. Alongside topical care and product advice, we encouraged our clients to live relaxed, enjoyable, and low-inflammatory lifestyles nourished with natural and minimally processed foods, robust digestive systems, and low-stress, active and restful lives. Every diet trend, fad, or life "hack" that has come out over the years seems to be some interpretation of these same principles.

In 2023, we changed our name to With & Within, expanding our offerings of self-care to include more than just skincare: enhancing one's quality of life through nutrition, daily life stress management practices, and travel. When a healthy, happy, and fulfilled mind and body are in harmony, clear skin is sure to follow.

With all this said, my goal with this book is to make everything I've learned about acne accessible, actionable, and effective for everyone, everywhere. Most of what's in this book is educational, technical, and practical, none of which is particularly brand-specific. You'll learn tools to shop for skin products, and at appropriate times, I will mention our skincare products in passing as examples of what to look for when shopping.

This book was written to give you the power to clear your skin on your own terms. Everything I know and think about acne is here for you to utilize. I'm so excited for you, your journey, and your future! With us, I hope to help you rediscover the intuition that lies Within to heal, thrive, and to enjoy life.

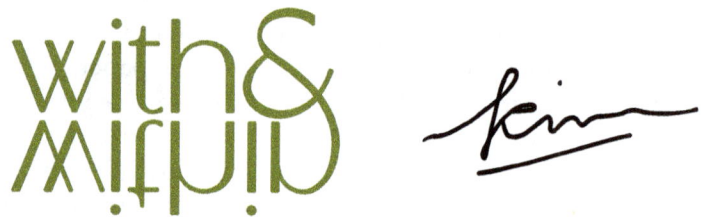

How to Use This Book

You're probably wondering what you're getting into. What exactly do you need to do to get clear skin? There's a lot of information in this book, but we'll take it one step at a time. Changing up your products to purge existing and prevent new acne from forming may be all you need to do to clear up. But if this first step improves your acne without totally getting rid of it, the wisdom that lies in the rest of the book is here for you.

The content in this book and the With & Within skin clearing program are unique, comprehensive, and, with your dedication, incredibly effective. I'll teach you about how skin and acne work, how the body works as a whole, and the precise lifestyle and dietary factors that can contribute to and aggravate your unique acne experience. You'll learn what products should do for the skin and how to assemble and properly use a truly effective and acne-safe skin clearing regimen.

You'll also receive informational tidbits to help you better understand both the skincare and natural holistic health world. I'll help you determine whether or not you have a possible hormonal or digestive system imbalance that's keeping your skin from being its clearest. We'll also highlight how different the With & Within approach is from traditional skincare programs (spas, dermatologists' offices, or on your own in a drugstore or upscale skincare aisle), and how to find a professional to help (should you need one).

Most people will see a marked improvement within the first four weeks and achieve true clarity around the three-month mark. For some with more stubborn cases, it can take up to six months, possibly with the help of a local esthetician. Just remember to be gentle, honest, and patient with yourself as you diligently follow the acne-safe lifestyle until you finally clear up.

The work is simple but not necessarily easy. Before we get into the practical side of things, I'd like to share some pragmatic tips to set you up for success and let you know what to expect.

The sage, the student and the cup

The student traveled far to consult with the wisest of teachers. Atop the highest mountain, in a humble shack, the student found the sage. "Tell me the purpose of your visit," said the teacher, pouring the student a cup of tea.

"I have apprenticed myself to the world's best instructors, read volumes, memorized every lesson, and tested my skills against the brightest minds," the student replied. "I know the laws of nature, man, and the universe. What can I learn from you—an old hermit?"

As the student spoke, the teacher poured... and poured...and poured...until the tea overflowed onto the table, then the floor.

"Stop!" cried the student. "Can't you see that the tea is overflowing?"

"Yes, I see," said the sage, "that I cannot serve you, because your cup is already full."

- Zen proverb

Begin by Emptying Your Cup

I learned of this story from an acupuncturist in San Francisco, and it really resonated with me. Most clients who came to With & Within for help were so desperate for clear skin, they did everything we told them to do and cleared up beautifully. These are what I considered to be the "easy" cases.

After just a few months of their hard work, their skin cleared up quickly—and stayed that way with lifestyle maintenance, and for some, seasonal skin treatments.

Maybe after all you've been through, you're now wondering, "Will this work for me?" My toughest clients were in the same boat. At first, they were skeptical (and sometimes even resistant) of the lifestyle advice we'd give them based on their past disappointing experiences. But when *they finally emptied their cups* and became more consistent with (and held accountable to) our suggestions, they started to see the results they were looking for all along.

Think of this book as a lifestyle change guide toward healthier, acne-safe living; a chance to empty your cup and start over with a new perspective on your skin and overall health. As you go through this process, there will definitely be an adjustment period while you swap your old acne-causing lifestyle habits for these new acne-safe ones. But before you know it, all the practices will become second nature. That is the essence of *Wu Wei*, a practice that we'll be using together to establish habits that will nourish you and starve your acne.

Wu Wei

I first learned about Wu Wei through an Instagram post. It was a video of a guy in a street stall somewhere in Asia, making hundreds of perfectly stuffed, folded, and shaped dumplings with masterful ease. He was in a rhythmic flow state, pumping out one dumpling every six seconds, all without getting his fingers sticky, in perfect ergonomic posture, without exerting much effort—or even attention—at all.

This 15-second video communicated exactly what I've tried to tell my clients when they are met with all the "dos and don'ts" of acne-safe living. Like anything new or different, all the new information might be intimidating and possibly upsetting at first, but with some practice (and mistakes) you'll eventually get the hang of it, and it will all become second nature. Before long, you're able to fold all the little acne-safe lifestyle pieces into your daily life without having to think about each detail.

Wu Wei is a multi-faceted concept from Taoism, of which a main tenet is about achieving an easy flow state where you're eventually "non-doing." This concept centers around the idea of doing something so much that it becomes second nature: an unconscious habit, like driving home without consciously thinking about the directions to get you there. Having habitual abilities like this can seem like a gift. However, when it comes to changing old habits to new ones, it is often difficult and overwhelming at first. Yet, with patience, diligence, and your eye on the prize of clear, healthy skin, all these healthy habits will soon become a regular practice of your daily life.

Disclaimers

I am not a doctor; I am a licensed esthetician. I don't know *everything* there is to know about acne and the skin, especially with all the new technology that's come out since I started With & Within in 2008. However, what's in this book is what I've seen work time and time again on my many clients over the years. For the majority, going "back to the basics" that you'll read about here has done the job of clearing their skin, and I'm confident that it will for you, too. Everything in this book is a combination of:

Techniques I learned from my teachers: Laura Cooksey of Face Reality Skincare and Dr. James E. Fulton Jr., co-creator of Retin-A, stabilizer of benzoyl peroxide (BP) for the treatment of acne, and a dedicated, lifelong dermatological chemist and researcher of acne.

Observations from the thousands of case studies within my adult-acne skincare clinic, With & Within, since 2008.

My personal research, education, and experience in alternative, healthy-lifestyle practices guided by multiple holistic health practitioners.

Before implementing any of the lifestyle changes suggested throughout this book and especially if you are on any medications or have any healthcare concerns, please check with your doctors to get their okay and supervision.

Below are a few key things I'd like you to consider before we jump into the work.

1. Let go of perfection

Acne is more about management than control. This doesn't mean that you'll never get another pimple again, even if you follow everything in this book 100%. It means that though you will for the most part clear up, if and when you do occasionally break out, you will likely know the cause (by reading this book), what to do about it, and what informed decisions (or compromises) you want to make. This bag of bones and flesh we exist in is an ever-changing organism, so we must embrace our bodies by celebrating what it can do and take good care of what we've got. Give it the time, grace, and space to be the mercurial miracle it is.

2. Nothing is going to work 100% for everybody, 100% of the time

We all have different bodies and skin, and there are so many variables to consider: our diets, our lifestyles, how our pores behave, and the products we use, among many others. How do we get you on the best path for excellent skin health? Thankfully, what's in this book has helped the majority of our clients through the years with consistently good results. If you stay committed to the suggestions in this book, the chances are very high that the process will work for you, as it has for thousands of clients before you.

Of course, through the years, there were a few for whom our program didn't work due to a variety of factors—medical conditions or prescriptions, chronic unmanaged stress, or basic program compliance. Sometimes the reasons were more uncommon: one client took all our suggestions but didn't clear up because they discovered their gluten allergy was causing all the breakouts.

It's unlikely you won't see *any* improvement, but if this is the case for you, let what you learn in this book be a baseline starting point for further investigation, should you have a more complicated scenario in which acne is just a stubborn symptom.

3. Every "body" is the same...but different

Acne doesn't care who you are, where you come from, or what you do. Your race, gender, sexual orientation, profession, or how many zeroes you have in your bank account doesn't matter. Excess skin cells, oils, and other debris accumulate in the pore and form acne in the same physiological and systematic way regardless of your political, socio-economic, or religious stance. Acne is an equal-opportunity hater, period.

But this acne is also your body's way of trying to communicate possible internal imbalances that can be and look different on each person. For example, sugar is generally inflammatory for everyone, but when taken in moderation by someone with a healthy gut, is typically well tolerated. However, someone who has a Candida yeast imbalance can suffer grave consequences by eating the same thing because of their compromised digestive system.

Candida

> Candida yeast imbalance: a common yeast that in excess causes problems like resistant acne and frequent infections, which thrives in the digestive tract, mucous membranes or the skin.

Some will experience more inflammation than others. Some will have painful, inflamed, "pizza-face" acne, some will have tiny but bumpy Braille-like acne. Some are temporarily reacting to medications they're taking, some are breaking out longer-term because of their stressful lifestyle. Some will clear up faster, while others take a bit more time.

However it manifests, the process for treating acne is the same for everyone: identify and eliminate acne-causing factors, reduce inflammation, consistently use the right products for your skin type to clear up, and, if you need to, get professional help.

4. Get your mind right, ready, and prepared

There are potentially big changes you'll make, so here are some ideas to mentally motivate yourself to stay on course.

Affirmations: How great will you feel once your skin is clear? What kind of life will be unlocked? Writing these thoughts down can help reinforce the positive end goal of clear skin, as well as become a theme over the next couple of months as you acclimate. "I'm investing in my clear-skinned future," "my skin is improving every day," or "I am doing my self-care best today."

Sticky notes: Create little love notes to yourself from the affirmations exercise above. Try posting them in places where you'll see them often… and maybe in places you find yourself tempted to swerve off-course: bathroom mirrors (where you want to pick at your skin), refrigerator (where you want to reach for your roommate's leftover birthday cheesecake), or the door (so you can see it as you leave for work or come back home). Think of these as visual cheerleaders keeping you on track to better health!

Deep breathing: Stop what you're doing. Right. Now. Take this moment to close your eyes (if possible) and take three long, slow, and deep breaths. This is an incredibly effective practice to ground you through tough moments, as well as to take in and appreciate good ones. Repeat as often as possible throughout the day.

Mind break meditation: Take a pause from the task at hand to refresh your mind and perspective with meditation. There are many ways to meditate. Here are a few:

- Guided: I love the Simple Habit meditation app for their case-specific one- to five-minute meditations, which have rescued me from many a meltdown over the years.
- Moving the body: Going for a quick walk around the block always helps to revive my brain, energy levels, and mood. Inner Walk (which you can do most anywhere) is a practice I've enjoyed. Dancing to music, gentle stretching, or doing twenty-five jumping jacks. Anything quick and easy.

- <u>Observation:</u> Cultivate a sense of being present by simply sitting in a sunny spot and counting how many dogs or windows you can see. Or sitting in your chair, carefully observing what it feels like to have the breeze passing through your hair or your points of contact between your body and the object supporting it. Notice how your skin feels brushing against your sleeve and the pressure of your arm on the armrest or your lap.
- <u>Nature.</u> Get outside. But opening up a window and looking at the sky counts, if that's all you can do!

<u>Community support:</u> Let your friends and family know that you are embarking on a new lifestyle plan to get healthy, especially if you live with people sharing the same space. It will be really helpful for those around you to know what you're up to so they can be supportive and also considerate of your new lifestyle.

<u>Clear skin buddy:</u> It would be awesome to have a friend or community you can lean on to share your recipes, breakdowns and breakthroughs with. Maybe one (or a few!) of your friends will join you on this lifestyle shift, or at least can be a source of support for you to call on as you move through the process.

<u>Self-compassion:</u> This is a big one. In today's normalized capitalistic society, almost all of us are extremely hard on ourselves and don't give ourselves enough credit for our efforts. You're likely not going to get this perfect right away (if at all), so allow yourself the grace and compassion as you fall off the wagon, brush yourself off, rest, rejuvenate, and get back on track.

<u>What to Expect...</u>

The biggest concern for our new clients is what exactly is going to happen to their skin and when they'll see results. There's sometimes an expectation that all pimples will stop appearing the day they start working with us, which isn't true. Here's what you can really expect:

<u>Initial improvement.</u> Most clients see quick improvement by changing their products alone, noticing the quality of their skin improve, sensitivity reduce, and moisture levels balance out. Blemishes continue to appear but they start to calm down, becoming smaller and healing faster than usual.

<u>Be prepared for the purge.</u> Purging occurs when "old" acne that's started forming weeks or months ago (before those acne-safe lifestyle changes) works its way up to the surface of the skin to be extracted. The amount,

intensity, and duration of this acne eventually decreases with time as the acne purges out of the skin, so long as no other acne-causing habits are still occurring. Because of the skin's delayed response, this process takes an average of two to three months to get through.

Luckily for most, this purge isn't worse than a bad day of acne our clients have already had. However, for some, the skin might get worse before it gets better. But don't worry, the anti-inflammatory ideas I reiterate in this book will help reduce the severity of your breakout period.

Purging is an annoying but expected part of the process to long-term skin clarity but it will be worth it once it's over with. You get out of the program what you put into it, and the more effort, diligence, and patience you put in, the more benefits you can expect. Stay the course!

<u>Different outlook.</u> As the acne-safe lifestyle becomes a habit, you'll likely notice a sense of ease about how your skin is behaving, your relationship to it and your daily choices and practices connect it all. Perhaps even a feeling of wholeness and acceptance.

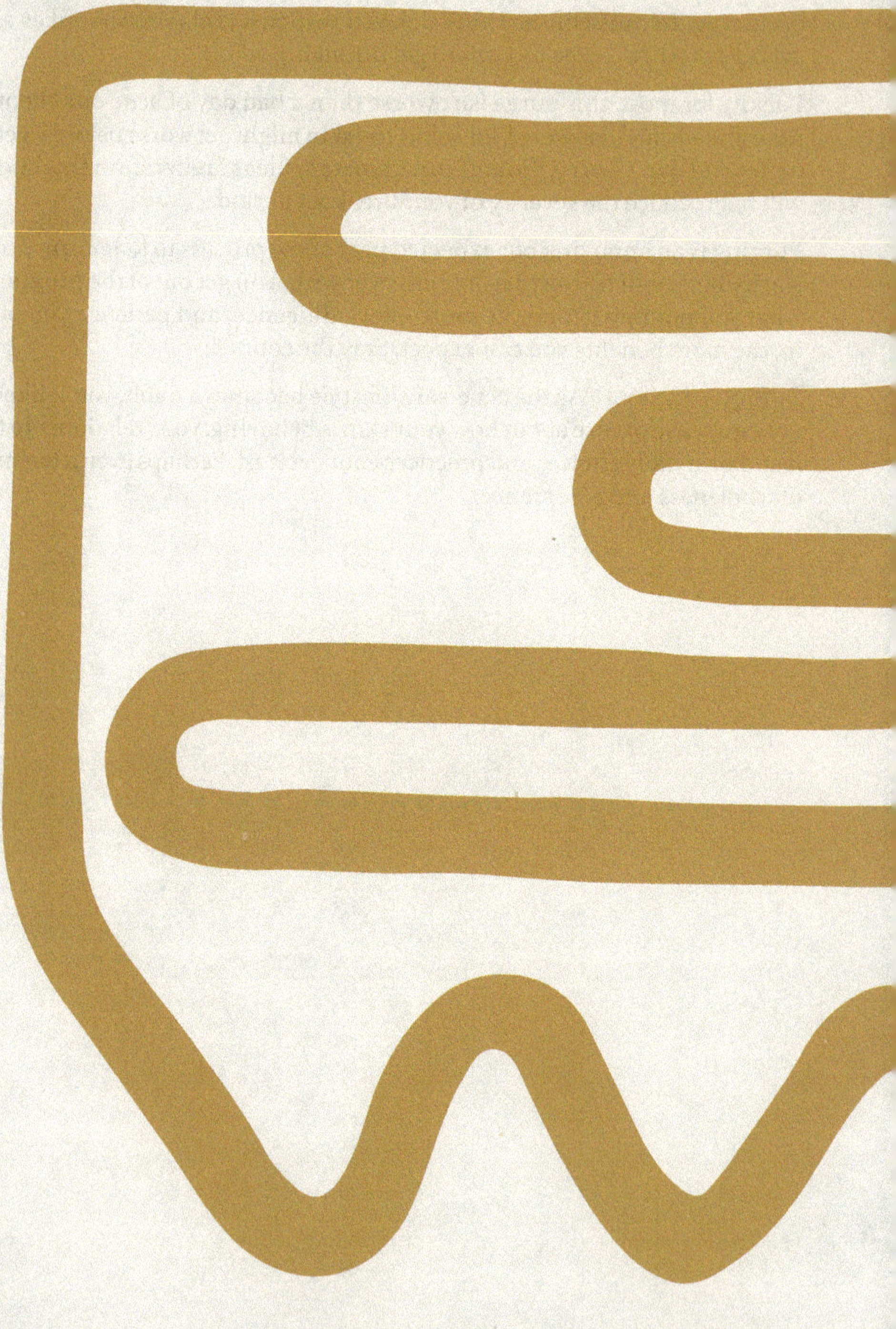

SECTION 1

Start with the Obvious -
Your Skincare Face Regimen

Plan Overview

When I talk about clearing up someone's acne, I always start "from the top down." This means let's start at the top layer of the body—the skin—which also happens to be somewhat easier to control (switch your products!) before working our way skin-deep toward body, diet, lifestyle, and so on.

Here, you'll learn about the "top layer" basics so you can get to know how your skin and products work. You'll learn how to audit and curate your skincare regimen to ensure they prevent (instead of induce) new acne from forming, jump-starting the clearing process. We'll then go deeper by reviewing your lifestyle so you can discover the root causes of your acne and learn what new changes to integrate to treat and prevent acne internally. Finally, in case you need the extra help, we'll troubleshoot by discussing some common roadblocks you may encounter and look at possible solutions.

This action plan will help you to do the following:

- Learn how your skin and products work so you understand what needs to happen to clear up your acne
- Assemble, properly use and maintain an active and acne-safe skincare routine
- Identify and reduce your acne-causing triggers (which will also reduce systemic inflammation and prevent new acne formation)
- Emphasize healthy digestion and elimination
- Observe and keep written and photographic records of your progress
- Achieve and maintain skin clarity

Learn the Basics

As you read this book, you'll soon understand what acne actually is, why your skin needs to purge, and what products *actually* work. Even the smallest steps will have a positive effect.

Here are our five basic steps to successfully purging and managing acne:

1. Figure out what's going on your skin and/or in your body that's making you break out and what to do about it. Use only acne-safe (and active exfoliating, if your skin can tolerate them) skin products properly and regularly, adjusting as needed. No comedogenic (pore-clogging) stuff!

Section 1 - Start with the Obvious - Your Skincare Face Regimen

2. No picking at your skin or pimples. Use ice instead (more on this later).
3. Optimize your diet and digestion. A healthy, whole food diet *and* mindful eating that's free of acne-causing or inflammation-inducing foods and stress is key.
4. Keep inflammation down with your daily lifestyle, diet, and stress management. You'll soon uncover possible triggers and learn how to correct them, reducing the acne-causing and inflammatory load on your body.
5. Stay the course. Keep pressing on through the process and even after clarity is achieved; clear skin takes maintenance because it's a lifestyle.

Icing

Gently applying ice directly onto the skin provides topical anti-inflammatory support, speeding the healing of existing acne and improving product penetration.

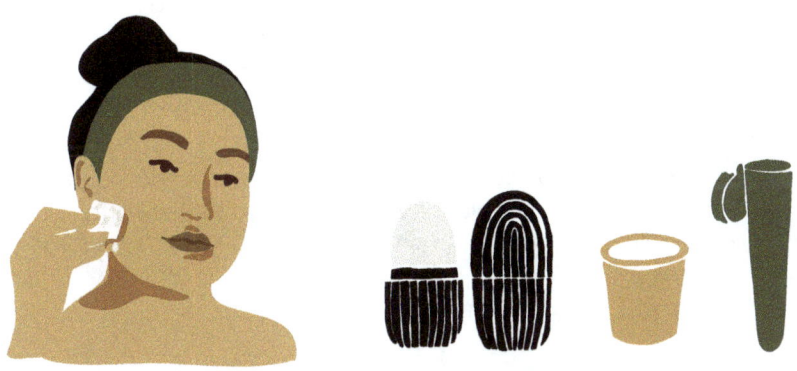

Ideally icing happens twice a day, after washing and before toning both to treat and prevent acne. Depending on how inflamed your acne is, we recommend icing up to 30 minutes each time using a silicone ice mold, a paper cup filled with water then frozen, or a popsicle mold.

Understand Skin Types and Conditions

Acne Overview

Acne is uncomfortable in more ways than one, but it's helped my clients and my team practice good skills like trust, patience, and being gentle. We also learned to see these bumps as little communicators, alerting us to an imbalance that needed to be addressed within our bodies or regarding our lifestyle. Like life, dealing with acne is less about controlled perfection and more about curiosity and management. Learning what's what and then making the best choices you can, as much as you can, consistently, is all it takes. Life will happen, your skin will react, you'll know how to manage it and eventually your pores will mature, outgrowing your acne. To begin tending to the physical skin, we must first figure out what skin type you have.

Acne seed

At the root of every blemish, breakout, eruption, lesion, pimple, or zit is an accumulation of dead skin cells, oils, comedogenic ingredients, and sometimes hair that's clumped together within the base of a pore, forming what I call an "acne seed." This causes an obstruction of the pore's natural detoxing function, resulting in what is commonly known as acne. These seeds must be extracted thoroughly in order for the pore to completely clear. Treating the skin on a topical level is important and will offer quicker visible changes, but for long-term results, we've got to go holistic.

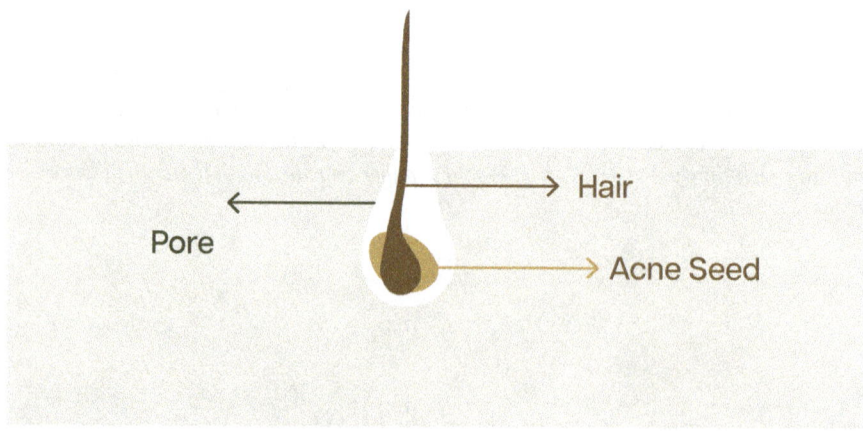

Section 1 - Start with the Obvious - Your Skincare Face Regimen

Skin Types

The skin is the largest living organ our bodies have, so it's important to take good care of it. Our skin does SO MUCH for us: it holds us together, serving as the ultimate waterproof jacket, protecting all our organs inside. Its flexibility has accommodated our growth through life. And no matter your gender, ethnicity, or age, skin will come under one of three skin types: oily, dry, or somewhere in the middle, a combination of both. Using this principle as a baseline to assess each individual's skin and needs, it's my opinion that there is no real need to distinguish different skincare in terms of different skin genders, tones, or ethnicities.

It's true that there are some characteristics we observe in some groups more than others. For instance, lighter skin tends to burn more easily in the sun, men's skin is generally oilier and thicker than women's, and darker skin tones tend to get more inflamed during extractions than lighter skin tones. You can use any product you want regardless of whom it's marketed to so long as it's acne-safe, appropriate for *your* skin type and used correctly.

Most people have a combination of both oily/dry skin, where folks are slightly oilier in the T-zone (forehead, nose, and maybe chin) and drier on the cheeks. That said, it's totally normal for your T-zone to be a bit shiny or oily at the end of a workday.

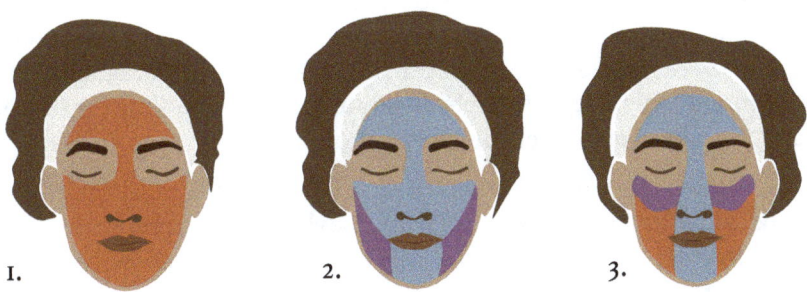

1. Dry skin is generally dry and tight all over (red), with very small pores.

2. Oily skin is generally very oily all over but especially on the forehead, nose and chin (t-zone) where the pores are the largest, and might be slightly drier or neutral along the jawline (purple).

3. Combination skin is exactly that - a mix of an oily t-zone (blue), neutral on the upper cheeks (purple) and drier on the lower cheeks (red).

Dry Skin

What it looks like: Truly dry skin is usually thin and fine-textured with very small to invisible pores, including those on the T-zone. There is very little, if any, oil present on the skin, even on the T-zone. Sometimes the skin is so dry, one might see superficial wrinkling or a rough texture, which is usually relieved with extra moisturizing along with a break from active products—anything with acids, retinols, scrubs, scrubby things, or drying things like benzoyl peroxide or clays.

What it feels like: After washing, dry skin might feel tight, look wrinkly, and may even start to slightly flake in areas (particularly around the mouth or eyes) within an hour of not moisturizing. Sometimes, if the skin is really dry, applying moisturizers can sting, even if they contain no active ingredients in them. Dry rough spots are also common and applying makeup over them can result in uneven coverage, accentuating dry skin.

What to buy: You'll want to look for non-foaming cleansers (lotion or cream textured, like our Hydrating Cleanser) and moisturizing creams (like our Hydrating Cream). If you need more moisture, add a product like a moisturizing serum, acne-safe oil, or hydrating mask to your regimen for as long as you're still extra-dry (like our Hydrating Gel or 100% Shea Butter). Once your skin recuperates, try backing off these products to see how your skin maintains its moisture levels. Using products that are too moisturizing for your skin, even if acne-safe, can make you break out, too.

Active product tolerance: Dry skin can tolerate some exfoliants, but start slowly and carefully watch your skin's behavior to monitor any trouble. Because there is little to no oil in the skin to create a buffer against these active ingredients, they penetrate deeply and quickly, making the dry skin easier to get over-exfoliated, dehydrated, or sensitized.

Seasons/climate: Warm, humid weather is usually the most comfortable for this skin type, as the moist heat helps the skin create more sebum. In dry or cold weather seasons, you will likely need even more moisture support. You can do this by:

- Doubling up your cream or lotion application, allowing the first layer to soak in a minute or two before applying the second.
- Using a sunscreen that does double duty by moisturizing. Our Safeguard SPF 45 is a favorite.
- Applying an additional layer of moisture under your cream or lotion, such as our Hydrating Gel, A Natural Difference's Rejuvenation Concentrate, a few drops of acne-safe oil, and/or some

Section 1 - Start with the Obvious - Your Skincare Face Regimen

100% shea butter. Experiment with layering to find what works best for you.
- Incorporating a moisturizing treatment mask, like the SkinScript Goji Berry mask, a few times a week. You can also massage a quarter-sized amount of Hydrating Cleanser onto your skin, leaving a thick layer on for several minutes as a moisturizing mask before rinsing off.

Oily Skin

What it looks like: Oily skin is usually thick with visible pores that are largest on the T-zone and smallest on the cheeks closest to the ears. Sometimes, tiny drops of oil can be found coming out of each pore! Sebaceous hyperplasia is also common with oily skin. This is a type of enlarged sebaceous gland where extra skin cells have "erupted," overflowing out of the pore and causing a raised bump. Sometimes when the skin is dehydrated or over-exfoliated, the skin can appear to be both dry (flaky skin) and oily (oil on top).

What it feels like: Immediately after washing the face, the skin will feel comfortable—neither dry nor oily. Within an hour, though, the skin will start to feel oily, and a sheen might develop. If you wear glasses, your eyeglasses are often greasy, and the skin feels oily to the touch all over the face. Makeup can often slide around and melt off instead of staying in place on the skin.

What to look for: For most mild to moderately oily skins, a gentle foaming cleanser (like our Charcoal Cleanser) and a lightweight moisturizer with a lotion consistency (or a light layer of our Hydrating Cream) are ideal.

If you're *really* oily (oily to the touch all over the face within one to two hours after washing), use an even more drying foaming cleanser that contains clay or benzoyl peroxide (like the Beyond Complexion 10% BP Wash).

TIP: Using BP as a treatment mask

You can also use this BP cleanser like a mask for extra drying and anti-inflammatory action by foaming it up, applying it to the skin, and waiting a few minutes before rinsing off. This is a great technique to use if you are inflamed, sensitive, or dry but still need some anti-inflammatory support or have rosacea.

Even though you're already oily and it seems counterintuitive, you should still moisturize to keep the skin's protective barrier healthy in between the time you're done washing and your skin produces that oil naturally. A hydrating gel or serum alone may be enough to moisturize the oiliest of skins. Mineral sunscreens in a loose powder (like the LaBella Donna SPF 50 powder) or non-moisturizing liquid or gel form (like the Tizo 2 and 3 SPF 40) work best since the minerals naturally and gently help absorb oil, leaving a matte finish.

Active product tolerance: Oily skin can generally tolerate stronger exfoliants because the oil "floats" the actives at the surface, preventing them from being absorbed into the skin. So, just a bit of drying is needed to absorb this excess and allow the active products to penetrate the pores in order to work. However, oily-skinned folks who overdry their skin can cause dehydration, resulting in the skin overproducing oil in an attempt to (over)compensate for the oil you dried up.

Seasons/climate: Warm weather usually makes this skin type more oily, making the colder and drier climes more comfortable. However, you may still need to moisturize even a tiny bit to support the skin during changes in weather and to prevent dehydration. You'll want to look for cleansers that foam up because any foaming action is inherently drying (though a well-formulated one shouldn't overdry or strip), serums, gels, and/or lotions to moisturize the skin (creams will generally be too oily for this skin type). Mineral-based sunscreens are inherently slightly drying, so they might be a good choice for oily-skinned folks (our Tizo Sunscreens are our oily-skinned clients' favorites).

Combination (Normal Skin)

Most people fall under this category, which is a mix of both oily and dry. Skin types are usually not an either/or proposition. This combo can change daily and is subject to the weather, climate, or medications you may be taking. The classic combination skin is usually a little oily in the T-zone and a little dry on the cheeks.

Products to look for: I personally have combination skin that veers slightly on the drier side, so I keep two cleansers on hand (the foaming Charcoal Wash and creamy Hydrating Cleanser) to switch between, depending on how my skin is feeling that day. Then, I'll use our Hydrating Cream or 100% Shea Butter (suitable for most skin types), with our Safeguard SPF 45 on top. If I'm feeling dry, I'll layer them (shea first, then cream on top), or apply the cream twice for extra moisture. If I'm extra dry and the Hydrating Cleanser and Shea Butter and Cream aren't enough, I'll sneak a few drops of safflower or sunflower oil onto my skin after toning and before the cream.

Section 1 - Start with the Obvious - Your Skincare Face Regimen

Learn What Skin Type You Really Are

Your skin may be imbalanced because of your current regimen. For instance, if you're using a ton of drying and exfoliating products that are irritating your skin, you may think your skin is dry and sensitive. Or if you're oil-cleansing and moisturizing with a heavy cream, you may think you have oily skin when it's actually the products you're using that are making it greasy. Oftentimes the skin seems confused: the skin is somehow both dry and flaky, but also greasy and slippery (which is often dehydrated or over-exfoliated skin).

To start rebalancing your skin, stop all your active skin products and stick with one non-active cleanser, one day moisturizer with SPF, and 100% shea butter as your night moisturizer to create a very bare-bones, acne-safe baseline skin regimen.*

Then, we can refine your regimen to help curb any natural dry/oiliness for optimal acne-clearing action.

> ## *TIP: Use shea until you find your SPF
>
> Since 100% shea butter will likely be much easier to find than an acne-safe SPF, you can use that morning and night until you find a suitable SPF for the day. Try to find a safe SPF quickly though, you'll need the protection.

For the first couple of weeks, the goal of the regimen is to normalize your skin so that it can be as dry or oily as it *naturally* wants to be. From here, we can truly see your skin as it naturally exists, and safely build out the active part of your regimen. See how your skin reacts for one to two weeks with your chosen cleanser and moisturizer(s). If your skin feels comfortable (meaning not too oily or dry), you've likely found the right combo for your skin during this season/climate. If not, the strategies below may help. Try one idea for a few days before folding in another.

- If you're feeling oily, try using a foaming cleanser (if you aren't already); switching to a lighter moisturizer; using a lightweight lotion or dry powder physical block sunscreen (the minerals are inherently drying).
- If you're feeling dry, try switching to a more moisturizing, non-foamy cleanser; using a richer moisturizer; applying a second layer of your current moisturizer; adding a few drops of acne-safe

safflower or sunflower oil or a layer of 100% shea butter to your skin before your cream or sunscreen.

After you have a good cleanse and moisturizing baseline (preferably including an acne-safe sunscreen), you can then carefully add in active exfoliating products to begin the corrective acne purging, prevention, and maintenance phases of your skin program.

Sensitive vs. sensitized skin

It's well known in the professional skincare community that clients almost always say they have sensitive skin, which isn't truly the case. In all my years of practicing skincare professionally, I've seen thousands of faces and have only seen a handful of *truly* sensitive skin. The rest were simply *sensitized*. What's the difference?

Sensitive Skin

People with *sensitive* skin are born with it or have developed/survived a condition that is either genetically inherited or the result of an autoimmune disease, cancer, or past major allergic reaction. Their skin is reactive to many products or ingredients, especially active ones that contain acids, vitamins, or scrubs. Some clients have been so sensitive that they couldn't use anything but water and shea butter on their faces. In these cases, it took us weeks or months to get their skin to *slowly* acclimate to using things like cleansers and moisturizers, let alone exfoliants. This usually manifests as skin that easily turns and stays red, commonly experiences uncomfortable sensations when using products or exposed to weather elements (like stinging or burning) and takes time to heal from external aggravators like products, treatments, weather, or the sun.

These folks likely also can't tolerate fragrances, skin products, or weather conditions that most others can, and often are more prone to other conditions like eczema or rosacea.

Sensitized Skin

People with *sensitized* skin experience irritated skin for a temporary period of time as a result of an external factor: something they did or used that irritated their skin. It's uncomfortable for a short while, but eventually, their skin heals and returns to normal. For example, after a sunburn, your skin is sensitive for that week until it fully heals. Another example would be if you fried your face by using every exfoliating product you found online in the same week, multiple times a day.

Isolating and eliminating these irritants should allow your skin to heal up within a few days, regaining its strength and resiliency.

Section 1 - Start with the Obvious - Your Skincare Face Regimen

Exfoliation

Exfoliation is when dead skin cells are removed from the surface of the skin, exposing newer, clearer, and generally brighter skin underneath. Exfoliants are products meant to gently induce this reaction, but when the skin starts to visibly peel or become irritated, the skin may be over-exfoliated.

Over-exfoliation vs. dehydration
Dry, flaky, maybe itchy and irritated skin can happen, and it's important to figure out what's causing it to treat it effectively. Take the time to visually inspect what's happening so you can take proper care of your skin. For example, it might be a mole requiring some medical attention.

Over-exfoliation
If your skin is peeling only in certain areas and your products *don't* sting or burn when using them (yet; with enough time it can) you are probably over-exfoliating. Peeling skin is happening because the exfoliants are doing their job, causing visible flaking. A change in weather can cause your skin to dry out, allowing your exfoliating products to penetrate into the skin more easily, causing flaking or rough patches.

In this case, try toning your skin less aggressively. People understandably often rub their toner pads more firmly on trouble areas or around their nose and mouth, causing the exfoliating acids to penetrate deeper, inducing flaking of the skin. Skip the areas that are still peeling and tone everywhere else. You can resume toning once the flaking has stopped.

Dehydration
If you are feeling dry, tight, and flaky all over and/or the active products you are using are a little stingy or burny, you are most likely dehydrated (in need of water) and/or are lipid-dry (in need of oil or sebum). Skin dehydration should be treated topically as well as internally. Dehydrated skin can also look a bit crepey, with a shiny and wrinkled, tissue-like texture on the surface of the skin.

CASE STUDY of all of the above: Sensitive, over-exfoliated and dehydrated.

I had one memorable case where a 27-year-old female client had one of the most intense acne bouts I had seen. Despite this, her spirit never wavered, and she trusted us to help her get clear. At her first visit, based on a visual estimation, we determined that only about 45% of her face was clear, and the rest was congested with acne. Her skin was so dried out that it was painful for her to eat a banana. The first thing we did was immediately put her on a strictly healing and hydrating skin regimen with no exfoliants, BP, or drying agents. In six days, the soreness around her mouth had gone away. On day ten, we had her start exfoliating with a very gentle acid toner just once a day. Along with regular extractions, over the next few weeks we slowly increased her exfoliation with the toner and worked BP gel into her regimen. This helped to dry out and calm down the inflamed, cystic acne she had. In ten weeks from her first visit, she was all cleared up—the same woman but with a much different outlook on life.

Understand Products

With gazillions of products on the market, it's hard to tell what's good, what to use, or even what they are supposed to do. Although you will need to use enough product for your skin to clear, in general, use as few products as possible to minimize chemical exposure as well as for ecological reasons. Skin, hair, and body products eventually wash away into our oceans, affecting wildlife and the environment. We also want your skin to breathe, so wear as little makeup for as short a time as possible each day.

There are tons of products on the market, and most are not going to be safe or effective for acne-prone skin. Products may contain good active ingredients in them but aren't formulated well or don't have enough of that active ingredient within the formula to have much of an effect. Often there's also a lack of detailed explanations on how to use the products together safely and effectively. But the biggest problem is comedogenicity.

Comedogenicity

Comedo = clogged hair follicle +
Genic = producing, forming

also: cloggy, pore-clogging, comedogenic

If a product is comedogenic, that means it's going to clog your pores and create new acne impactions or "seeds." "Non-comedogenic" is a term not regulated by the US Food and Drug Administration (FDA), so unfortunately, this term has been merely a marketing gimmick used willy-nilly on products whether or not they are truly acne-safe. I can't tell you how many products I've seen over the years that said "non-comedogenic" on the front of the bottle and had several pore-clogging ingredients on the back. By diligently using our ingredient list and carefully testing it yourself, you can be your own advocate and avoid falling victim.

Comedogenicity is tricky because you won't know if the products are actually safe until you test them on your skin. Similar to the food industry, comedogenic ingredients can be secretly ushered into a product under an umbrella ingredient like "fragrance," much like "flavoring" or "caramel" are used to conceal often-toxic chemicals and preservatives in food.

Products that foam like toothpaste, face washes, and shampoos tend to congest the skin almost immediately—within a few days to a week. Things that stay on the skin, like makeup or creams, tend to take three months or more for new breakouts to surface.

If you are acne-prone, definitely avoid comedogenic ingredients and products. You can use the product checker search tool[1] on our site to audit your own products and access these ingredient study papers from Dr. Fulton[2].

Look Beyond the "Proof"

Many popular brand name products, including those specifically targeted at treating acne, contain comedogenic ingredients no matter their price point or sales channel (online, drugstore, high end retail, natural spa or conventional medical offices). The skincare industry uses marketing terms like "doctor-tested and recommended" or even "non-comedogenic" to describe and sell products that we have found to actually be comedogenic.

Every so often, you'll see a product that's labeled as "comedogenically tested", but without industry standards to adhere to, the results of these tests may not be so reliable. Products developed for the face are often tested on the backs of lab test subjects, who may or may not have acne-prone skin in the first place and don't have the acne-safe lifestyle in practice to rule out non-topical breakouts.

"Miracle" Products

Though some products can seem to "work overnight," what actually is more likely to be happening is that the product is making the inflammation temporarily calm down (which you can do for free with ice), making the skin appear clearer. But with the acne seed still stuck inside the pore, you aren't really clear because once an inflammatory situation returns to your skin, that same seed will flare, causing that pesky inflamed zit to resurface.

Another reason some products seem to work so quickly is due to their low pH. Long-term use of low-pH products will eventually damage the protective barrier of the skin, rendering it sensitive (and the product ineffective or giving plateaued results) and susceptible. The skin can tolerate the occasional use of low-pH products (like a chemical peel, for instance) because it will eventually recover, given proper post-treatment healing skincare.

SPF

Sunscreen gets a bad reputation for causing breakouts. However, with a keen, acne-safe eye and some experimentation, they don't have to! The overarching principle to keep in mind is that regardless of what kind you use, the most important thing is to find one you like and to use it regularly and as directed.

What Does SPF Mean?

SPF is an acronym for Sun Protection Factor, a mathematical formula that helps determine how long you can be in direct sunlight before you start turning red (and burn) without any sunscreen on. SPF measures protection from UVB rays only, not UVA ones.

Let's say you can stay in direct sunlight without sun protection for a maximum of ten minutes before you start turning red. This means that if you wear a properly applied sunscreen lotion with an SPF of 15, you should theoretically be able to stay out in the sun for (10 minutes x 15 =) 150 minutes before your skin starts to turn red or burn. However, any time the SPF comes off your skin somehow (you get wet, sweat, swim, or rub the sunscreen off on a towel), you should reapply immediately or else risk sunburn.

What Exactly Does Sunscreen Protect Me From?

The sun emits different types of light rays in relation to skin/sun damage: UVAs are the aging rays, UVBs are the burning rays, and UVCs are the cancerous rays of the sun. When you get a sunscreen that says Broad Spectrum Protection, Multi Spectrum or UVA/UVB on it, you know you'll be getting protection from both ray types (UVAs and UVBs). As the ozone layer is increasingly depleted, we will likely be more exposed to UVCs (to date, there are no sunscreens that specifically target or can claim to protect

Section 1 - Start with the Obvious - Your Skincare Face Regimen

from UVCs). This is where I suggest using an antioxidant serum to try to protect what the SPFs do not.

SPF Myths

Chemical SPFs are more irritating than physical SPFs.
This is a gray area answer. In general, physical SPFs are more popular and considered more sun-stable than chemical ones in North America, while in Asia and Europe, chemical SPFs are more popular. There are some explanations for this.

According to Dr. Vivian Bucay, MD, at the Bucay Center for Dermatology and Aesthetics in San Antonio, Texas, as of 2019, the FDA has not updated its list of approved sunscreen ingredients in years, currently comprised of much older and fewer (16 approved at the time of writing) ones than Europe or China (27). In the US, SPFs go through inspections as a drug (a long, slow, and expensive process). The US FDA is not only slow to approve new ingredients and formulas but is also lax about existing standards (UVA protection, for example). This results in a smaller range of products legally available in the US but also limited efficacy.

So the adage that chemical SPFs found in the US are more irritating than physical block ones may be true for formulas found within the US, but not necessarily outside of it.

> *"We are terribly behind the rest of the world in approving sunscreens that are superior to those we have,"* says Dr. Bucay. *"Sunscreen formulations undergo a standardized testing method to determine what degree of protection it offers."*

I'm dark so I don't need to wear SPF.
Wear SPF even if you are darker skinned. While it's true that darker skin tones are less sun sensitive, skin cancer is still a risk and can be even more lethal for those with darker skin tones.

SPF in your makeup counts as SPF.
This is not totally true because your makeup isn't applied all over your face, ears, neck, and chest like one would apply an SPF lotion or cream. It's best to layer protection by applying your SPF lotion/cream of choice all over, then mineral makeup on top.

I stay inside all day, so I don't need SPF.
If you can see the sun, it can affect you. Sunlight comes in through windows and reflects off mirrors, and you'll also be exposed when you leave

the house. There are also some murmurs that blue lights from electronic devices count as UV exposure.

SPFs always make me break out.
Now that you have access to our product checker, you can find safer choices and hopefully find a formula that works for you. SPF ingredients aren't inherently cloggy, but the formula base can be.

Silicones and dimethicones: proceed with caution

A small percentage of folks are reactive to silicones and dimethicones, ingredients often used with mineral SPFs for improved spreadability. If you are affected, try a powder mineral sunscreen like La Bella Donna's Minerals On-The-Go SPF Powder Brushes instead to get the mineral protection without a potentially clogging liquid, lotion, or cream base.

Sunscreen Types

There are two different sunscreen ingredient types: physical and chemical. Here's info on both, based on what's available in the US.

Physical Sunscreens (aka Mineral Sunscreens)

These types of sunscreens use two active ingredients—zinc or titanium dioxide, both natural minerals from the Earth. They work by reflecting sunlight and heat off the skin. You can think of physical SPFs as being made up of rocks that are ground up into a super-fine powder suspended in a lotion that's then spread across the skin, dispersing the powder to reflect light rays from the sun. Even though minerals are natural ingredients, the FDA calls them "inorganic sunscreens."

Physical sunscreen pros
- Has much more comprehensive protection, naturally defending against UVA/UVB rays with fewer active ingredients.
- Known to be a better choice for those who tend toward hyperpigmentation (red or brown dark spots left behind after a pimple or other skin trauma has healed) or rosacea because of the slightly higher degree of heat reflection.
- Minerals are inert ingredients, making them more stable and less likely to irritate sensitive skin.

Section 1 - Start with the Obvious - Your Skincare Face Regimen

- No waiting time needed between application and sun exposure (but it's best to apply a few minutes ahead of time anyway to allow the formula to settle onto the skin's surface).
- They have great staying power as the minerals are formulated to adhere to the skin in order to protect it. They are less likely to rub or wash off before you're ready to remove them with a thorough wash.

Physical sunscreen cons

- Essentially made up of very finely ground minerals, these formulas can often leave a whitish cast on the skin if they're not rubbed in thoroughly or if the sunscreen is not as refined a formula as it can be. Our Safeguard SPF 40 is honestly the best physical block formula I've tried for small areas like the face; however, some cast is left behind if used on larger body areas or darker skin.
- Can take extra diligence to completely wash off. Use a cleansing washcloth to help.
- Most physical sunscreens on the market are formulated within a comedogenic base to make the ground-up rocks easier to spread across the skin. Commonly used are oils like coconut or soybean, or silicones and/or dimethicones. Silicones and dimethicones, though acne-safe for most, can be comedogenic for a small percentage of people.
- Many "natural" formulations also tend to include seaweed extracts that offer some sun protection and anti-redness properties but can cause iodide acne to form, a type of acne induced by excess iodine found in foods and skin products.
- Because minerals are inherently porous and absorbent, you may find physical sunscreens to be a bit drying. While this can be desirable for oilier skin, drier-skinned people may need to use a moisturizing mineral SPF or add a layer of hydration under their sunscreen or mineral makeup to make sure they don't dry out.

Chemical Sunscreens

These include all the other sun protective ingredients you'll see on labels like avobenzone, oxybenzone, and octinoxate, as well as almost all other ingredients ending in -zone and -xate. Labeled as "organic sunscreens" by the FDA, these work by absorbing sunlight and heat.

Chemical sunscreen pros

- Thanks to their thinner texture, these are very easy to apply and spread across the skin.

- They leave no whitish cast, so are especially desirable for darker-melanated or tanned skins to use.
- Very easy to find, as they're the most common type of SPF manufactured in the US.

Chemical sunscreen cons
- They aren't as stable as standalone mineral SPF ingredients, so they need to be combined with several other SPF ingredients and thus may be more irritating for sensitive skin.
- Not great for humans: many studies suggest that chemical sunscreens induce endocrine dysfunction of the reproductive and developmental systems.
- Not great for the environment: tropical locales like Hawai'i, the US Virgin Islands and Mexico have banned chemical SPFs because they damage coral reefs.
- Don't protect as quickly: you should wait at least 10-15 minutes to allow it to start working before sun exposure.
- Don't protect as long: they break down with direct sun exposure faster than mineral SPFs do.
- Because chemical sunscreens absorb slightly more sunlight and heat than physical SPFs, the chances of hyperpigmentation formation with chemical SPFs are potentially higher.
- They can also make skin and eyes sting, especially when sweating.

Although the Skin Cancer Foundation site does not seem to identify the difference in sun protection in chemical versus physical sunscreens, in the American professional skincare industry, physical sunscreens are generally preferred over chemical.

How Strong Should My SPF Be?

According to the American Skin Cancer Foundation, anything after SPF 50 starts to increase only by a fraction of a percentage:

- SPF 15 protects you from 93% of UVBs
- SPF 30 protects you from 97% of UVBs
- SPF 50 protects you from 98% of UVBs

No matter what SPF rating you get, you still need to reapply every two hours or as needed/directed.

Other Important Factors

Regularly applying sunscreen is just one part of a well rounded sun protection regimen. Here are additional ideas to incorporate:

Avoid the sun at its strongest, usually between the hours of 10 a.m. to 4 p.m. Be especially mindful when you are in a new climate, as the sun can be much stronger than you're used to (higher elevation or tropical zones closer to the equator).

Seek shade. Cooler temperatures found in the shade can help prevent overall inflammation, along with heat-induced rosacea and hyperpigmentation.

Physically covering up with large hats, long sleeve shirts, long pants and sunglasses are also protective. The World Health Organization (WHO) recommends loose-fitting and colored fabric. Some fashion brands like Uniqlo, Solumbra, and REI use modern technology to builds SPF into their fabrics. Large-framed sunglasses with polarized lenses are great for protecting the eyeballs themselves from the sun, along with the skin around the eye area by helping to prevent squinting (which can cause eye/brow wrinkles over time).

Sun exposure is also not always obvious. Foggy days can still expose you to sunlight, which, in some cases, is actually magnified by the water content of the atmosphere. Basking in the sun with a constant breeze that keeps you feeling cool is still sun exposure, and you can end up getting a surprise sunburn because of that deceivingly cool wind. People who drive or work indoors next to a window are still exposed to the sun. In fact, the American Skin Cancer Foundation says those who drive in the US get more skin cancers on their left side, and those who drive in opposite-driving countries get them more on their right sides (and car windshields supposedly have more sun protection than side windows).[3]

Always be mindful of your sun exposure and practice appropriate safety measures.

Which SPF is the best?

Ideally, you'll find one that's acne-safe that you like enough to use regularly, is suitable for the activity you're going to use it for, and also moisturizes. I personally prefer physical block sunscreens because of their inherent UVA protection, staying power, and tendency not to sting my eyes like chemical sunscreens do. Physical block ingredients zinc oxide and titanium dioxide (the only two mineral SPF ingredients on the market) protect from UVAs. The only other US-approved chemical ingredient that does this is avobenzone. Avobenzone breaks down quickly in the sun, lasting only thirty minutes, and is usually combined with other chemical SPFs (which are known endocrine disruptors) to increase stability and longevity.

Exfoliation

Exfoliation is the removal of dead skin cells accumulated on the upper layers of the skin to reveal smoother layers underneath. This can be done either physically (by scrubbing with a product that has scrub particles suspended in a cleanser, cream, or oil base; electronic cleansing brush, washcloth, microdermabrasion) or chemically (with acids in serums or peels) or with enzymes. You can exfoliate at home with products or devices or in a skin clinic with a licensed professional using stronger products and devices.

First commercially introduced in US markets in 1993, exfoliants have been used throughout history. Many foods, fruits, vegetables, sugar cane, and sour milk contain naturally occurring non-toxic exfoliating acids. Aged red wine was used in France; lemon and other fruits were used in Hungary and Europe. Cleopatra, known for her beautiful skin, is said to have bathed in milk. Ancient Egyptians' early acne treatments included using drying clay masks, which would dry the skin so much that it caused the skin to peel, essentially exfoliating it.

Some skin experts will suggest you exfoliate only a few times a week, avoiding daily exfoliation at all costs. However, this truly depends on the type and strength of exfoliant used, your inherent skin condition and tolerance, and what your goals are.

The 4 Exfoliant Types

Enzymes are usually papaya- or pineapple-derived, found within cleansers or masks and used often in the treatment room to prepare the skin for extractions. They work by digesting the glue that holds dead skin cells together. Enzymes are generally the most gentle of the lot, yet still quite effective.

Physical exfoliation like scrubs, washcloths, or brush devices physically scrub dead skin off the surface. This method works quickly but only at the surface level of the skin and can be abrasive, irritating, and inflammation-inducing. This should be fine for healthy, clear skin a few times a week but may increase inflammation for those who are sensitive or acne-prone. Physical exfoliants can put too much pressure on fragile, inflamed follicles, ultimately making inflamed acne worse, while also opening pimples and spreading the bacterial pus around. Physical exfoliation is NOT recommended for inflamed acne. However, if you can get the inflammation under control, you can try to slowly work it into your routine to enhance your chemical exfoliation's penetration. This can be particularly beneficial for body acne and ingrown hairs, but exercise extreme caution and restraint for the face.

Chemical exfoliation done with acids found in cleansers, serums, toners, creams, and professional-strength peels are what I like to call "controlled wounding." Essentially, acids are gently burning the top layers of your skin (the wounding), stimulating your skin's immune response to regenerate new skin cell growth and collagen production. The great thing about chemical exfoliants is that you can infuse additional active ingredients like brighteners and antioxidants within the same formula. Treatments can range from various products you apply at home, a peel you'd get at a medical spa or a deeper procedure that requires general anesthesia from a plastic surgeon. (Tip: Hyaluronic acid is not an exfoliant but a moisturizer, and is ok to use anytime.)

BHA, aka Beta Hydroxy Acid, aka Salicylic Acid: BHA is oil-soluble, so it seems to do a better job of digesting sebum and acne-impacted pores than AHAs. Salicylic acid has been untested for this and thus is ruled NOT safe for pregnant or nursing people.

AHAs, aka Alpha Hydroxy Acids: While there is only one type of BHA (salicylic acid), AHAs come in many forms. These are generally regarded as safe for pregnant or nursing people, but always check with your doctor. Here are a few:

- Glycolic: The most common type of AHA, originally found in sugar and fruit. This small molecule penetrates quickly and deeply, can often tingle or sting, and has brightening properties.
- Lactic: Originally found in milk and honey but nowadays more commonly derived from corn or beets. Glycolic's more gentle cousin, lactic's small molecules can still burn and thus need to be neutralized. It also has moisturizing benefits.
- Malic is naturally found in apples, citric in citrus fruit, and tartaric in grapes.
- Mandelic: Originally found in bitter almonds, it is antibacterial, viral, and fungal. It purges non-inflamed acne and brightens hyperpigmentation without aggravating inflammation.

Retinols technically count as chemical exfoliants but behave slightly differently than their counterparts. Vitamin A-based, they stimulate collagen growth and brighten the skin but can also aggravate inflammation in some sensitive skin types. Dr. Fulton recommended that the patient first condition the skin with BP gel for two to four weeks before introducing a retinol or vitamin A skin product to reduce any inflammatory effects. This is contraindicated for pregnant and nursing people.

Benefits of Exfoliation

- Allows other products to penetrate deeper into the skin, improving their efficacy
- Assists in the accelerated purging action of acne seeds from deep within the pore
- Prevents acne by eliminating dead skin cells before they have a chance to clump up and form acne seeds in the pore
- Softens and prevents fine lines and wrinkles
- Brightens hyperpigmentation
- Stimulates collagen production, which in turn stimulates the skin's immune/healing response, and smooths the skin
- Improves elasticity
- Can reduce and prevent textural scarring

Possible Side Effects of Exfoliation

- Skin irritation: Don't use products that are too strong or used incorrectly or too frequently. Stinging or burning at home is typically not okay. Ideally, you never feel more than a 2 or 3 (on a burning sensation scale of 1-10, with 1 feeling like water and 10 feeling like fire) for longer than thirty seconds when using said product.
- Sun sensitivity: Wear sunscreen. The new skin that's revealed after exfoliation needs to be moisturized and protected.

Exfoliating at Home Versus With a Professional

Homecare exfoliation is part of the daily skin regimen that keeps your skin its clearest and healthiest. Professional exfoliation consists of using chemical peels with an esthetician or undergoing resurfacing laser treatments with a cosmetic dermatologist to clear your skin of dead cells.

The two combined will yield the best results, and professional oversight can also help optimize your homecare program as needed, as well as catch or prevent any other potential problems before they start.

With & Within's Philosophy on Exfoliants

Chemical exfoliation is our choice method via our Mandelic Toner before adding serums. There is less of a chance of inflammation with chemical versus physical exfoliation, with the efficient benefit of other added ingredients like antioxidants and brighteners. However, for skin that is completely clear or has strictly non-inflamed acne, physical exfoliants (like a scrub, using just the fingertips) can be helpful. Use caution and discretion and discontinue use if irritation or inflammation occurs.

Benzoyl Peroxide (BP) for Acne (and Rosacea)

Stabilized by Dr. James Fulton in the early 1970s, his BP formulation was bought out and distributed by Steifel, a GlaxoSmithKline company, by the trade name Panoxyl. When he combined BP with water, he found that it penetrated into the pores much better than prior oil-based formulations. He found that it exfoliated within the pore, loosening impactions and suppressed irritating fatty acids in sebum much better than oral antibiotic tetracycline—thereby relieving inflammation, sparing a healthy body from unnecessary prescription drugs and preventing the disruption of intestinal flora.

BP is one of our most powerful weapons: it's antibacterial through the oxygen it pushes down into the pore, eradicating the excess anaerobic *C. acnes* bacteria that causes inflammation. It has a drying effect, which reduces oil overproduction and effectively fights acne. It may also help prevent new acne from forming.

Many BP gels on the market today are often suspended within comedogenic bases, defeating the purpose of treating acne as the comedogenic bases create new acne impactions. If not used carefully, they can also overdry the skin, causing more acne to form. However, for very oily, stubborn, or inflamed acne, BP preparations that contain sulfur may be beneficial to further dry out the acne and calm the inflammation.

The best way to ensure that you know whether or not it belongs in your regimen is by trying out the basic regimen as is: icing your skin diligently and reducing your inflammatory/acne-causing factors for a month or so, or even working with an esthetician who can treat and evaluate your skin and track its progress. If after you've done all you can (icing, diet, stress management) for long enough (one to three months) and are still inflamed, adding BP can help. Due to its drying nature, it can help speed up the clearing of oilier skins, absorbing the excess sebum that blocks the penetration of active products, rendering them less effective than they could be.

When, Why, and Who Should Use It

Several factors determine whether BP is necessary, including inflammation levels, oil production levels, and, of course, a client's tolerance to BP. We find most clients don't need it so long as they switch to an acne-safe regimen, ice religiously, and maintain a low-inflammatory lifestyle.

Generally, if you are over twenty-five with mild to moderate acne and/or are not very oily, the basic acne-safe regimen should clear you up. If after four to six weeks of inflammation or excess oiliness still persists, integrate BP to further control it.

To keep the skin comfortable and curb any acclimating dryness or peeling that might occur when first using BP, use a hydrating gel or serum, not creams that can deactivate it. After a few days, if you are still dry, adjust your regimen further: switch to a non-foaming, moisturizing face wash (like our Hydrating Cleanser) for a few nights, stop using BP, and just moisturize at night instead. Continue with these adjustments until your skin's moisture levels are restored, and slowly reintroduce BP gel as tolerated. BP is generally considered safe for pregnant or nursing women (check with your doctor).

We typically only have clients use BP if:

- The acne is very active, with lots of new and stubborn acne constantly appearing. Often, these clients are in their teens or early twenties, have active hormonal situations like pregnancy, are taking hormone therapy/birth control medications, or have busy, high-stress lifestyles.
- The client has a highly inflammatory response that's visible on the skin, like stubborn, inflamed acne or skin that welts immediately after a minor scratch.
- The skin is very oily. Excess oil keeps the exfoliants from penetrating through the skin's surface, rendering them not as effective.
- Dense congestion (many blocked pores packed closely together) is present. Some inflammation is inevitable while all those pores are purging at the same time.

How to Use BP

Using BP is an excellent anti-inflammatory tool that you don't have to use forever. Use it consistently when first purging your acne, and once clear (of even non-inflamed acne, not just inflammation), you can gradually decrease your use of it over the course of several weeks.

In general, we had clients use BP gel only in the evenings. After four weeks, if the acne was still inflamed or the skin extremely oily (thus interfering with the penetration of exfoliants), we'd increase their usage to both day and night (taking care that the client avoids sun exposure and does not

Section 1 - Start with the Obvious - Your Skincare Face Regimen

dry out). They may apply sunscreen after letting the BP gel penetrate for at least thirty to sixty minutes. Using BP twice a day was very rare, though.

People with balanced, non-reactive skin should easily be able to use BP in the evening with the Hydrating Gel to curb any dryness they may experience. Those with sensitive or dry skin can acclimate to using it by washing, icing, applying the BP gel all over the face and wearing it like a mask for fifteen minutes before thoroughly washing it off, then proceeding immediately with toning and moisturizing every night. Eventually, you'd leave it on longer and longer each night (thirty minutes for two nights, sixty minutes for two nights, ninety for two nights, working up to 120 minutes) until you're able to wear it all night without removing it, with no irritation or dryness. While your skin is still acclimating, you can wash the BP gel off, then tone before moisturizing. Once you're wearing the BP gel all night, be sure to tone first. Another option is to alternate BP gel and Hydrating Gel layered together on one night and then only Hydrating Cream the next night, alternating the two until you can wear the BP gel and Hydrating Gel combination every night with no problems.

For people who are too sensitive and/or dry to start with the BP gel but need inflammatory support or who suspect an allergy to BP gel or have rosacea, make sure to conduct a patch test (see below) before using any BP products. If you successfully complete the patch test, try starting with a BP cleanser by foaming it up, massaging it into the skin, and quickly rinsing it off. You can eventually leave the cleanser on the skin for longer periods of time (a few minutes at most) before rinsing to enhance the product's effectiveness while building your skin's tolerance to using it.

If your skin tolerates the BP cleanser and you still need extra anti-inflammatory action, try introducing the BP gel at night once or twice a week, layering it with Hydrating Gel as needed and tolerated. If your skin is sensitized, avoid using any active products until it's fully healed, then carefully reintroduce BP as above.

First-time users of BP should always use BP gel with Hydrating Gel underneath or on top of it. You can substitute pure aloe vera gel in place of our Hydrating Gel, so long as it's acne-safe. It's optimal to put the BP on the skin first and then the Hydrating Gel on top to maximize the BP's efficacy. But if you are dry, create a moisture buffer by applying the Hydrating Gel first and the BP on top, as well as using Hydrating Cleanser to moisturize the skin while cleansing.

Special Note: No creams or lotions are to be used with BP gel! Doing so could stop the BP from working.

Clear Skin for Everyone

BP acclimating calendar

Day 1	Day 2	Day 3	Day 4
15 min	15 min	15 min	30 min
Day 5	**Day 6**	**Day 7**	**Day 8**
30 min	30 min	60 min	60 min
Day 9	**Day 10**	**Day 11**	**Day 12**
60 min	2h	2h	2h
Day 13	**Day 14**	**Day 15**	**Day 16 onwards**
All night	All night	All night	All night

To acclimate to using BP gel: Wash, ice, apply the BP gel for the specified amount of time before rinsing off, toning and moisturizing for the night. When wearing BP gel all night: Wash, ice, tone, apply BP gel and Hydrating Gel if needed.

Section 1 - Start with the Obvious - Your Skincare Face Regimen

A Few Important Notes About BP

If an allergy is suspected, discontinue use on the face and do a patch test behind the ear (or on the neck) for three to seven days. If a reaction starts (even if it's before the testing time period of three to seven days), discontinue use and consult a doctor.

BP bleaches fabrics, so take care to wash your hands thoroughly with soap after applying. Be mindful of what may come in contact with your hands and face when you apply it. This is another reason why wearing it at night is more suitable to avoid ruining your fashionable daytime wardrobe!

BP is drying not only for your acne but also for your hands, so again, wash thoroughly (perhaps with a moisturizing, acne-safe hand soap) and consider moisturizing afterward with an acne-safe product like our Body Lotion.

The areas around the eyes, nostrils, and mouth can easily get dry and irritated from too much BP exposure. Avoid using BP too close to or directly on these areas, and if needed, occlude and protect these spots with a sparing application of 100% shea butter.

BP and eye creams don't mix! Using both at the same time can cause the BP to bleed into the eye cream, causing dryness and irritation around the eyes. Apply eye creams in the daytime when there's no BP on your skin.

Overzealous applications can rub off the face and into the eye via pillowcases. If your eyes are irritated, try applying less product farther from your eyes and changing your pillowcase regularly.

BP can sting and burn when you raise your internal heat, so do your regimen *after* your physically exerting activity (like exercise or going out dancing). Applying it right before going to sleep, along with staying dry and cool through the night, is best.

BP cleansers take at least thirty seconds on the skin to activate. For best results with using a BP face or body wash, massage it on and allow it to remain on the skin for at least a full minute before very thoroughly rinsing away.

If BP is a part of your regimen, it's extremely important to use it as directed and that you continue to do so for several months after you clear up (or for the longer term if you are younger and/or your acne is still active). BP often works better as a preventative measure, so while it may seem that skipping BP applications doesn't seem to impact your skin in the short term, remember that it takes one to three months for pimples to form, which is when you are more likely see the impact of missed BP applications down the road.

Lastly, wear sunscreen in the daytime to avoid sunburn![4]

How to Start the Clearing Process

Things to Do Right Now

Document your baseline starting point, visually and introspectively.

Visually

Take several clear, well-lit pictures and videos of your clean, bare-faced, and moisturized skin as you start the program, and again every week or two to track your progress.

When taking your videos and photos, get as close up and focused as possible, filling the screen with your face. Use indirect light (natural is best, but indoor is okay; whatever accentuates textures and pigment is ideal), preferably taken in the same spot at the same time of day. Capture all the texture and any pigmentation at multiple angles for a detailed starting baseline.[5] And remember, these are taken for reference only, so quickly make sure the images are clear and sharp, then archive them away. We want you to be aware of but not feel bad about your skin, so there's no need to get obsessed over these pictures.

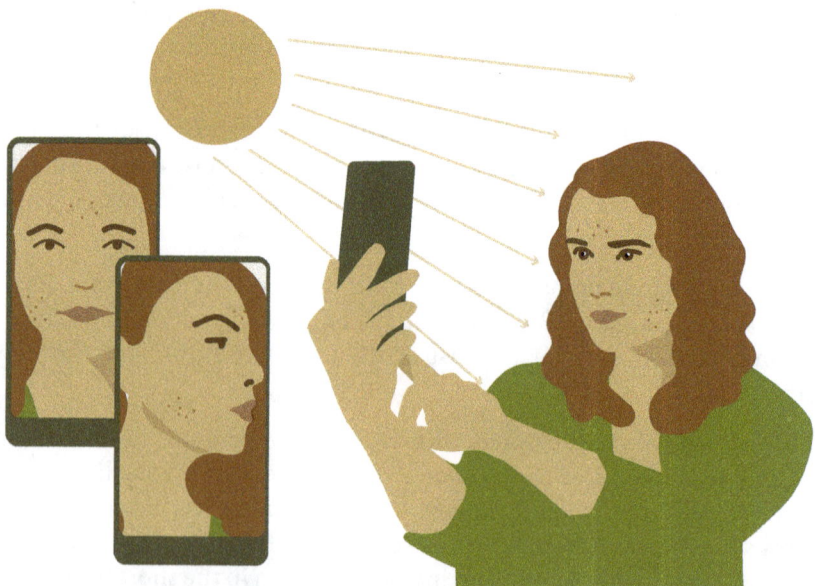

Use the front camera on your phone to take your selfies. Or, use the back camera by facing a mirror, using the reflection as your guide and touching the phone screen to focus the camera, ensuring a clear and sharp image.

Section 1 - Start with the Obvious - Your Skincare Face Regimen

They also serve as empowerment tools. I've had many clients come in for their maintenance treatments feeling down because of a recent crop of pimples that have popped up from a stressful time with a careless diet or from travel. Then we pull up their old "before" photos, and they are instantly reminded of how much better off their skin is now, not to mention how much more empowered they feel knowing what their triggers are and how exactly to fix them.

Introspectively

For some, it might be helpful to keep a journal. This can help you make sense of a breakout that happens weeks later. Take a few minutes to answer some questions to see how you feel about your skin now and again as the weeks go by:

- On a scale of 1-10, how much do I think about my acne?
- On a scale of 1-10, how painful is my skin?
- On a scale of 1-10, how confident do I feel?
- On average, how much time do I spend getting ready in the morning, taking care of my skin, or putting on makeup to cover up my acne?
- What things in my life do I feel my acne has held me back from? Personally—dating? Professionally—being taken seriously and getting that job I want?
- How in control do I feel over my acne?
- Do I know what my acne-causing triggers are?
- Do I know how to clear my skin?

Check your products

We'll go through this in more detail shortly, but you'll want to check the products you use on your skin as well as what foods you keep in the kitchen for acne-causing ingredients. Once you've checked your skin products, do the same process for your kitchen. The most common dietary aggravators for acne-prone skin are coffee, soy, dairy, and sugar (especially sodas), as you'll learn in Section 5. If you only keep acne-safe foods in your house, you'll be less tempted to indulge in foods that may cause problems for you. If you live with other people, try to separate your acne-safe food from non-acne-safe food.

Eliminate variables

To prevent interference with the clearing process as well as avoid potential over-exfoliation, we recommend that you abstain from skin treatments and products (including prescriptions, with your doctor's approval) other than what we outline in this book. We want to eliminate variables that may complicate your clearing process so we can clear you up as quickly as possible.

Do your regimen completely at least twice daily

Using the right skin products correctly and icing to keep inflammation down is the best first line of defense against acne. Once you're clear, keep up with the regimen twice a day to maintain. Some people *may* be able to get away with doing their regimen once a day, preferably at night, to wash off the day's grime and makeup (making sure to wear SPF during the day), but only when you get clear will you see what you can (and can't) get away with.

Let it go

Refusing to get rid of the expensive (but cloggy) products you still have a lot of and "want to finish up" will only prolong your acne and ultimately can make the purging process more expensive. In-clinic, we had a few clients unwilling to divorce their $60 shampoo but ended up spending hundreds of dollars on treatments to clear up the acne it gave them.

Check Your Skin Products

During this part of your skincare adventure, we've arrived on a two-lane road. You might take the more "scenic" slow lane of auditing your stash and salvage what looks safe to use. You may be able to save some money by using what you have and brighten someone's day by donating the ones that won't work for you (to friends if they've been opened, to shelters if unopened). This way takes more time and patience. Or you can take the fast lane by using With & Within products. This path allows you to eliminate the guesswork, time, and resources involved in experimenting otherwise. If you choose this route, you can skip to the next section, *What to Expect During the Clearing Process*.

In our clinic, most clients came to us using all kinds of random skincare products that often contained pore-clogging ingredients, exacerbating or prolonging the very problem they were trying to eliminate. This is how the product audit was born.

By auditing what you're currently using, you'll have a more educated stance on whether or not the products you have now are going to help or hurt your skin. You'll likely discover products in your arsenal that were making you break out in the first place. This audit will help you because you'll see a dramatic improvement (or even achieve complete clarity) by switching to only safe products.

Section 1 - Start with the Obvious - Your Skincare Face Regimen

You'll want to check every product that touches the skin on your face and body *directly*, like:

- Cleansers, toners, serums, moisturizers, treatment masks, sunscreens
- All kinds of makeup, primers, powders, sprays
- Body washes, scrubs, washes, lotions, creams, butters
- Other products like chafing gels, bug spray, medications, ointments, wipes

You'll also want to check anything else (products, clothing, etc.) that touches your skin indirectly. It seems obvious that you'd audit the products you use directly on your face, but looking at what you use on your hair, hand cream, or even your toothpaste can be the last puzzle piece to skin clarity. Check your:

- Hair cleansing, conditioning, and styling products
- Lip and oral care products
- Laundry detergent (pillowcases, towels, washable PPE masks)
- Product rubbing off other people onto you (babies, pets, make-out partners)
- Helmets, headbands, protective masks, eyeglasses, yoga mats, sports equipment
- Unwashed clothing residue (new or vintage)

Prescriptions, to use or not to use?

Clients who were new to us and still on medications to control their acne were often apprehensive about stopping them for fear their faces would majorly break out (which rarely happened). In fact, more often than not, these clients didn't notice much, if any, difference after stopping the drugs, which were usually oral antibiotics or spironolactone. Clients with severe inflammation might have opted to continue taking the oral antibiotic while first integrating the skin and lifestyle changes we taught them, eventually weaning off of them as their inflammation came under better control. Birth control is trickier, though, because of the hormones' more direct, intimate, and erratic skin effects and prolonged acclimation time.

We suggest stopping topical prescriptions when switching over to your new active and acne-safe skin regime, but make sure to discuss this with your doctor first.

Step One: Check + Confirm, then Copy + Paste (First-Round Ingredient Check)

Compare the ingredients on your bottle to the list you find online[6]. Make sure it matches, since oftentimes ingredient lists online are different from what's on the actual bottle. Then, use the With & Within product checker to do a quick preliminary check on what acne-causing ingredients are in the products you're researching by copying and pasting the ingredient list into our search box. If a product passes this first look, then it gets to move on to Step 2.

Step Two: Carefully Analyze, Then Keep or Toss

This is where you double- and triple-check your findings from Step 1 to make sure there are no misspellings or alternate names in the ingredients you are researching. For instance, botanical plant names in Latin are very common; we found many seaweeds this way. I suggest you use the same product checker page and use the text scanning function on your computer to make searching for each ingredient one by one easy.

Products with ingredients rated 0-2 are safe to use; 3s might be best to avoid, and 4s and 5s you'll definitely want to steer clear of. Not all products

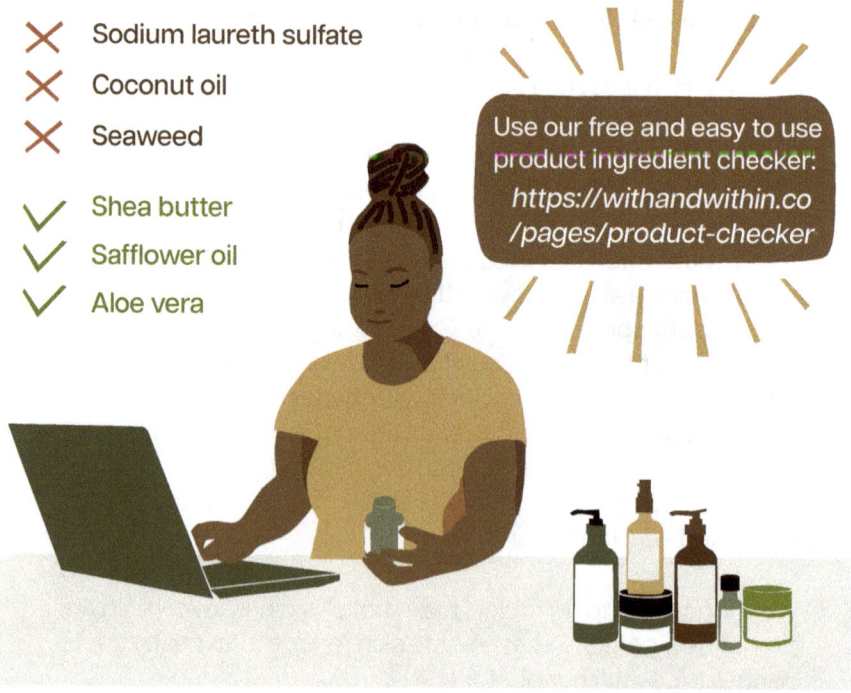

with 3s are bad; it's just that you won't know if and how bad until you are on Step 3 to test them.

> ### TIP: Mostly acne-safe might be ok
>
> If you have trouble putting together a regimen of only acne-safe products, use whatever acne-safe products you can find and fold in one product that's questionable or cloggy. The majority of acne-safe products and exfoliants may "cancel" out the rare cloggy ones.

Step Three: Carefully Test

Congratulations! If you made it here, that means you have products that made it through Step 2 and can now test them on your skin to see if they are truly acne-safe. Ideally, you are using only one "not yet tested" product at a time. This way, if you are breaking out, you can easily match the new acne to the particular product you're testing out.

Test the chosen product on your skin while carefully looking for any negative reactions from using it. Three months is optimal.

Step 3 testing requires lots of patience and time, especially if you test for the optimal three months. The products we sell in our shop are proven effective and will save you this time.

Product Shopping Tips

In addition to detergent foaming agents (sodium lauryl sulfate, sodium laureth sulfate) and thickeners (isopropyl myristate, or cetearyl alcohol used in the same formula with ceteareth-20) rampant in most mass-produced products, there are a few others that commonly pop up which require some extra attention.

Vitamin E or Tocopherol

Often included in skin and food products as a preservative, vitamin E, also known as tocopherol, is usually derived from cloggy soybean oil, though recently, more companies are sourcing it from acne-safe sunflower or safflower oils. Soybean-derived vitamin E can be a problem when ingested. I had a client who mostly cleared up but kept breaking out on his neck until we discovered he was taking soybean oil-based vitamin E capsules. Once he discontinued taking them, he cleared completely.

Oils

Thanks to our in-house research, we found that most oils used topically are comedogenic, given enough time, especially if used undiluted directly onto the skin or hair or are higher up in a formulation's ingredient listing. According to Dr. Fulton's research, safflower, sunflower and mineral oils are the only ones rated with a super-safe zero. In the clinic, we also found 100% shea butter and shea oil to be safe. We shy away from mineral oil because it's a highly processed and refined petroleum product and we prefer to use healthier, non-toxic oils. You can read more about oils for both topical and dietary use on our lifestyle library blog post here.

<u>Oil pulling</u>: A new trend to the West with roots in centuries-old Ayurveda in which edible oils are swished around the mouth (much like mouthwash) for several minutes to promote improved oral and whole-body health. Proceed with caution if using any other oils besides safflower and sunflower. Repeated and constant exposure to other oils may exacerbate acne formation around the mouth, upper lip, and chin.

<u>Oil cleansing</u>: Using oils to cleanse (wash) the face: A big fat no. Despite all the marketing claims, this has led to many greasy, broken-out faces walking into our clinic. Though these cleansing oils may be okay for non-acne-prone skin, if you are acne-prone but need more moisture, find an acne-safe, non-foaming moisturizing cleanser to use instead.

<u>Oil as a moisturizer</u>: This could be okay if your skin really needs it after exhausting the other moisture-adding tricks, and even then, literally only two to three drops for the entire face per application. Use acne-safe oils sparingly, only when and where you need them, and "seal" them into the skin with an acne-safe cream on top to lock in that moisture.

Fragrance

Fragrance is most likely going to be the most common comedogenic ingredient with a 3 rating that you will find. However, "fragrance" is an umbrella term used for several hundred ingredients, many of which are comedogenic. For this reason, as much as possible, avoid using products that contain fragrance unless that fragrance:

- Has been tested to be acne-safe, preferably on actual acne-prone folks by an institution like With & Within, or at the very least passes our product checker OR is verified by the company as to what exactly is included in the ingredient they call "fragrance."
- Is composed of only essential oils and is disclosed as such on the ingredient label. Fragrances labeled "natural fragrance" are still questionable. If you're really vested (and have the patience), contact

the manufacturer to make sure this is true before using a product, and reference our blog post for pointed guidance.

Products that are fragrance-free, have a more "natural" or minimalist packaging design, and/or are sold in health food stores or natural care aisles have higher chances of being acne-safe, but they can still be cloggy. "Natural" formulas can contain cloggy ingredients like coconut oil, cocoa butter or seaweeds. "Eco-" and "green"-looking packaging can make the product appear simple and acne-safe when it's actually not. Always check the ingredients.

The Most Common Comedogenic Ingredients to Avoid

Although there are hundreds of ingredients to watch out for when shopping acne-safe, the most common ones are mentioned in the next few pages. In order to access the full list, use our free and easy product checker tool.[7]

The following items are commonly found in products located in conventional medical and mass retailers internationally sold in drugstores, supermarkets, department stores, and as prescription medications.

- Sodium lauryl sulfate
- Sodium laureth sulfate
- D&C colors like D&C red #30 (or red #30); artificial colors derived from crude oils
- Myristic acid
- Fragrance

In stay-on products like lotions, creams, makeup, and powders:

- Glyceryl stearate SE
- Isopropyl myristate
- Cetyl alcohol
- Cetearyl alcohol and Ceteareth-20 (both must be in the same product, but may not necessarily show up right next to each other on the ingredient list; Cetearyl alcohol on its own is fine)
- Ethylhexyl palmitate
- D&C colors like D&C red #30 (or red #30); artificial colors derived from crude oils
- Fragrance

Dimethicones, silicones, and petroleum-derived ingredients like paraffinum liquidum. These are commonly found in sunscreens, makeup primer gels, hair smoothing products, and creams targeted toward dry skin. Dr. Fulton says they are safe, but I've seen them break out 5-10% of our clients.

"Natural" formulations are commonly found in health food stores or smaller boutique brands. Avoid the same as above plus:

- Oils: coconut, argan, soybean, algae, wheat germ, jojoba, olive, sweet almond
- Cocoa butter
- Iodide-rich ingredients like sea salt and seaweeds like kelp, algae, and spirulina (they can reduce redness but can induce iodine breakouts/rashes)
- Vitamin E (usually soybean oil-derived, but sunflower-derived is okay)
- Fragrance

Demographic- or Region-Targeted Brands

Asian skin brands

Avoid the same as above and most commonly:

- Myristic acid is found in virtually every cleanser in this market, foaming or not. The Asian market is big on moisture, so for the most part, creamy cleansers are the norm, as is layering several moisturizing skincare and makeup products to achieve a dewy (read: greasy) look.
- Silicones, dimethicones and comedogenic oils are very common in leave-on moisturizing products.
- Fragrance is definitely rampant in formulations from this area, so it can be difficult to find products without it. In general, products with the most minimalist-designed packaging are the likeliest to be fragrance-free or at least less aggressively fragranced than their counterparts.

Black skin brands

Same as above and most commonly:

- Coconut oil
- Cocoa butter
- Black soap made from coconut oil
- Most oils and butters in all products, especially moisturizers and hair styling products
- Many thick, curly, kinky hair products are used very closely or directly on the skin

Hispanic skin brands

Same as above and most commonly:

Section 1 - Start with the Obvious - Your Skincare Face Regimen

- Highly drying cleansers and alcohol-based toners
- Thick mineral oil or petrolatum-based moisturizers, often highly fragranced

European skin brands
Same as above and most commonly comedogenic oils like argan, soybean and coconut oils.

Textured hair
Taking care of textured hair using the least amount of hair products possible would be the best way to keep the skin its clearest. Hair styling products will still likely be needed, but products used for intense hold, smoothing, waterproofing, etc. don't allow the skin to breathe, complicating things. Most oils and butters are also comedogenic, the residues of which transfer easily to scarves, pillowcases, and hats, which can create acne. Also, try not to touch your hair to avoid the same acne-inducing residue transfer.

Assembling Your Regimen

Order of Product Priorities
In a perfect world, every single product you use is acne-safe to rule out any topical acne-causing factors. Once we make this change, we can likely attribute any remaining breakouts to other triggers like diet, lifestyle, or body health. Acne-safe products will prevent new acne from forming, and active products (like exfoliants) will help flush out existing acne while preventing more by sloughing off dead skin cells before they get a chance to create new acne seeds. Our first step is to find acne-safe products to wash, moisturize, and sun-protect our skin with before adding an active anti-acne product.

Testing "Maybe-Safe" Products
The thing with experimenting with products that aren't vetted is that an ingredient list could look good and safe, but you won't really know for sure until you actually use the products on your skin. Foaming products (like cleansers and shampoo) will usually clog you in days, making for easy test results. But testing products that are designed to stay on the skin (like moisturizers and makeup) are trickier because they take more time to clog and patience to gauge.

The best way to test these is to apply them only on one side of the face, the same side of the face, for several weeks and/or months at a time. It's really important to test only one product at a time because if you are using many and you break out, it will be very difficult to tell which is the problematic one.

How to Determine What Products are Good

Cleansers

A good cleanser should remove daily oil and grime along with lightweight makeup, leaving your skin feeling balanced (neither too oily nor dry) after rinsing. Waterproof or long-wear makeup or SPF can be removed with a soft cleansing washcloth or perhaps will need a separate makeup remover product.

We put our clients on either the With & Within Hydrating Cleanser or Charcoal Cleanser, depending on how dry or oily their skin is. If after a month or so they still needed extra acne-fighting support, we might give them a mandelic acid cleanser (for brightening and anti-bacterial support) or BP cleanser (for drying and controlling inflammation).

It's common for people to alternate cleansers depending on the season or climate. I personally like to have both cleanser types so I can choose which one is best for my skin that particular day.

Moisturizers

A good daily moisturizer should keep your skin feeling supple, soft, and comfortable, not too oily/greasy or tight. If you'll be exposed to harsh weather elements, applying extra layers of moisturizer and sunscreen on the skin may help to prevent windburn and chapped skin. Warming your fingertips and hands prior to application will help facilitate more even product distribution.

Sufficient moisture in the skin is very important to help the skin's healing and purging process, as dehydrated skin can result in a rougher texture and acne that's harder to purge. Even if you are oily, you'll still likely need some kind of hydrating product to balance out the active products in your regimen.

In our clinic, we infused moisture into our clients' regimens with the appropriate moisturizing sunscreen for the daytime and the With & Within Hydrating Cream for nighttime. If the client was using BP gel at night, we'd have them layer it with the With & Within Hydrating Gel since cream could deactivate BP's activity. Sometimes (especially during cold, dry-skin months or climates), we'd have clients alternate evening treatments: Hydrating Cream one night and the Hydrating Gel & BP combo the next.

If you don't have access to these products, shop using the With & Within product checker OR try these:

- 100% safflower or sunflower or shea oil; three-ish drops for the face should be enough

Section 1 - Start with the Obvious - Your Skincare Face Regimen

- 100% shea butter (used alone or, if extra moisture is needed, on top of the oils above and under your Hydrating Cream)
- Dr. Fulton says 100% mineral oil is also acne-safe, but I prefer plant-derived oils instead

One hundred percent purity of oils and butters is necessary, as blends often contain pore-clogging carrier oils and other ingredients.

Using oils

For the oils, use a bottle with a dropper. No more than three drops for your face, and more if you are doing your neck and chest, too.

Do NOT directly touch the dropper to squirt product onto the face! This introduces outside bacteria and sebum into the entire bottle of product, contaminating it.

To properly apply oil, dispense the three drops, one each onto your ring, middle, and index fingertips, return the dropper back into the bottle, then touch the same fingers on the opposite hand. Distribute all over the face using tapping motions all over the face. This may not seem like enough product, but oil spreads easily. Within a few seconds, you will feel the entire surface of your skin evenly moisturized. If not, you may need to tap a bit more all over the face or add just one drop more of oil.

You can do light massage movements once the oil is distributed all over the face to promote absorption. If you are clear and have no inflammation, using a *gua sha* (using a smooth-edged massage tool to scrape the skin, inducing blood circulation and lymph detoxification) or jade rolling may be incorporated into this step.

Using shea butter

Scoop out a small pea-size of product with a spatula (or a clean finger) and rub it between the fingertips of both hands (or entire hands) to warm and completely melt it into oil. Doing this will make it much easier to apply than in its solid state. Massaging the butter into your fingers/hands until it's almost all absorbed before moisturizing your face with them will help keep the butter from getting too oily.

Clear Skin for Everyone

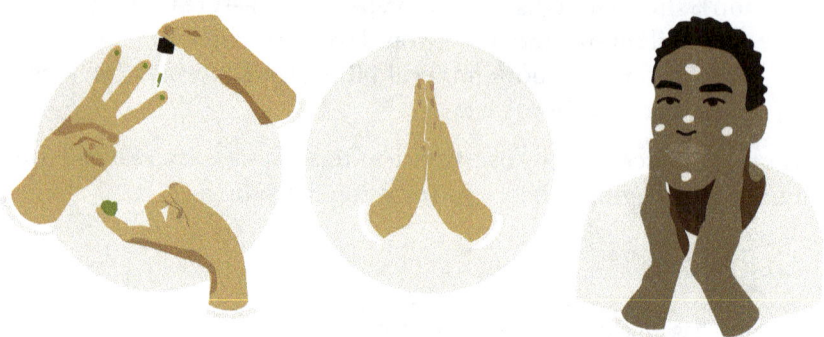

Dispense oil one drop at a time onto each fingertip, or scoop out your cream in one swoop. Touch your fingertips together, and dispense the product evenly all over the face.

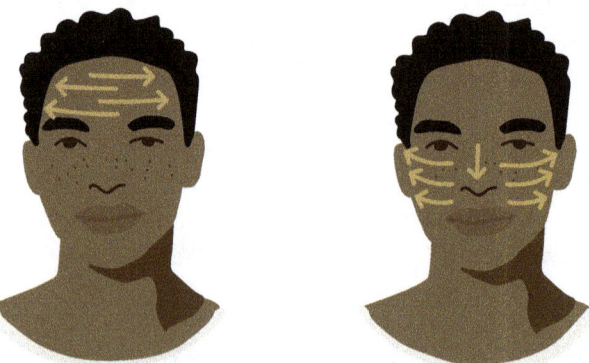

Using the length of your fingers and working from the center of the face out towards the ears, gently massage the product into the forehead, down the nose and the cheeks. (This technique is also recommended for applying toner.)

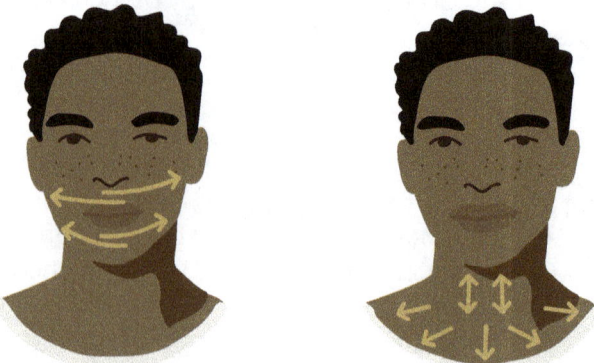

Proceed working in your product above and below the lips, onto the chin and jawline, finishing with the neck and chest.

Gently pat your shea butter-moisturized fingertips or hands onto the skin, evenly distributing the product all over the face, neck, and chest. Rub the excess butter into your hands, then go back over and massage the product into the rest of the face with your now dry hands.

"Drying Time": Both the oil and shea butter may make you feel a little greasy for about five to ten minutes but should be absorbed fully after that. If you're still oily after the "drying time," you're likely using too much, so just gently pat off the excess with a clean, dry towel or tissue and use less the next time.

Note: A grainy texture is a natural characteristic of pure shea butter as a natural response to temperature changes. Warming the jar of butter to its liquid state (by placing the container in the hot sun with a dish or cloth underneath it to catch drips, or gently warmed in a bowl of very hot water, stirring the contents as it melts) and allowing it to cool and harden overnight at room temperature should smooth everything out.

Sunscreens

Now that we've got your face cleaned and moisturized, sunscreen is next. Proper sun protection is crucial for many reasons, namely skin cancer prevention and its aging effects: pigmentation, inflammation, and burning. Having a proper and reliable SPF will allow you to safely incorporate active acne-clearing products.

Sunscreens have come a long way in terms of usability, but unfortunately NOT comedogenicity. Using our product checker (https://withandwithin.co/pages/product-checker) will help guide you to safer options. Although safe for most people, dimethicones and silicones commonly found in SPFs can break out a small 5-10% of acne-prone skin, so take caution if you are super sensitive and acne-prone.

In the clinic, we use sunscreen as the main source of moisture within the regimen. We recommend the following sunscreens, in order of most to least moisturizing:

- With & Within Safeguard SPF 40: Our most moisturizing and protective formula in a cream form.
- Clear Choice Sport Sun Shield SPF 45: Suitable for most normal and combination skin types in a lotion form that spreads and absorbs easily.
- TIZO 2 and 3: No moisture at all, which can be great for oilier skins that need mattifying oil absorption. You can also layer moisture

underneath it where needed. It has a velvety finish that many like for under makeup, which can also be used on its own.

If you don't have access to these products, use our product checker to see if what you've found locally is safe for you to try.

SPF under makeup is a must

While it's better than nothing, using makeup that has SPF in it on it's own is not an adequate substitute for sunscreen because you wouldn't be covering areas like your neck, chest, or ears. Applying a broad-spectrum SPF all over first and applying makeup on top offers the best coverage. A mineral powder SPF is a good option for reapplying protection and touching up makeup throughout the day.

Minerals and moisture

Minerals in makeup and SPF products are inherently drying, so you may need to hydrate extra, compensating for the dryness minerals may cause on your skin. You can try using a hydrating, non-foaming cleanser, applying a drop or two of moisturizing oil, shea butter, or moisturizer during your routine and letting it fully absorb before makeup or spritzing rosewater after your makeup application and throughout the day to hydrate and refresh.

Makeup

We generally recommend mineral makeup over conventional dye makeup, as synthetic colorants are commonly comedogenic. As a general rule, loose mineral powder makeups are more likely to be acne-safe than pressed, liquid, cream, or hybrid formulas. It's the base and binders (often silicone or coconut oil) that are problematic, not the minerals themselves. Make sure to check the ingredients of the specific and individual product you are interested in to make sure it's safe. Find more details about makeup later in this section.

Other Products

It's best to get you on a clear-skinned baseline before inviting possible pore-clogging and irritating variables into your regimen. Accessory products like skin treatment masks, treatment lotions, and potions can wait.

Reintroducing "Cloggy" Products

If you really must, once you're completely clear, slowly work in these questionable products *one at a time*, preferably one new product for three months, carefully looking to see if they make you break out. Starting with a clear face will make it easier to see what works and what doesn't.

Formulations Change Often

Manufacturers will often change their formulations (or sell different ones in different areas), so what may have been acne-safe the last time you bought it may not be the next time you refill. Even without an obvious rebrand or packaging change, do your due diligence and check those ingredients.

What to Expect During the Clearing Process

With proper adherence to the program, our clients cleared up in an average of three months. During this time, our priorities were to purge existing acne, keep inflammation down to keep the purge as quick and low-inflammatory as possible and prevent new acne from forming with products and lifestyle for long-term clarity. Here's a rough idea of what to expect while these changes occur simultaneously:

Your Skin Acclimates and Rebalances

Depending on your starting baseline, it might take your skin about two to four weeks to adjust to your new regimen. During this time, light irritation like slight peeling, flaking, or redness may happen but usually goes away in the first one or two weeks. As long as your skin eventually comes back to normal, this is all expected and temporary.

For some, your skin may feel greasier than usual because your formerly dehydrated skin is acclimating to being naturally moisturized. This is also normal. Give it a couple of weeks to rebalance before adjusting your regimen. You'll eventually notice the texture of your skin start to improve and will be less confused as its moisture balance will start to normalize (i.e., not be so dry or so oily or both).

TIP: Acclimating sensitive, irritated skin

If you experience severe irritating side effects that don't resolve within two or three days, stop the active part of your regimen right away. To help calm your skin, stick with basic and gentle washing, icing (if tolerable), and moisturizing for a few days. Your skin should normalize within a week.

Once your skin is back to normal, slowly work in one active product at a time. For example, use a toner once a day, building up to twice a day over the course of one to two weeks. You may want to do a test patch, too; say, starting with one cheek or behind the ear versus the entire face.

Your Inflammation Starts to Come Down
You'll also notice the inflammation starting to diminish, especially if you switch all your skin products and start icing regularly at the onset. With your skin being more balanced, it will be less irritated and thus less sensitive and inflamed. If you're "doing all the things" and are still inflamed, you probably need to ice more (or maybe need some BP).

Your skin purges
You'll continue to break out as you move through the purge, which usually lasts around two or three months, with the acne tapering off toward the end, becoming smaller and healing faster than usual. As the purge progresses, we start to see a slowdown in new acne formation. This is a sign that your skin is close to being done purging and is on its way to finally getting clear.

Clarity and maintenance
Months three to four and onward bring clarity and maintenance. Continue with your acne-safe lifestyle and use only acne-safe products to maintain your clarity. The number of active products—like acids and benzoyl peroxide—may be reduced depending on how active your acne is and what your skin can tolerate now that it's clear.

Finally, you'll reach the meeting point where your old acne is done purging, and your skin is clear because your acne-safe lifestyle choices are coming to fruition. This usually happens at around the three- to four-month mark.

Purging

There are a few things to consider and expect over the following several weeks while your skin starts the clearing and purging process. Just like cleaning house, things may get a bit messier before they get better—but have no fear! With the right management tools in place, this acclimation and purging period will be over before you know it, and your clear skin will soon become a reality.

As you start your new regimen, your skin will feel healthier, more moisture-balanced, and less sensitized within two to four weeks, and inflammation will be significantly reduced within four to six weeks (with the homecare alone, before a full treatment even happens). The overall quality of the skin improves; however, it will still "break out" for the first month or two. I'd now like to introduce a concept called "purging."

Learning about and managing your expectations around purging is super important. You might get frustrated with the process, think the program doesn't work, or maybe even give up before the actual changes take effect. This purging—along with the acne-safe lifestyle—is what makes the difference between a quick temporary fix and long-term clarity.

Purging is when old acne seeds (that started forming *before* your acne-safe regimen and lifestyle changes) are making their way out of the skin—for good. Since it takes several weeks for acne to form, it also takes at least several weeks for it to go away. The amount and intensity of this acne eventually decrease with time as the seeds purge so long as no other acne-causing habits are still occurring.

Allow for the purge

So even after starting your new active and acne-safe skin regimen, don't expect perfectly clear skin overnight or even within a few days or weeks; allow for the purge. You'll definitely see improvements, but still expect to break out for a little while longer as everything comes together. And ice more than you think you need to!

Let's Walk Through an Example of Purging in Action:

- You do something that causes acne (drink milk and eat cheese).
- You make an acne-safe lifestyle change (stop consuming milk and cheese and instead use active, acne-safe products).
- Time passes, allowing for the old milk and cheese acne to purge, the skincare products to work, and the new lifestyle changes' preventative actions to take effect.
- The pimples become smaller, heal faster, and become sparser as the skin eventually clears.

Important points related to the above:
- All the dairy you consumed up until the change had already started to create acne seeds.

- Your skin may also still be exhibiting an inflammatory response for days or even weeks as a secondary response to that same dairy you consumed.
- Because of the skin's delayed response, it can take 1-3 months for all that dairy acne to purge.

For most folks, the purge isn't worse than a bad day of acne our clients already had. But for some, the skin may get worse before it gets better. This can be a slower or more intensely inflammatory purge. This book will offer all the anti-inflammatory tools I know to help reduce the severity of your purge. Seeking professional help from an esthetician to administer peels and extractions or a doctor to inject cortisone shots or prescribe anti-inflammatories may be necessary.

A More Difficult Purging Process Can Be Caused by Largely Unavoidable Factors Such as:

- Really deep pores (longer distance for that seed to travel)
- Really tight pores (the pore opening is so tight at the surface that it bottlenecks the seed underneath, keeping it stuck inside; exfoliants alone likely won't make them jump out, so you might need some extractions)
- Highly inflammation-prone skin that makes product penetration or extractions difficult
- Extremely oily skin, which can prevent active product penetration and efficacy
- Skin that is slow to regenerate, heal and/or purge
- A second or third purge; rarely, some folks experience this if they have a lot of congestion and/or their skin is slow to heal, but each purging round should be better than the previous ones. If the acne persists with the same ferocity even with program compliance, this is a sign that a larger underlying systemic issue is at play. Seek a holistic health practitioner's help.
- Folks with really tight pores or super-inflamed acne will likely need an esthetician to get the seeds extracted or purged via chemical peels.

An extended purging stage can also be caused by lax compliance with the acne-safe lifestyle and/or regimen or by picking.

At our skin clinic, we supplemented our extraction and peel appointments with LED (light emitting diode) treatments that effectively encouraged the skin's natural healing and anti-inflammatory responses. If done well,

Section 1 - Start with the Obvious - Your Skincare Face Regimen

thorough acne treatments can help to alleviate, treat, and prevent some of the potential inflammation associated with the discomfort of the purging, speed up the skin-clearing, and prevent scarring.

But if it's been at least three months and you swear up and down you're doing all the things, your acne really isn't getting any better and is maybe occurring at the same rate as before you started, you may be dealing with new acne forming instead of old acne purging. Identifying and eliminating the acne-causing sources causing the new breakouts will finally clear the skin.

Why does the old acne seem bigger and/or there's more of them?

Imagine your face is a garden bed and that the acne you have are carrots in various growth stages. Some are tiny seeds that have yet to germinate, some are just starting to sprout, and others are straight up full-grown carrots ready to be picked.

Through the years, you've planted some seeds yourself (for example, used cloggy products or ate a ton of acne-causing foods) that germinated and grew (into pimples). Over time, you've had your share of bountiful and random "harvests" bursting out all over. But now, you're sick of the constant new growth. It's time to clear things up for good! Using this analogy, you can see how the older the vegetable seed is, the bigger the carrot is.

It can seem like those acne seeds are getting bigger, multiplying in quantity, and/or increasing in frequency (carrots maturing!) as they more quickly rise to the surface of the skin. As these seeds make their exit and with the right tools in use, the remaining bumps that follow should decrease in size, severity, and eventually, quantity. The skin's texture gradually improves and eventually clears all the way up!

Keep in mind, though, that if your acne is persistently or increasingly red, swollen, and painful, you have an inflammation problem that should be addressed immediately.

How to Wash Your Face and Use Your Products

Use separate towels to dry your face rather than what you use for your hair and body, especially if you have inflamed acne that may open up when washing or using hair styling products. This helps to keep your skin its cleanest possible, avoiding cross-contamination from dirt accumulated on the body and hair, along with any possibly cloggy body or hair stuff you may be using.

Make sure that you are washing your towels with acne-safe laundry detergent and no softener, as the residue left behind from detergents (and laundry softeners) can also aggravate acne. Change your face towels often, especially if you have oily skin and/or inflamed acne.

Use WARM water to wash your face—not hot, not cold. Hot water will dehydrate and irritate, and cold water isn't as effective with foaming and rinsing the cleanser off your skin (similar to unsuccessfully washing greasy dishes with cold water).

Don't wait too long in between steps while doing your regimen, as even the short standing time between steps can dry your face out. Washing your face and waiting more than a few minutes to moisturize is too long. However, if you feel you *have* to wait between each step for products to dry before applying the next thing (especially your toner), you might be using too much product. Follow the product directions to ensure you are using the right dosage. Aim for a thin layer of each product all over the skin that easily absorbs on its own within thirty seconds or so.

The total cleansing and product application (excluding icing) should really take only around two to three minutes to complete.

Step 1: Get Ready to Wash Your Face

Now that you've got your house in order and everything within reach is acne-safe, it's time to start using your products and purging. Having the right skincare, haircare, and body care products is half the battle, and the other half lies in using them properly *and* consistently.

Go to your freezer and grab your ice so that it's within easy reach as soon as you're done washing your face. It'll melt a little while you wash your face, but that's okay. Make sure to bring enough cubes with you to last a full icing session (or better yet, use one of the silicone ice molds from the With

& Within online shop; it's essentially one big ice cube in a silicone tube that helps to keep it from melting too quickly).

Now, take your jewelry off. Daily grease, grime, dust, and skincare products get into and stay within the grooves of jewelry filigree, around stones and settings, and in between crevices. This means your rings, necklaces, and big hoop earrings. Tiny earrings you keep on 24/7 should be fine, but they should still be regularly removed so you can clean that area of your body for general hygiene and gain access to the skin if you tend to break out there. If you're breaking out on your neck, definitely remove your necklaces so you can wash both your neck and jewelry. You might even want to abstain from wearing necklaces until the skin has cleared up.

Tie back your hair. Wet hair can seep styling products onto your clean face, which is all the more important if you don't wash your hair every day. This way, you can concentrate on cleaning your face and not moving your dirty hair around. If you wear bangs, it's best practice to at least wash them (if not all your hair), especially because they rest on your face. When washing your face, get into the entire hairline. Gingerly washing your face to avoid getting your bangs wet will result in a cleanse that's just not very thorough.

Wash your hands. Once all your jewelry is off and your hair is tied back, wash your hands with an acne-safe hand soap or body wash.

Remove your makeup. For the most part, all makeup should come off with your regular face wash, maybe with the help of a face-cleansing washcloth. However, greasy and transfer-proof lipstick and waterproof mascara are really tough to remove with acne-safe cleanser and water alone. Use a tissue to remove your lipstick so you don't smear it all around your face.

Waterproof and longwearing makeup

If you wear thick layers of waterproof mascara or other transfer-proof makeup that needs to be taken off with an oil-based remover, use a dry toner pad afterward to gently remove the excess oil.

Dr. Fulton says mineral oil is mostly acne-safe even though it's not the environmentally "cleanest" product to use regularly (it's made from crude oil). I've tried alternative acne-safe oils, but they don't do as good a job as mineral oil. Feel free to experiment with safflower and sunflower oils or shea butter. Oil-free makeup removers aren't going to do anything for this type of makeup.

Don't use a regular terry washcloth to forcibly remove this makeup because it will sensitize the skin as it's a form of mechanical exfoliation. Wet and soft microfiber face-cleansing washcloths with a little cleanser work really well in a much gentler way.

Brush your teeth. Always brush your teeth before you wash your face. This is important for three reasons:

1. Toothpaste residue around your mouth clogs pores if you are using comedogenic toothpaste (which is pretty much all of them), so shop carefully. SLS (sodium laureth or lauryl sulfates), coconut oil, and carrageenan are common comedogenic ingredients that are found in toothpaste and should be avoided.
2. You'll dry your face out in between having washed your face (but not moisturized it yet) and brushing your teeth. Just those few minutes in between can be enough to dehydrate your skin, making it flaky and sensitive to your active products. It's best to brush before washing in case your oral hygiene regimen takes a long time.
3. Keep the active products on your skin. You don't want to wash off the skin products you just put on, which is particularly important if you break out around the mouth.

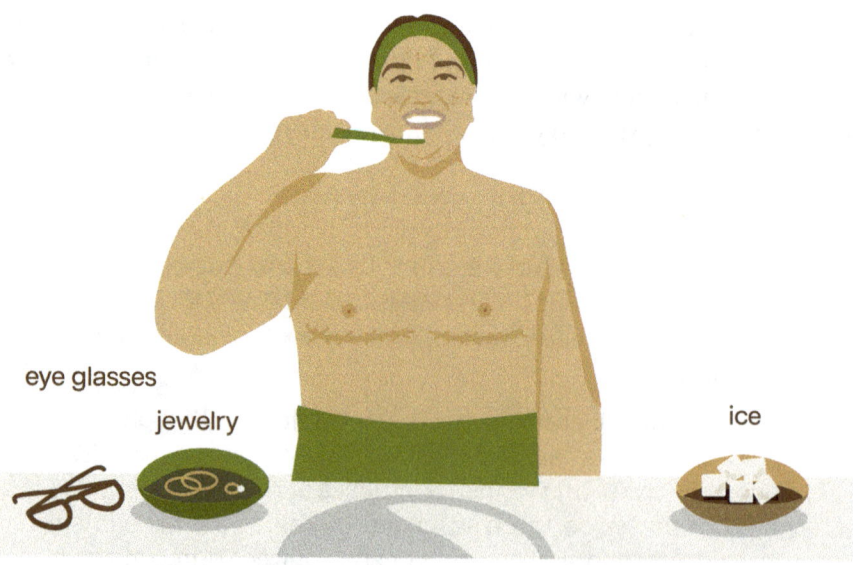

Prepare to wash your face by first tying your hair back, removing your jewelry, brushing your teeth and having your ice ready.

Section 1 - Start with the Obvious - Your Skincare Face Regimen

Step 2 — Wash Your Face

Always use warm water, never cold or scalding hot. Cold won't foam up a cleanser properly nor rinse it away completely, and hot is going to burn, sensitize and dry out your skin. Your face is a living organ, so treat it with care. Get into a rhythm of gently yet thoroughly massaging your face while you cleanse to ensure you are getting to every spot on your skin several times.

Foaming cleansers

Foaming cleansers need some water to lather up and get sudsy, just like when you're doing your dishes. Foam it up on your hands alone, with a plastic foaming net or shower pouf, or lather it directly on your face.

To foam in your hands, wet them and squirt a one-inch circle-sized amount of cleanser onto them. Rub your hands together slowly, adding small splashes of water as needed to get a good foam going, and then apply it to your wet face.

Or apply the cleanser to your wet face, and wet your hands and rub your face, repeating this wetting and rubbing motion as much as you need to get a foam going. Add the water a little bit at a time to your hands—not splashing your face—so as not to over dilute and wash away the cleanser.

You should end up with a foam that is light, soft, and bubbly, not as thick as how the gel originally came out of the bottle. If the texture feels thick and isn't foaming much, it's probably because you haven't diluted the cleanser with enough water. If the cleanser isn't foaming at all, you may have over-diluted it and need more cleanser. Then, start the foaming process again.

Once you get some good foaming action going, use the entire surface of both your hands with a circular motion to make sure you're getting into every nook and cranny: into the hairline, around the ears, underneath your chin…repeating this cycle several times all over the face.

If you're breaking out on your neck and chest, you'll want to get these areas too, though it may be best for you to do this in the shower. Don't forget around and behind your ears, especially if you are very oily skinned or are breaking out here. Hair products often get caught in the crooks of the ears, causing blackheads and pimples to form inside and around them. These areas are more easily and thoroughly washed and rinsed off in the shower.

If you need to get a bit more action from your active cleansers (cleansers that have exfoliating acids or drying agents in them), work them into the skin, and before rinsing off, leave them on the skin for a few minutes to allow those active ingredients to work. Just take care to keep your eyes clear from any drips to keep them safe from eye irritation.

Non-foaming cleansers

These cleansers do not foam, so you won't need water until you rinse them off. In fact, using water will dilute the moisturizing features of these cleansers. Dispense a one-inch circle-sized amount of cleanser onto your fingertips, touch them together in a prayer-like fashion to get it evenly distributed to both hands, and then apply it all over your *dry* face to evenly distribute. Applying the non-foaming cleanser to dry skin will allow your skin to soak up the moisturizing ingredients in it without water dilution getting in the way.

Once your cleanser is evenly distributed all over the face, start your gentle-yet-thorough cleansing facial massage. Just like with foaming cleansers, I use the lengths of my fingers with a circular motion all over, making sure to get every nook and cranny: into the hairline, by the ears, and underneath your chin, and repeating this cycle several times all over the face.

If you are experiencing dryness, you can use your non-foaming cleanser as a moisturizing mask by leaving it on the skin for a few minutes after having massaged it in. You can also try dispensing a bit more of your moisturizing cleanser and/or adding a drop or two of sunflower or safflower oil to it and extend your cleansing facial massage for extra moisturizing benefits. Once you're done with your facial cleansing massage, you can either rinse off thoroughly or use a wet microfiber makeup-removing cloth to wipe away the makeup and sunscreen, making sure to rinse very thoroughly afterward.

Rinse thoroughly

Splash your face with warm water at least ten to twenty times, using your fingers and hands to work that water into the face, completely rinsing off the cleanser. Make sure to rub thoroughly into your hairline and sides of your face to wash away any cleanser that may have gotten into your hair and under your chin. Cleanser wiped off versus rinsed off, even if acne-safe, can result in breakouts.

Step 3: Ice Your Face

Now it's time for the cryotherapy part of your skin regime: icing your face. Since ice is wet, you don't need to dry off your skin in between washing and icing, but don't dilly-dally in between your regimen steps lest your face dry out, getting dehydrated and irritated.

The bigger cubes you can use, the easier to hold onto, the more icing surface area you'll have to work with and the longer you'll be able to do it. The silicone ice molds we sell in our online shop are perfect because they are a

Section 1 - Start with the Obvious - Your Skincare Face Regimen

great size, each cube lasting about fifteen to twenty-five minutes, and the silicone tubes keep your fingers from freezing. You can also use small paper cups to use like a push-up popsicle.

1. Straight from the freezer, run your ice underneath some water to safely remove the cap and take the dry chill of the ice off, avoiding frostbite. (Think of licking a metal signpost in a snowy climate and your tongue gets stuck to it; not a good idea.) If you bring your ice to the bathroom with you before you wash your face, the slight melting of the ice during those few minutes should make the ice wet and safe to apply to your skin.

2. Immediately after washing your face, lightly rub the ice directly onto your face, cold and water dripping everywhere. This is best done over a sink or a towel draped around your chest to catch those drips, or even in the shower. There is no need to apply pressure, but keep moving the ice around on your face to distribute the cold and prevent frostbite or ice burn.

3. Rub the ice all over your face and spend extra time on areas where the skin is most inflamed (or feels like it's going to be), and start your icing distraction routine, whatever that is. Watch your favorite show, dance along to a short playlist, or use it as a time to deep breathe and meditate twice a day.

4. After you're all done, gently pat your skin dry with a clean towel and proceed with the rest of your regimen *immediately* after drying off. The next steps are usually your toner, followed by your treatment serum and/or your moisturizer or SPF. Don't take too long after drying your face to finish the rest of your regimen. Your face will dry out, making it susceptible to dehydration and sensitivity to your active products.

Redness and flushing after icing are totally normal and expected. Your skin will normalize within at most a half-hour after icing, but usually much sooner. Unless your skin is super-sensitive or you iced too much/incorrectly, your skin should return to normal by the time you walk out the door to start your day.

TIP: Icing for pretty much everything

This icing trick also works for ingrown hairs, mosquito bites, healing scabs, or anything itchy anywhere on your body!

How Long and Often You Should Ice

Icing twice a day, anywhere from three quick rounds all over the face for maintenance, at least five minutes for mild acne and up to thirty minutes each time for more inflamed cases is an incredibly important part of your clearing program. Start slow and work up to longer if needed, and take breaks if you get too cold or your skin turns too red or irritated. Once you start to clear up, you can back off the icing a bit, but I do recommend keeping it up at least a few times a week to maintain your clarity and prevent any new pimples that may pop up.

How Does Icing Work?

It is now common knowledge that inflammation is the root cause of many health issues, and acne is no exception. While it is critical to manage inflammation with diet modifications and stress management, you can also reduce inflammation topically by icing your skin (aka cryotherapy, using cold to slow down blood circulation in specific areas, relieving inflammation and swelling).

The benefits of icing are manifold. It:

- Helps prevent inflammation before it sets in.
- Relieves existing inflammation (much like alleviating a swollen ankle), speeding healing, thus reducing scarring and pigmentation.
- Creates micro-fissures in the most superficial layers of the skin. Dr. Fulton saw that it allowed corrective products to penetrate more deeply, allowing them to work more effectively and efficiently.
- Is free and/or cheap—anyone can do it anywhere.
- Keeps fingers busy and reduces picking.

While its effectiveness (and low cost!) make icing worth it, some people do find it uncomfortable. Try to distract yourself while icing and get through it; it's a game-changer for people with acne, *especially* the visibly inflamed kind.

Icing: How You Might Be Doing It Wrong

As good and simple as icing is, you can still do it wrong. Here are some pointers to keep it on the beneficial side! Do not:

Press hard on the inflamed lesions with the ice. This actually causes more irritation and, thus, inflammation. It's not the pressure that makes the ice work, but the direct cold temperature.

Keep the ice stationary in one spot, allowing for a kind of frostbite.

Ice for longer than thirty minutes at a time (or even less, depending on how sensitive your skin is). If you finished doing your regimen a half hour ago and your skin is really red or you see broken capillaries, you've taken it too far. Start slowly and gradually increase your timing as your skin can tolerate *and* as your acne needs.

If you don't think icing works, it may be because you're not icing long enough. Set a timer and aim for just two to five minutes longer than you usually do (thirty minutes total maximum) to be sure you're really getting it in.

Are you applying the ice directly to the skin? The ice should literally be melting on your face, getting it wet. You'd be surprised at how many clients were applying the silicone tube to their face with the ice melting *inside* it and not *on* the skin.

If you are really doing all the things and you're still inflamed, it may be time to do a once-over on the diet and stress management side of things to make sure you're good on those systemic inflammation-inducing fronts and possibly incorporate some anti-inflammatory supplements like Zyflamend (a natural formula with tons of herbs to help alleviate inflammation) or Optizinc (zinc monomethionine, zinc, and copper; the copper aids in zinc absorption). Always check with your doctor and obtain your current vitamin levels before starting new supplements.

After you're done icing, gently pat (not rub) your skin dry with a clean towel. In case you need to *very quickly* stop and do something, it's best that your skin remains wet. Once it's dried off, dehydration starts to set into the upper layers of the skin, which can set off a series of negative effects.

Icing for rosacea

I recommend taking it very slow or maybe even skipping icing altogether, depending on how sensitive your capillaries are. A quick one-time swipe of ice on the skin may be okay, but just know that too extreme temperatures (especially when directly applied to the skin) can break more capillaries, exacerbating your rosacea. You can try instead using splashes of cool water or applying a cool compress or a cool, wet towel directly onto the skin for a few seconds or minutes as your skin can tolerate. We want to cool the skin down but not get it super cold as we would with icing to preserve your tender capillaries and prevent breakage. Consult your esthetician or dermatologist for the best advice.

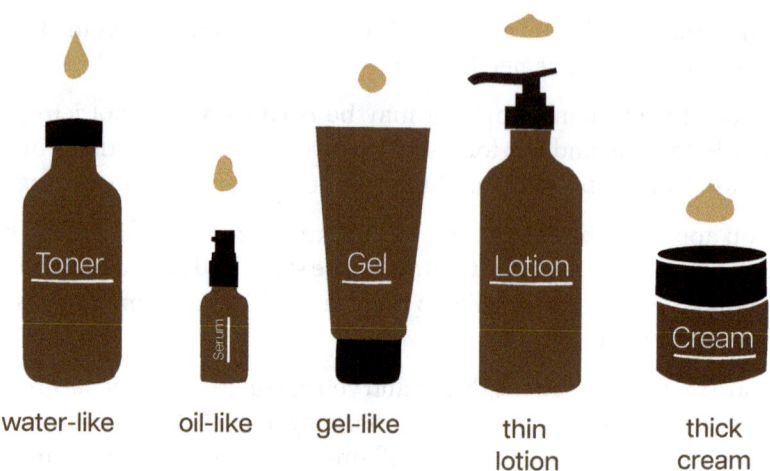

water-like   oil-like   gel-like   thin lotion   thick cream

Apply your skin products in order of thinnest to thickest in texture: watery toners first, followed by serums, gel and/or oil (in that order), finished off with your moisturizing lotion or cream.

Step 4: Apply Your Products

Using the right products in the right way is imperative for good results. Here are some best practices to get the most of our skincare regimen.

Order of Product Layering: Thinnest to Thickest

The general order of applying skin products is from thinnest to thickest. You want to apply the products with the thinnest consistency first and the thickest consistency last for the best efficacy. For example, toner is like water, so apply that first. Serums are like gels, so apply those next. Lotions and creams are the thickest textured, so apply these last.

Use Enough, But Not Too Much

Use just enough of your products to work their magic on your skin. Too little will render the product ineffective; too much will likely render your skin sensitized. Erring too far on either side of the spectrum will elongate the clearing process. You should feel a cool sensation as the product glides across your skin, which dries completely in about thirty seconds.

Chest and Neck Acne

If you're breaking out on your chest, the topical treatment approach is relatively simple: simply bring your face regimen down to your chest. This

Section 1 - Start with the Obvious - Your Skincare Face Regimen

means whatever toner and serum situation you have going on up top, just do the same down below.

You'll probably need to give some extra attention to detail when cleansing this area, though, since washing your chest over the sink is not as easy to do. You may get better results by washing your face and chest in the shower, making sure to turn the water temperature down when working on your face and chest.

In-clinic, we've seen chest acne commonly associated with digestive gut imbalances like excess Candida yeast or H. Pylori bacteria. It could also have to do with the gym, necklaces, supplements, or medications (like birth control), or be a case of Mallorca Acne (a condition that's triggered by the sun's UV rays and oils in sebum and heavy creams). You can eliminate additional topical aggravators by using acne-safe laundry detergent, hair, and body products like washes, scrubs, lotions, and perfumes and bringing your skincare regimen down to the chest diligently twice a day. You can also try using a mandelic acid cleanser for the body.

If you're breaking out on the neck, take care to thoroughly cleanse and dry the skin here and exercise caution using active products, as the neck skin can be more sensitive. If you wear necklaces, scarves, starched or high-neck shirts, these may aggravate your acne here.

Toner

Once your skin is dry, apply your toner (or if you're skipping toner, apply your serum). There are two ways to apply toner onto your skin depending on whether it's moisturizing or exfoliating/active/treatment-focused: with toner pads or with your hands.

At the clinic, we have non-woven toner pads that are used quite commonly in the professional facial treatment room. Made of synthetic materials, these are designed to dispense the toner onto your skin instead of absorbing it, resulting in your needing to use less product for it to work. Swabs and pads made from cotton are more absorbent, so the product ends up in the trash instead of on your face, where it should be. Reusable toner pads are available, though shopping around for one that works just right may be challenging.

If the toner is a moisturizing formula, you can apply this directly to your face without using a toner pad so long as you aren't spraying it into your eyes. Alternatively, you can spray it into your hands, touch them together palm to palm, and then pat the toner gently all over your skin, neck, and chest. Using a toner pad will ensure thorough and even application.

Let the products do the work

Many clients breaking out on the lower half of the face are often a bit overzealous with the application of their toner to try and get the acne off of it. Yes, this practice would help speed exfoliation, but it is also important to keep the skin comfortable and to keep the moisture barrier intact, which helps facilitate healing and clearing of the skin. Let the acids in the toner do their work. No need to rub extra hard! You can tone around the peeling/sensitive areas, and when those areas heal and are back to normal, you can begin toning here again.

How to tone—face first, neck and chest last

The goal with toning (and applying any skin product, really) is to ensure a light, even coat of the product all over the skin. One or two passes over the entire face, neck, and chest should be enough.

Dispense about two one-inch circle shapes (dots) of the toner on the pad by removing the bottle cap, placing the toner pad over the orifice, and turning the bottle over. Repeat this to create a figure eight on the pad. This should be enough to swipe all over your face and feel the toner's "wetness" on the skin.

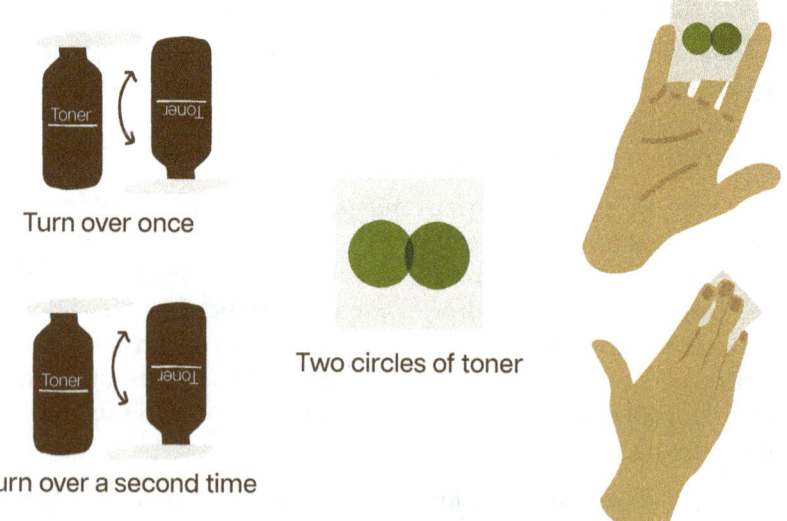

Turn over once

Two circles of toner

Turn over a second time

After dispensing toner onto your pad, slip the pad between your fingers as shown, so you can use the surface of your middle and ring fingertips to evenly press and distribute the toner onto your skin.

Section 1 - Start with the Obvious - Your Skincare Face Regimen

The skin on the forehead is a lot thicker and generally more tolerant of active products thanks to its more active oil glands, so you'll want to start there. Work your way down the sides of your face, including into the hairline, then the nose and cheeks, finishing up around the mouth. If your skin isn't sensitive, you may do a second pass before moving down to the neck and chest. Save the neck and chest for last because chances are your face is cleaner than these areas and you don't want to cross-contaminate. If you are experiencing acne on the chest, you'll want to use a new toner pad to dispense more toner and apply it there. *See page 62 for a diagram on the sequence of applying toner to the face.*

TIP: Watch for over-exfoliation

It's common to want to vigorously rub your active products over trouble areas. This is okay if you are trying to create a chemical peel-like effect on your skin, but it's imperative that at the first sign of peeling, redness, or irritation, you back off and let the skin heal from the over-exfoliation. Doing this every day is absolutely not recommended because your skin will perpetually be peeling, dried out, and irritated, which is not what we want.

Remember, if you are already peeling from exfoliation of any kind—an active product, a professional treatment, dehydration, or sunburn—*do not apply* exfoliants or scrub these areas. Use your healing and moisturizing products until these areas heal, and then slowly work the active products back in.

Serums

These can be great additions to any skincare regimen so long as you are using the right kind for your skin goals, skin type, and in the right order. The general rule is to apply the serums onto your fingertips, pressing the lengths of your fingers together to distribute it and immediately pat it all over your face.

The neck tends to be a sensitive area, so you may not need to apply your treatment serums here every day or night. It's totally okay to skip this area if you experience any irritation but do make sure to bring your face care regimen down to your chest to prevent breaking out and premature aging here; a sun-protected face with a sun-damaged chest might look funny. No need for BP here; be gentle as the neck and chest skin can be sensitive to actives and exfoliants.

Do's

Making sure your hands are warm, clean, and well-hydrated will do you well for this step of your regimen. Dry hands will absorb the serum instead of getting it onto your face where you want it most. The warmth will help ease product distribution and increase penetration.

If your skin is sensitive, apply your moisturizing serum first and active serum *on top*, creating a protective moisturizing buffer for your skin to better tolerate the more active serums to follow. Yes, it will slightly dilute the serum's activity, making it work in a gentler way, but it's better to maintain your skin integrity than to abuse it, which would slow down the clearing process.

Don'ts

Touching the dropper onto your face contaminates the whole bottle. It also doesn't make for an efficient application as the product tends to run straight down your face and off it, unless you quickly catch it with your other hand and spread it around, difficult to juggle while you are trying to place the dropper back in its bottle. Squirting it into your palm is also wasteful (especially if your hands are dry) because your palm ends up absorbing the product instead of your face.

Antioxidant serums are meant to protect your skin against free-radical damage like the sun, so I would strongly suggest using these types in the daytime; nighttime is okay, too, if you want to boost your antioxidant levels. Some popular antioxidant ingredients include:

- Vitamin C (usually combined with vitamin E). Note: a small percentage of acne-prone folks are sensitive to vitamin C and will break out from it, so exercise caution.
- Spin traps
- Coenzyme Q10 (aka CoQ10)
- Alpha-lipoic acid (not an exfoliating acid but an amino acid)
- Ferulic acid
- Some naturally high-antioxidant fruit extracts such as mangosteen, blueberries, açaí, and goji berry

I would recommend using exfoliating treatment serums at night to avoid the harsh sensitizing and results-reversing effects of the sun. Less exposure to the sun while simultaneously using active products on your skin will help reduce the chances of irritation. Active ingredients commonly found in these serum types include:

Section 1 - Start with the Obvious - Your Skincare Face Regimen

- Vitamin A
- Retinol
- Retinoic acid
- Retinoids
- Alpha-hydroxy acids, aka AHAs
- Glycolic acid
- Lactic acid
- Malic acid
- Mandelic acid
- Beta-hydroxy acid (aka BHA, aka salicylic acid)
- Benzoyl peroxide
- Peptides

Some notes

Hyaluronic acid is not an exfoliating acid but a moisturizing humectant, meaning it binds water from the atmosphere into the skin. It's safe to use both day and night.

Other ingredients such as niacinamide, peptides, and collagen should all be okay to use both day and night.

Make sure your products are acne-safe by using our product checker and carefully testing it.

With any active product, make sure to introduce using it slowly to mitigate any possible acclimation irritation. Using a new exfoliant once or twice a week, slowly building up to every other night over the course of two to three weeks, is a good way to do this. Change the frequency of use as your skin can tolerate and needs.

Watery liquid serums like vitamin C

You'll need to work *very quickly* with these precisely because of how watery they are. Squirt a dropperful directly into your tightly cupped fingertips, quickly flip your hand over into your other hand's tightly cupped fingertips to share, then lightly pat the length of your fingers all over your face to distribute. Once it's all distributed, you can gently rub it into both sides of your face simultaneously. After you're done applying the serum to your face, repeat the process for your neck and chest.

Creamy gel serums and oils

You'll have more time to work with these since they have body and are less likely to run through your fingertips. Dispense them onto your fingertips, pressing the fingertips of each hand together in a prayer-like fashion, and then gently pat all over your face to equally distribute before massaging it in simultaneously on both sides of the face. Repeat the process for your neck and chest.

Exfoliating serums as a spot treatment

You may apply a tiny dot-like amount of extra exfoliating serum to any inflamed pimples (or ingrown hairs) that you may have currently active at this time before you apply your moisturizer all over. Use the tip of a cotton swab to keep your serum dropper clean and your hands off your pimples. (I cut my cotton swabs in half, so I can utilize both ends of the swab and sit them in a little shot glass in my bathroom cabinet, minimizing waste.) Applying benzoyl peroxide as a spot treatment can be okay too; just be careful not to bleach your clothes or sheets while you have it on. If the skin stings or burns upon application of any active product, immediately wash it off and moisturize the skin to prevent irritation.

Benzoyl Peroxide

We find that most don't need to use benzoyl peroxide to calm the inflammation down so long as they ice their skin and implement a low-inflammatory diet and lifestyle. Make sure that it's a truly acne-safe formula by checking the ingredients using our product checker tool.

Think of using BP as a preventative. Its main function is to get the inflammation down by killing excess bacteria and drying out the skin's excess oils. Be sure to apply BP *all over the general affected area* (i.e., the entire cheek) versus spot treating (i.e., the one pimple on your cheek). This is especially important while you're purging.

Most people will only need to use BP at nighttime. You need to protect your skin during the day with SPF, and using BP twice a day isn't necessary for most skin; in fact, it may be detrimentally drying and sensitizing. If you are super oily/inflamed, you can use it during the day as well, but watch out for intense dryness or irritation. Also, BP bleaches, so be sure to wash your hands well and watch your linens and clothing.

Don't put hydrating or moisturizing creams over the BP because it will stop it from working. (Different skincare labs will say creams are okay. Feel free to experiment if you wish.) If you are using too much or applying it too close to the eyes, you may experience dry eyelids or irritation as the BP rubs off the pillowcase onto your eyes. If any stinging or burning occurs, wash the BP off with an acne-safe cleanser and moisturize with hydrating cream or gel. Let your skin heal up completely before trying it again. Sensitive-skinned folks may want to perform a patch test first before applying it all over the face; a small amount behind the ear, on the neck, or on the inner arm for three to seven days will suffice. If there is no reaction, try using it on the face.

Moisturizing Lotions or Creams

The last step is to seal in all the treatment product goodness we've applied onto the skin and protect it by maintaining its moisture and, if in the daytime, sun protection. Protecting the moisture barrier on the skin is important for all, but especially for darker-skinned folks, to help prevent hyperpigmentation scarring.

Using a clean finger or spatula, remove a 1-2cm bean-sized amount of moisturizer from your jar (or pump) onto your fingertips and touch your hands together in a prayer-like motion, distribute all over your face, and then gently massage the product in thoroughly. If you are particularly dry, you may reapply a second layer of moisturizer or switch to your hydrating non-foaming cleanser the next time you have to wash your face. Take all the cream you need from the jar in one swoop with a clean finger (or use a spatula) to avoid double-dipping, which introduces bacteria into the container.

For thicker creams that may be more difficult to spread, warm the cream prior to applying it by rubbing your fingertips together for a few seconds to get the texture to soften. Warmed-up product will help it blend into your skin much easier, which is particularly helpful when putting on something thick like a physical sunscreen cream.

How to Adjust Your Regimen

The meaning of a balanced skincare regimen will be different from person to person. Your regimen may be customized to prevent dryness while someone else's keeps their oiliness in check. However, all proper acne regimens should work to loosen impactions, making for easy removal of acne seeds—either to be exfoliated out of the skin on their own or removed manually by an esthetician's extractions—without throwing off the skin's natural moisture balance.

If you experience an imbalance, chances are that the products you're using are *too much* for it at any given time; they might be too drying, too moisturizing, too harsh, or maybe not active enough. You will learn to assess your skin's condition and tweak your regimen to remedy it. For example, using an insufficient amount of moisturizer can dehydrate the skin, which then causes it to produce too much oil, overcompensating for the lack of moisture. Drying out the skin also constipates the pores, leaving acne seeds stuck inside, unable to purge themselves as efficiently as lubricated pores.

Products that are too harsh can sensitize the skin so much that it won't be able to tolerate the exfoliants or treatments needed to purge the acne seeds. Here are some skin symptoms to watch out for.

Regimen is Too Drying (Dehydrated, Lacking Natural Oils/Lipids)

Your skin feels tight or flaky throughout the day, even after moisturizing your skin. (Some tightness immediately after washing might be normal if you are using an active cleanser, but don't wait too long in between regimen steps.)

You may notice superficial wrinkles on the surface of the skin; this often has the look of a crinkled-up piece of paper you try to smooth out after it was bunched up in your pocket for a day.

Flaky skin that feels a bit rough to the touch in small areas or all over.

Regimen That Is Too Moisturizing (Greasy, Too Moisturized/Oily)

Your skin starts to break out superficially. Even if you're using acne-safe products, you may start to get tiny white pustules (they look like pearls that have pus in them). This usually starts on your nose and/or the rest of your T-zone (which is a naturally more oily part of the face).

Your face feels greasy, especially on the cheeks, within one to two hours of washing your face. If you touch your skin with clean, bare fingers before lunchtime, a touch of oil residue is left on your fingers.

Regimen That Is Too Harsh or Active (Products are Too Strong for the Skin or Climate, Peeling Skin, Stinging, Burning)

You may notice some flaky skin or rough spots in certain areas, especially if you're rubbing extra where you're broken out.

The products might not sting or burn at the beginning stages of over-exfoliation, but with prolonged use, they can start to do so either in isolated areas or all over the face.

You might start to feel like your products sting and burn all over the face, even ones you've used for a long time. If this is happening, back off the active products and/or prep dry skin by using a few drops of acne-safe oil to create a protective barrier on it before cleansing and moisturizing.

If the irritation persists, your skin can start to look red and get irritated.

Section 1 - Start with the Obvious - Your Skincare Face Regimen

Not Active Enough (Skin Doesn't Seem to be Getting Any Better)

Some clients may only be using moisturizing, nurturing, or basic cleaning/maintenance products and are lacking an active exfoliating product that would actually make a noticeable difference in the skin.

Start using an exfoliant to start the purging process. After using an acne-safe *and* active regimen for at least four to six weeks, you should notice a difference in your acne. You should notice a reduction in inflammation, a balancing of oiliness/dryness, smaller pimples that heal a lot faster than before, and generally clearer skin.

Common Problems

Waiting too long

Waiting in between your regimen steps for the products to "dry" will dry out the actual skin, making it sensitive, peely, and flaky. Also, if you're feeling the need to wait in between steps, you're probably using too much product. Use just enough product to cover the whole face for them to work, but not so much that you have to wait several minutes for one product to "dry" before applying the next.

Overzealous over-exfoliation

Overusing active products will cause over-exfoliation, which can escalate from minor symptoms to larger ones, including stinging and burning that lead to irritation, sensitivity, and dryness. This complicates and prolongs the clearing process, requiring healing time before you can focus on clearing.

Let the acids in the toner do their work. There's no need for elbow grease here! You can tone around the peeling/sensitive areas, and when those heal, you can begin toning here again, gently. A thin, light layer of any product is all you need to treat your skin successfully.

Underusing products

Skipping days or trying to stretch out your active products to make them last longer also isn't great because the skin needs a certain minimum amount of product for it to actually work. Use the product-dispensing guidelines in this book and on your product labels for good starting points.

Using products that are too strong to use every day, so you actually end up not exfoliating enough (i.e., using a very strong product once per week vs. slow, constant, daily exfoliation), is also not good. The goal is to exfoliate the skin just enough to purge and prevent acne without causing any irritation, flaking, or dryness of the skin. People with active acne should exfoliate gently twice a day, every day.

Washing multiple times a day

There's typically no need for someone with acne to wash their face more than twice a day (unless they exercise, wear professional stage makeup, or very rarely, have such super-oily skin that needs extra drying action to get it under control).

If you sweat in the middle of the day or you need to wash multiple times a day, you still shouldn't be exfoliating more than twice a day. Use your active products when they are able to stay on your skin the longest.

Doing too much

We know it's difficult not to want to physically push products into the skin deeply or scrub away the acne, but seriously, let the products do the work for you—there is no need to be too aggressive with them. Be gentle with your skin. There's also no need to keep "checking" a pimple all day by poking at it to see if it's still there or getting any better. The pores are tiny, and every poke is likely to aggravate the sensitive and tiny ecosystem that's going on inside.

If you're feeling sensitive or dry in certain areas, just avoid using your active products (exfoliating toner and serums, BP, all active acidic products) directly on those areas. You may continue to work around them. The crooks of the nose and expression lines around the mouth and eyes are common areas affected. Conversely, you can apply more hydrating gel, cream, or sunscreen on dry areas that need them. For example, you don't need to apply extra cream all over the face when it's just your nose that's extra dry.

Post-treatment (especially after a chemical peel), it's normal to experience dryness around the eyes, mouth, and nose, and occlusive products (like shea butter) will help while your skin heals. This should only be a temporary solution until the skin heals.

If you are still experiencing uncomfortable dryness, you may need to adjust the rest of your regimen.

Weather and the seasons

These can affect the skin's moisture levels. It's very common for clients to adjust their regimen according to the weather or season they're in. Observing your skin and knowing when it's dry or oily will allow you to tweak your regimen as needed to accommodate the dryness/oiliness. A cleanser you've been using during the fall in coastal San Francisco may not be moisturizing enough for the same time of year in the dry deserts of Death Valley, and a winter regimen may be too greasy for the same complexion in the summertime. Summertime is generally warmer, so the skin's natural oil production is usually higher, resulting in the need for a slightly more drying cleanser and/or lighter moisturizers. The wintertime is colder, and indoor heating can create very dry air that dehydrates the skin, so humidifiers and products that are more moisturizing will help moisturize and rebalance the skin.

Maintenance mode

If you're already clear and in maintenance mode, you aren't going to see much of a difference in your skin as far as acne is concerned because you're already clear! Take a look at your before pictures and humble yourself. But at this point, if your skin goals change (i.e., you want to focus on brightening spots from acne that's healed), you can integrate those targeted products to boost your regimen. See *Section 10, Maintaining Your Clear Skin*.

Supporting Dry Skin

You'll want to opt for products that offer more moisture than what you're currently using. Choose creamy, non-foaming cleansers, moisturizing creams (versus lotions or gels, which can be layered under your cream), and maybe even add an acne-safe moisturizing face serum or mask to your weekly routine. Try one or two things first to see what works best, folding in more as needed over time, or else risk over-moisturizing and getting acne as a result (even from acne- safe products).

Humidifiers can help moisten the air of a dry indoor environment; there are even portable ones you can use anywhere, including cars! If you don't have a humidifier, you can try gently simmering an uncovered pot of water on the stove. This helps the dryness of the inside air and, when combined with essential oils, naturally infuses natural anti-bacterial herbal and calming power into the air, which is particularly soothing during the cold season. Different oils have different therapeutic effects: eucalyptus globulus for clearing and cleaning the air, lavender for calming, rose for soothing, and citrus or lemongrass are just a few examples.

To further support hydration internally, see *Section 5 - The Digestive System, Diet and Acne*.

Balancing Oily Skin

For internal causes of oily skin, try checking your diet for and reducing androgen-rich and oily foods, like lots of red meat (especially conventionally raised, as growth hormones in them yield bigger harvests), nuts (especially peanuts), oily or fried foods, and sugars. Stress has also been proven to induce sebum production in the skin; in fact, severely oily skin is a precursor to *pyoderma faciale*, an extreme type of acne rosacea. Integrating stress management techniques into your daily routine can also help, along with other resources (therapy, faith, support groups, and moderate and regular exercise). On that note, extreme sports training has also been shown to increase oil production (and inflammation), so combine high- and low-impact routines, taking care to experiment and see what works best for you.

Consider getting your reproductive hormones checked. Excessively oily skin is commonly accompanied by excess facial and body hair growth and for people with ovaries, Polycystic Ovarian Syndrome (PCOS). Seeing a doctor can offer clarity at the root of the imbalance instead of just endlessly treating it at the surface level.

External fixes for oily skin include using products that are more drying for the skin. Opt for foaming cleansers, moisturizing lotions, or gels (not creams), and perhaps try using benzoyl peroxide (in the form of cleansers and/or leave-on gels). Try one or two things first to see what works best, folding in more as needed, or else risk over-drying and getting acne as a result (even from acne-safe products). You might also benefit from doing your full regimen a third time of day, possibly including the exfoliation part, especially if you are still breaking out.

Using blotting paper can offer an immediate and satisfying fix, but regularly stripping the skin of oil like this can actually induce more oil production in the long run.

Body and Hair Care in the Shower

General shower temperature: turn the heat down! Hot water used for the body often leads to very dry skin, which some clients scratch all night, creating rashes, instead of just turning the water temperature down. Warm is best.

In addition to washing towels with acne-safe laundry detergent, use a separate towel for your face and your hair and body. This is especially beneficial if you have inflamed acne (that can open up and ooze onto your towels), use hair products, or are active (keeping pollutants, sweat, and toxins from your body away from your face). Washing your face in the shower is great because you can really get into the hairline, have easy access to other body parts that are breaking out and get a really thorough rinse. However, the water tends to be too hot for these gentle areas, so you'll want to make sure that you turn the water temperature down when caring for them.

Products

Use only acne-safe products while showering, including your hair products, even if you are only breaking out on your face and especially if you are breaking out on your back or body.

As tempting as it may be to use gym- or hotel-supplied toiletry products, they are often comprised of comedogenic ingredients, especially products that foam, even "natural" and "organic" ones (which may not contain SLS but may have cloggy oils, fragrance, or seaweed in them). You may get away with using it once or twice if you forgot to bring your acne-safe stuff, but you'll likely notice breakouts in your scalp, the back of your neck or hairline. Keep a travel-sized kit of essentials that you refill from your full-sized bottles at home to keep acne-safe as much as possible while on the go.

Body Washes and Bar Soaps

Pretty much everything on the market that foams up is cloggy, thanks to sodium lauryl (or laureth) sulfate, fragrances, or specialty ingredients (like coconut or argan or avocado oils, to name just a few). Use the acne-safest products you can find, and be very diligent about this if you're breaking out on your body.

Body Scrubs

Scrubbing the skin can be great, so long as you don't have any active inflamed acne, sunburn, or another form of compromised skin. Skin should be strong and healthy prior to any scrubbing. There are a ton of ways you can do this: with a cream, sugar, or salt scrub, mitt, sponge, or brush. Physical scrubbing alongside chemical exfoliation may actually help purge non-inflamed acne from the skin a bit faster. Physical scrubbing can also be a great pre-shaving step to ensure a smoother shave.

A simple scrub you can make yourself is to combine your acne-safe face or body wash with something like our biodegradable scrubbing powder. You mix the blend of finely milled walnut shells and baking soda with any liquid cleanser, adding as much or as little scrubbing texture you desire for use on both body and face. Just make sure that you are *not* scrubbing actively inflamed acne! For body acne, I suggest you use a benzoyl peroxide-based cleanser to help get the inflammation down before integrating a scrub.

Remember to moisturize after exfoliating to maximize the benefits of the scrub, and wear SPF.

Hair Washing and Conditioning Products

The tricky thing about hair products—cleansing, conditioning, and styling—is that even when they contain safe ingredients, they may still be cloggy because of their intended use: to stay on the strands to moisturize, smooth, and style the hair through sweat and humidity. These can also travel from your hair onto your face, body, and pillowcase, causing breakouts. Acne-safe shampoos for natural hair are easier to find than ones for dry, color- or chemical-treated kinds.

In the shower, cloggy shampoo, conditioner, and treatment masks will inevitably cause breakouts along your hairline (forehead, temples, sideburns), under your chin, neck, chest, and back as the cloggy suds run down your skin. For this reason, I suggest you wash your hair first *before* the rest of your body and rinse away from your face. However, if you *must* use non-acne-safe stuff *and* experience breakouts on your body, try washing your hair in the sink to avoid any possible product exposure to your skin.

Optimally, one pump (or nickel/quarter-sized amount) of shampoo should be enough to get the roots of your hair washed, and as you rinse it out, it will cleanse the length of your hair. Obviously, the amount of shampoo you'll need to use will depend on your hair length, type, how thick it is, how much styling product you use, etc.

Hair Conditioning Treatments and Masks

You can pretty much assume all these products are cloggy. What's great for the hair is oftentimes terrible for acne-prone skin. Use our product checker and try to use only acne-safe products for the clearest skin possible.

Apply the product to your hair and keep it tied up, away from touching your face. It's best if the shower is not so steamy to avoid the product running all over your skin (or into your eyes). Position yourself so that the cloggy hair product does not touch your skin, head upside down or to the side as you comb it through. Wrapping in a shower cap and rinsing in the sink may be a good option to avoid hair mask-related acne on the skin.

Non-daily Hair Washing

If you don't wash your hair every day, you'll need to take extra care in wrapping it up with a natural fabric scarf or headwrap and changing your bed

Section 1 - Start with the Obvious - Your Skincare Face Regimen

linens regularly to avoid product buildup and transference to your skin. Our natural oils can also build up and cause problems.

All the products you use every day build up on each other and, combined with heat and sweat, can set your skin up for disaster. Choose acne-safe products as much as you can and use as little of them as possible. Thoroughly wash your hands of product residue after applying it.

Make sure you're washing your face thoroughly by cleansing, rinsing, and getting the active products (toners, exfoliants) into the hairline and around the ears to help mitigate any breakouts that may happen here. Remember, these hair products travel and can break you out not only on your hairline but also your ears, neck, chest, and back, especially as they pass these areas when you wash it all out.

Order of Operations

FIRST, Wash Your Hair.

Take care to keep the hair products off the skin as much as possible and away from your face/breakout-prone areas. A handheld shower head may help with this, giving you more control over where the suds wash away.

For the best chances of clarity, wash your hair of styling products every night (even if they are acne-safe) before you go to sleep. The residue from built-up products plus natural sweat and oils can cause acne problems, and washing thoroughly will help prevent them.

If you aren't a daily hair washer, then at least wear a shower cap when showering, and when you're done, wrap your hair up with a new and clean natural fabric wrap before going to bed. This will help prevent product/oil/sweat buildup on your sheets. Change your pillowcases regularly, as residue from all of your styling (and face care) products transfer onto it and then onto your face while you sleep. By using a new side of your pillow every night and then replacing the whole case every other day, you'll be easily preventing new acne exposure.

SECOND, Wash Your Body.

Cleanse your body with an acne-safe body wash to get the daily oil and grime off, revealing a clean surface ready for your treatment cleanser or scrub (if you are going to use one). You may opt to use a gentle scrubbing mitt to help stimulate blood circulation, exfoliate, and thoroughly clean your skin. Using your treatment cleanser, massage it into your freshly cleaned skin, and try to leave it there for as long as possible, allowing the active ingredients some time to work. Carefully and thoroughly rinse off. Remember, active ingredients like benzoyl peroxide can bleach fabrics if not washed away thoroughly.

LAST, Wash Your Face.

Washing your face last helps to ensure residue from hair and body products aren't left behind. If not washed thoroughly off the skin, even acne-safe products can break you out. So turn the water temperature down, and always wash your face (and anywhere else you're breaking out) last in the shower. Be sure to get into the hairline, in and around the ears, neck, and chest, and rinse thoroughly.

FINALLY, Finish Up.

Complete your face regimen (ice, tone, serum and moisturize) before putting on your body and hair products to prevent cross-contamination.

Makeup

Learn how to make the acne-safest best of the vast makeup world until you clear up so much that you don't feel the need to wear it anymore.

Acne Safety—Even "Safe"-looking Labels May Lie.

My first big lesson on ingredient label transparency and trust was with a very popular mineral makeup brand that we'll call Brand A. Back in 2008, they sold their one original formula whose ingredient list appeared safe—there were only five ingredients that each checked out fine against our comedogenic ingredient list. However, my clients' skin still had trouble fully clearing.

As time went on, although they saw dramatic improvements from their baseline starting point, many of my clients seemed to plateau at an 80% clarity rate. As my practice grew, so did the demand for mineral makeup. Thanks to a client who found a powder that kept her super clear, I enlisted other clients to try that same product. After seeing these clients stay clear using the new (Brand B) mineral powder foundation, I signed up to sell it.

As I switched my clients over from Brand A to Brand B, many who were previously hovering at 80% clarity started clearing up even more, well into 90% and up. But, I still hadn't made the connection between the new makeup change and the increased rate of clarity in my clients until I had one of my clearest clients run out of her Brand B compact. Since it'd be a

Section 1 - Start with the Obvious - Your Skincare Face Regimen

couple of weeks before she could see me to restock, she found some Brand A leftover from before the switch and started using that. The next time she came back, she was broken out. After all the extractions that day, she went back to using her Brand B makeup and, by her next follow-up visit, was completely clear.

I had trusted the ingredient list I saw on the Brand A makeup, thinking that it was acne-safe and relegated any breakouts to my clients not being as compliant with the acne-safe lifestyle as they said they were. But after replicating the same results with other clients, it was clear there was something hiding within the Brand A foundation that seemed to be problematic.

Although it helped many of our clients, we eventually stopped carrying Brand B. They had a very limited shade selection, which made it difficult to find a match for medium and darker skin tones within their range. And I learned my second lesson about label transparency through their rebrand. For many years, Brand B did not fully disclose all ingredients in their products until the company was bought out and new packaging rolled out. We sold their acne-safe pressed and loose mineral foundation powders, along with their (unknowingly to us, not acne-safe) mineral powder sunscreen, blush and bronzers. Only at the training event they hosted to launch the rebrand did we find out that algae was hidden in these products. We stopped selling these products and found our clients who were using them cleared up after we isolated and removed the clogger.

With & Within shop

Checking ingredient lists is a definite must in order to evaluate whether or not a product is even worthy of trying. But physically testing the product for at least one to three months (alongside an acne-safe lifestyle) is where you really get to see if something is truly acne-safe. This is a hallmark of all the products I decided to sell in my shop; they all had to go through rigorous testing to make sure the product was pleasant to use AND acne-safe before it got on our shelves for sale.

Dyes in Makeup

Most color in makeup and general skin/body care products sold on the mass market are made possible by the use of pigment dyes that are largely derived from coal tar and petroleum. These show up on cosmetic (and food) labels as "FD&C" or "D&C" followed by a color name and number (i.e.,

FD&C Red No. 30 or D&C Violet No.2), or simply as the color and a number (i.e., Red 30 or Yellow 5). Lake colors, dyes, and pigments combine these dyes with metallic salt and show up on a label simply as "Blue 1 Lake."

These dyes not only pose a problem for acne skin, but many of them are also reported to have adverse effects on the body, such as carcinogenicity, heavy metal content, tumor formation, and general allergic effects.

Cochineal and carmine (for red) are acne-safe but are not as popular with animal rights groups to use, as they are, in fact, derived from female cochineal beetles (mostly from Peru). Other dyes include annatto (a seed, for orange/yellow), henna (a plant, for brown), chlorophyll complex (alfalfa, combined with copper for green), vegetable carbon (for black), and caramel (for brown, from burning sugars but also commonly from soy).

Mineral Makeup

To me, because of the reasons above, mineral (aka iron oxide) makeup reigns supreme. They are innately vegan, come in a variety of colors, and offer natural inherent sun protection. Essentially ground-up rocks, these minerals are inherently porous, which can make them slightly drying. Buffer their drying effects by moisturizing your skin underneath, using a primer of some kind to create a barrier, or set your makeup while moisturizing your skin by spraying some rosewater on top after you're done applying all of your makeup. I find the loose powder versions of these are the most acne-safe; the creams, lotions, and even pressed formulas have more ingredients and thus more likely to be comedogenic. If you can't find the exact ones mentioned below, use our With & Within product checker to see what looks safe for you to try.

> ### "Allergic" to mineral makeup?
>
> Bismuth oxychloride is an ingredient very common in mineral makeup and is the one that's usually responsible for the allergic reactions that people who are "allergic to mineral makeup" have. These people likely can still use mineral makeup but just need to find a formula that doesn't contain this one problematic ingredient.

Foundation

Illuminare (from Southern California) is a liquid mineral foundation we've sold with much success in the clinic for several years. It comes in three different formulas and has quite a forgiving color range, even though they only have five shades. A little goes a long way, and with a small brush, you can use it in small areas as a concealer, minimizing your makeup kit. You can also blend shades together for the perfect seasonal match.

Youngblood (Southern California) offers loose and pressed powder foundations and rice powders that are acne-safe. These "safe" pressed formulas do contain jojoba oil but did not seem to pose a problem with the hundreds of clients we had using them for several years. (Jojoba oil is problematic when higher up on an ingredient list and especially when used "neat" directly on the skin.)

Blush, Bronzer, Highlighters

Alima Pure (out of Portland, OR) is another mineral makeup-based company we used to sell in-clinic. Their loose mineral formulas (foundation, powders, highlighters, bronzers, eye shadows) are safe. You can mix these powders with an acne-safe cream, lotion, or serum to create a different texture to play with. You can also try using safflower oil, sunflower oil, or shea butter if you want to make a kind of acne-safe body shimmer product.

Eye Makeup

Comedogenic FD&C dyes are not allowed in eye cosmetics for safety reasons, but naturally derived carmine (a red bug that's dried and crushed for its red pigment) is okay to use around the eyes (and as blush) as it's acne-safe. We advise sticking to loose mineral powder makeup (use a wet brush if you want a sharper, longer-lasting look), as acne-safe eye pencils and (natural) mascara are very difficult to find.

Brow Makeup

Brow pencils and cosmetic products are notorious for having comedogenic ingredients, causing people to break out in their brows. One of our former estheticians discovered a workaround by using Alima Pure loose eyeliner powder and shea butter to create an acne-safe brow butter. Brush the eyeliner powder into the brow, then use a clean mascara brush (aka *spoolie*) to brush in some shea butter. To do this, take some shea butter warmed up between your thumb and forefinger, then pinch the mascara brush with those fingers, twirling the brush around to get the butter from your fingers onto the brush, then brush into the powdered brow. The look from this technique is natural, and the shea butter keeps the color and hairs in place and brows zit-free!

Lip Makeup

Acne-safe lip products can also be very difficult to find. Most often, the very ingredients that make any product creamy will be cloggy, especially in "natural" products: coconut oil, cocoa butter, soybean oil, and argan oil, just to name a few. Colorganics (out of Marin County in Northern California) is the only brand that we were able to find whose lipsticks and lip glosses were completely acne-safe. We still have yet to find an acne-safe lip liner.

Brushes and Sponges

Wash your makeup brushes and sponges at least weekly to keep your skin clear. Use an acne-safe face wash or unscented shampoo or body wash. Our Charcoal Cleanser is a perfect product for this, but any non-active, acne-safe foaming face wash should do the trick. It's often said that high-quality makeup brushes that are well cared for will last you a lifetime!

In a cup, squirt a bit of your face wash into some warm water. Take your brushes and dunk them upside down, swishing them into the water solution, foaming up the cleanser and loosening up the makeup that's built up within the brush bristles. Repeat this process with a fresh cup of sudsy water once or twice more or until the water emerges clean. Thoroughly rinse off your brushes in a cup of fresh, warm water sans cleanser to ensure all cleanser residue is washed off. Gently squeeze the excess water out of

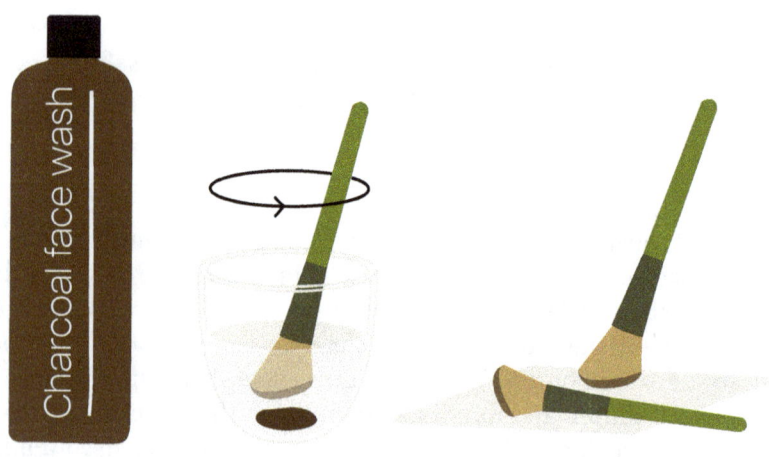

Watch our quick video on how to wash your brushes the acne-safe way on our With & Within YouTube channel: https://www.youtube.com/@withandwithin

the bristles with a clean towel by pinching the bristles dry with a towel and laying them flat to dry.

Laying your brushes flat to dry prolongs their life, as sitting the brush's bristles pointing up in a cup allows the water to drain into the brush barrel, loosening the glue that holds the whole brush together.

Brush-cleaning sprays can be used as a quick fix for absorbing excess makeup and oil in between full cleanses, much like what dry powder shampoos do for the hair on your head in between shampoos. Commercially sold brush-cleaning sprays are usually filled with all kinds of chemicals, colors, and fragrances and are also expensive.

> ### Homemade brush cleaning spray
> Make your own by filling up an empty spray bottle with rubbing alcohol, a few drops of lavender and/or tea tree essential oil and voilà—you've got homemade brush-cleaning spray.

In between brush washings, spray this alcohol mix onto a clean face towel, gently rub your brush over the sprayed area to remove the excess makeup and oils left behind from daily use, and deep clean your tools at least once every one to two weeks.

Primer
Some clients complained about the mineral makeup not staying on very well or separating due to the client's oily skin. When applying, press the makeup firmly onto the skin with a sponge after using the brush. If more support is needed, try using a primer (like Youngblood Mineral Primer) underneath the foundation and/or a setting powder (like Youngblood Rice Powder) on top.

Setting Spray
Spraying your skin down after carefully patting on your makeup can help prolong its wear. Our favorite is 100% pure rosewater, acne-safe with no other ingredients added, but try a few and see what works for you. Drier skins may benefit from rosewater with glycerin.

Photography, Wedding, Special Event Makeup
Long-time client and makeup artist Rachel Rockwood (Instagram: @rachel.rockwood.mua) recommends using makeup or sunscreen that

contains SPF 20 or less—either physical or chemical—to reduce the pale-faced flashback effect that often occurs when mineral makeup collides with flash photography (usually at night), where faces show up unnaturally pale in photos as the makeup reflects the flash.

You may have to succumb to using non-acne-safe makeup so that it will actually stay on and get you the look you want that's most suitable for photography. Do your best to live your best acne-safe lifestyle before the big event to minimize breakouts, and just enjoy the big day—acne-safe makeup or not! The acne from the makeup probably won't crop up until well after the festivities, anyway.

Hairstyling Products

If you're breaking out around the hairline, jawline, neck, or chest, find acne-safe substitutions as soon as possible! This includes shampoos, conditioners, masks, treatments, styling products, pastes, activators, gels, butters, oils, adhesives, all of it. Acne-safe hair styling products are difficult to find, especially if you are on the search for products suitable for very dry, textured, or curly hair. Silicone-based hair styling products may be okay for some clients and can break out others. Dimethicones/silicones are typically fine for most people, and 5-10% break out from it. Most hair products these days contain a multitude of cloggy oils and butters, so you'll be hard-pressed to find something skin-safe easily.

Cleanse and tone into your hairline and behind your ears. Use your facial cleanser and toner to prevent buildup, and make sure you are rinsing shampoo, conditioner, and facial cleanser thoroughly from these areas. Apply your corrective products here to clear any acne that may already be forming.

Style your hair after doing your face regimen so you don't rub sculpting paste residue onto your face. Having your hair tied back off your face and using no product is your best bet. Avoid using styling products to minimize exposure to potential skin cloggers. Resist touching your face after touching your hair.

Synthetic and natural hair extensions are sometimes coated with preservation chemicals. Try soaking synthetic hair in apple cider vinegar and washing/conditioning natural hair extensions prior to installation.[8]

Acne-safe Hair Product Tricks

Double duty. An acne-safe body lotion can double as a safe hair styling cream, as clients have done using With & Within Body Lotion or 100% Shea Butter for light hold and to smooth frizzies. An acne-safe body wash (like Shikai Moisturizing Body Wash) can also be used as a hair shampoo, as I've done for years.

Just a drop. Try adding a drop or two of acne-safe sunflower or safflower oil to your acne-safe hair products like shampoo or conditioner. Often, acne-safe products aren't very moisturizing, so adding a tiny bit of acne-safe oil might help.

DIY your own styling products. Crafty clients of ours turned us onto ones they made for themselves. Surprisingly easy to do, you can try making acne-safe flaxseed hair gel or sea salt spray (substitute acne-safe body lotion for the "natural conditioner").

Stick to the lightweight gels, sprays, and mousses. Fragrance-free water-based formulas are best. Waxy, oily, and greasy pomades and creams are the toughest to completely wash out.

Use our product checker while shopping and check our blog for product recommendations and updates.

Dry Shampoo

Dry shampoo sprays are almost always cloggy because of the fragrances, oils, and other ingredients within them—not to mention the often sticky residue they leave behind. These sprays also usually come in an aerosol can, which isn't super great for the environment. You can find a plethora of natural homemade DIY dry powder shampoo recipes online or find a company that makes one sans aerosol spray.

Heat Styling

The intense heat of blow-drying (and other heat styling) can be very drying to the skin. Using a flat iron doesn't directly blow hot, dehydrating air onto your skin. If you must blow-dry, a diffuser will help, as will a cooler air temperature.

High-quality styling tools should help to straighten or curl your hair without much (if any) need for product—even heat-protective ones. Be wary of drying your skin out, which can happen with the repeated use and exposure of hot tools so close to the face, and take care to monitor and moisturize.

If you find yourself needing to style your hair with heat tools most days, it may be worth it to go to a salon to get a longer-term hair smoothing treatment to minimize the daily use of tools. You might break out from your salon visit for a few days, but it might be worth the trade-off to not have to deal with your hair—and dehydrate your skin—as much on the daily.

Shaved/Bald Heads

You'll still want to cleanse, moisturize, and SPF to protect your scalp and neck. Find an SPF you like, use it, and keep covered with hats or wraps. Skin cancer on the scalp of bald and shaved heads is very common and often not detectable until later years of life.

Picking

CAUTION:

These techniques described here are only for acne that have already opened on their own. DO NOT attempt to extract any pimples whose pore openings are still intact!

Most everybody does it, but picking isn't good for acne-prone skin, no matter how good at it you think you are. It's very difficult to fully and correctly extract an acne seed from the pore, and the chances for further infection and permanent scarring are high. Extractions are best left to a professional who can get the right leverage and has the right tools and skills for a safe extraction.

When trying to find ways to manage it, we found it made a difference whether or not the picking was conscious or unconscious and learning what state of mind the client was in when initiating the behavior. Some had a more severe problem with it, diagnosed with skin-picking as a body-focused repetitive behavior (BFRB). Many overachievers—many of whom have acne—are perfectionists with brains that are difficult to turn off, so creating alternative activities to fall back on when the craving of picking comes on will be helpful. Figuring out if your picking style is conscious or not will help determine which management tools may be more helpful.

If you find yourself unconsciously picking while you're sitting in traffic or at the computer, would keeping fidget toys or squeeze balls in the car or near your workstation help? If you're doing it when you're tired or frustrated, what other stress-relieving activity can you go to when you feel the urge? Would covering your mirrors or changing out your light bulbs to dimmer ones in the bathroom help?

If you only pick at inflamed acne, pumping up your skincare regimen by emphasizing icing and maybe using benzoyl peroxide to bring down inflammation will be key. Or if you have a skin care professional that you like, perhaps seeing them more often for chemical peels will help you keep your hands off your healing skin and accountable for any skin damage. Picked skin that's scabbed over makes it very difficult, if not impossible, for a professional to successfully extract the acne seed. This also increases your chances of scarring, both permanent textural and (usually) correctable pigmentation.

Picking the Right Way (If You Have To)

All the guidance provided thus far was presented first in hopes that you wouldn't have to pick your own skin. The risk of doing this is you might break the skin and risk infection. Squeezing with bare fingernails and ripping the skin apart is ripe for a bacterial infection and permanent scarring. Also, you likely won't get it all out; perhaps draining some fluid but not fully extracting the seed will result in that same pimple getting inflamed all over again. When the skin starts to heal, you'll probably be left with a big scab that's more unsightly than the pimple itself—covering up the likely much larger inflamed pimple that still has the acne seed inside.

But sometimes inflamed pimples will unintentionally open up when you're washing your face. What do you do? I will share the best practices around this below. Practice restraint and proceed with caution.

Doing it Right

You'll know that you've properly extracted something if the next day, the skin directly over that pimple is flat and no longer feels sore. A scab may be present, but if it's flat and is no longer tender to the touch, you just may have extracted yourself successfully. Any inflammation or soreness (like the pimple is still there) likely means the seed is still stuck inside. At this point, the best option is to do what you can to get the inflammation down (icing) and spot treat (either with your toner, exfoliating serum, or BP gel).

Even the pros get help. Just because you have access to a pair of scissors and a mirror doesn't necessarily mean that you should cut your own hair. It's quite impossible to get the right angle, leverage, and visibility to pick your own pimples. In our clinic, it was obvious when even our own expert estheticians took matters into their own hands through their big(ger) pimples and expressed regret.

However, there is a way to do some squeezing, if done very gently, with much care, restraint, and intention. Picking becomes a problem when it's done haphazardly, which is usually when the person is tired or stressed out—not the best time to be doing anything, really. Or when it's done with reckless, frustrated abandon, without caution or care. When something opens up on its own while washing, though, this may create an opportunity to very carefully relieve some fluids that cause inflammation and pain—again, so long as it is done very carefully and gently.

A note of caution: Don't use metal tools on your face. The ones sold on the retail market are terrible for the skin, and for the most part, even professionals don't use them; and if they do, they are likely only using them for sebaceous filaments on the nose or chin, NOT for acne.

If you are going to pick, make sure you've been on your acne-safe and active skincare regimen for at least three to four weeks, icing twice a day (or more). Always use clean hands, cut your nails short and NEVER use your bare fingers or fingernails! As you combine what you've learned in this book and what you observe on your skin, learn to identify which pimples you can likely successfully extract and which ones you should leave alone. Finally, make sure you are doing this intentionally in a relaxed, calm fashion with plenty of restraint. We don't want you in a stressed, hungry, or tired frame of mind when doing something this delicate to your skin.

Step 1: Apply a Warm Compress

Soak a disposable toner pad in very warm water. Apply this over the already-opened pimple and see if it helps drain the fluids without any squeezing. Just place the moist toner pad over the skin and gently apply pressure. If you want to stop here, and it's totally okay to stop any bleeding with this step, ice once more (around, not directly on, it), apply your spot treatment (always use a cotton swab to gently dab either some of your exfoliating toner, a tiny drop of exfoliating serum, or a teeny bit of BP gel to dry it up). You can then proceed with the rest of your regimen.

If you want to go further, choose one tool and one method and *try no more than 3 times on your total extraction attempts!* Your skin will start to get more inflamed, and it won't do any good to continue to poke at your skin.

Section 1 - Start with the Obvious - Your Skincare Face Regimen

Step 2: Choose Your Tool

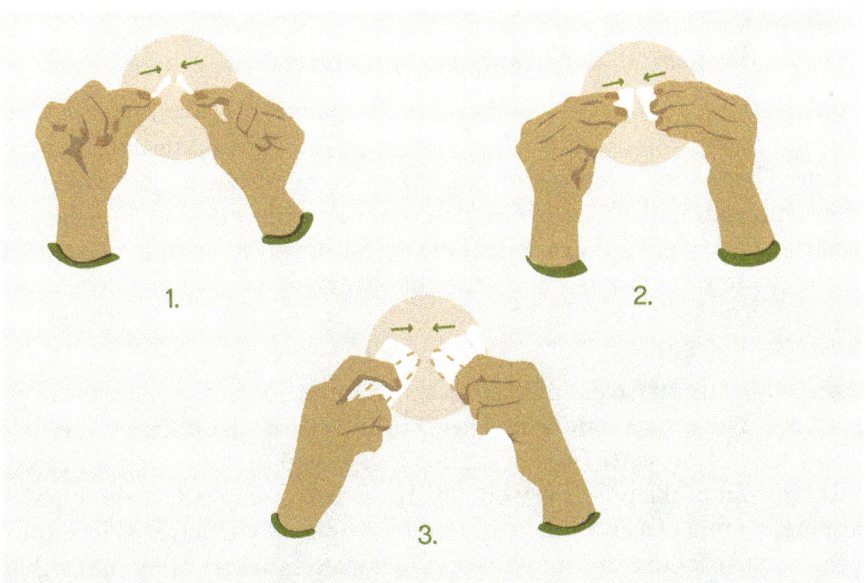

Tools to consider for at-home extractions:
1. Two cotton swabs, soaked in very warm water.
2. Folded or rolled up disposable toner pads, using the pointed ends to squeeze.
3. Carefully wrapped up fingers, index fingers under the tissue as shown with dotted lines (no nails!).

Tool one: two cotton swabs soaked in very warm (not hot) water.
If you have long nails, definitely use this tool.

This tool is best for a beginner because it's a bit easier to see what you're doing without your fingers in the way. It also has a bit more leeway because you can't apply as much pressure with cotton swabs as you can with your fingers.

Tool two: folded or rolled-up disposable toner pads
If you have medium or (preferably) short nails, use this method. Long nails will obscure visibility and pressure won't be as precise.

Take two disposable toner pads and soak them in very warm (not hot) water. Fold them up twice to create a square (if they're square-shaped) or fold in half and then roll them into a cone shape with the center poking out (if they're round) to create a kind of cushioned probing device that you can hold by pinching with your fingers. You will be using the tips of the pads, or pokers, to gently apply pressure around the pimple.

Tool three: carefully cushioned and wrapped-up fingers
Only for the most restrained and the very short-nailed!

Fold a clean disposable tissue over itself once and cover your fingers with the now four-ply tissue by poking your finger into the middle of the folded tissue. The tissue's purpose is to cushion and cover your fingertips so that they (and your nails) are *never* in direct contact with your skin. If the tissue starts to tear or get dirty or soiled, move your finger to another clean area of the tissue you are using to create a new working surface.

Step 3: Technique

Aim only to drain excess fluid from the pimples. Don't try to get the acne seed out. The actual acne seed doesn't usually come out unless you either apply a lot of pressure (which we don't want you to do), or if it's already bursting out of the pore, very obviously ready to come out. Only squeeze as much as you can and still keep your eyes open. If you have to close your eyes because it hurts too much, stop. Do not attempt to drain pimples that are larger than a quarter of an inch or near your eyes. Get professional help with these from a medical doctor or nurse.

Draining even just the fluid from pimples that opened up will help speed up their healing, along with greatly reducing inflammation and pain. However, if you happen to get some jelly or solid matter out, that's okay too, but stop there. Squeezing any more will risk damage, and even if you have a professional esthetician to visit afterward, they likely won't be able to do much because of the scab or compromised skin left behind.

Using pressure, type 1: V-shape, or volcano style
Apply pressure with the tools mentioned above, aiming downward toward the bone in a V shape, toward the root of the pimple. This will help create a kind of ricochet effect where you're squeezing underneath the skin, like trying to get a volcano to erupt from underneath the Earth's surface. This is the technique we found to be the most successful in the clinic when done correctly and when the pimple is ready.

Pressure type 2: Parallel to the skin surface
You may try applying pressure parallel to the skin's surface (pointing your tools toward each other, and not down toward the bone), but you'll need to leave quite a bit of space between your tools and the pimple to allow some leeway for the pressure to go. If you close in on the pimple too closely with

your tools, you'll likely just cause the pore to close in on itself, sending the seed and the fluids you're trying to drain further inside.

Know when to stop

Aim to try no more than three times on a single pimple. Sometimes, if the pimple doesn't yield on the first try, wait five to ten minutes to allow the skin's inflammatory response to possibly "float" the seed closer to the surface for an easier extraction. Once you've attempted the third time to drain it—whether it was "successful" or not—stop.

If the extraction was successful, you should eventually get to a point where any fluid drained is now clear. The area may still look inflamed, but it will likely start to flatten out in about twenty-four hours. If the pimple is particularly large, painful, is still bleeding, and/or has white or green pus present, it may be infected, so quickly finish up, apply a compress to stop the bleeding, and seek professional help.

Step 4: Ice, Clean Up and Spot Treat

Wipe the extraction site clean with a clean disposable toner pad saturated with a mildly active (or non-active) toner. Then, ice the area to relieve inflammation and soreness from your gentle poking. If tolerated, you may carefully and sparingly spot treat using a cotton swab to apply a tiny sparing amount of exfoliating toner, serum, or BP gel directly onto the pimple to finish off the extraction process.

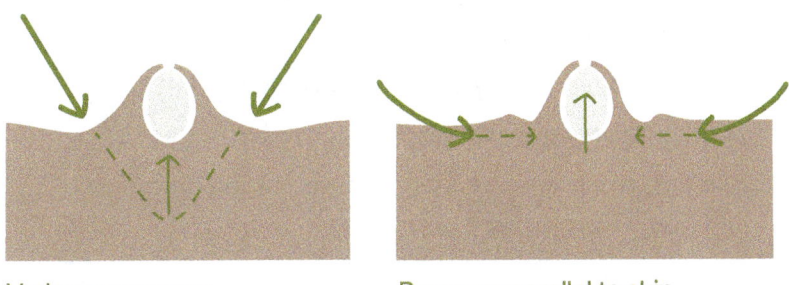

V-shape pressure　　　　　　　Pressure parallel to skin

When extracting, technique is paramount. The goal is to apply pressure (solid green lines) in order to create a ricochet effect (dotted lines), to avoid squeezing the pore shut (and driving the seed further inside). You can either direct the pressure going downwards in a V-shape (especially helpful for inflamed lesions), or parallel to the skin (for non-inflamed or seeds close to the surface), as illustrated here.

Aftercare

As the skin heals in the days ahead, it may scab up. Avoid scrubbing, exfoliating, poking at, or otherwise touching the area until it's fully healed. Leave the scab alone. The skin is healing underneath it, and the scab will fall off on its own when it's ready. Picking and peeling off dead skin or scabs will invite more complications, including infection and scarring. Gentle icing directly over the extracted area should be fine, but pay special attention, use caution, and keep it at a minimum as tolerated.

With the right practitioner, you'll have better chances of a complete extraction if you're able to see an aesthetic practitioner-trained doctor, nurse, or qualified practitioner at a medical spa who can, if needed, use a sterilized lancet or needle to open the pore, allowing for an easier and more thorough extraction. This can be especially beneficial for those with very inflamed acne or tightly packed pores.

Endnotes

1 *https://withandwithin.co/pages/product-checker*

2 *https://withandwithin.co/blogs/blog/comedogenic-ingredient-study-papers*

3 *https://www.skincancer.org/blog/driving-your-risk-for-skin-cancer/*

4 See also *https://www.ncbi.nlm.nih.gov/books/NBK537164/*

5 See also *https://withandwithin.co/blogs/blog/how-to-take-before-and-after-photos?* for more tips and a video

6 *https://skinsalvationsf.com/pages/product-checker*

7 *https://skinsalvationsf.com/pages/product-checker*

8 See *https://katleverette.com/* for more information

"Even beyond having skin I feel confident in, I never thought I'd be in a position where I can actually make informed choices and adjustments instead of wasting money on expensive BS at (prestige mass beauty retailer) and thinking, "I guess I just have bad skin." I now know how to navigate that process and feel confident that with a little research and patience, I'll figure it out. Thank you so so much."

- ET, client since 2017

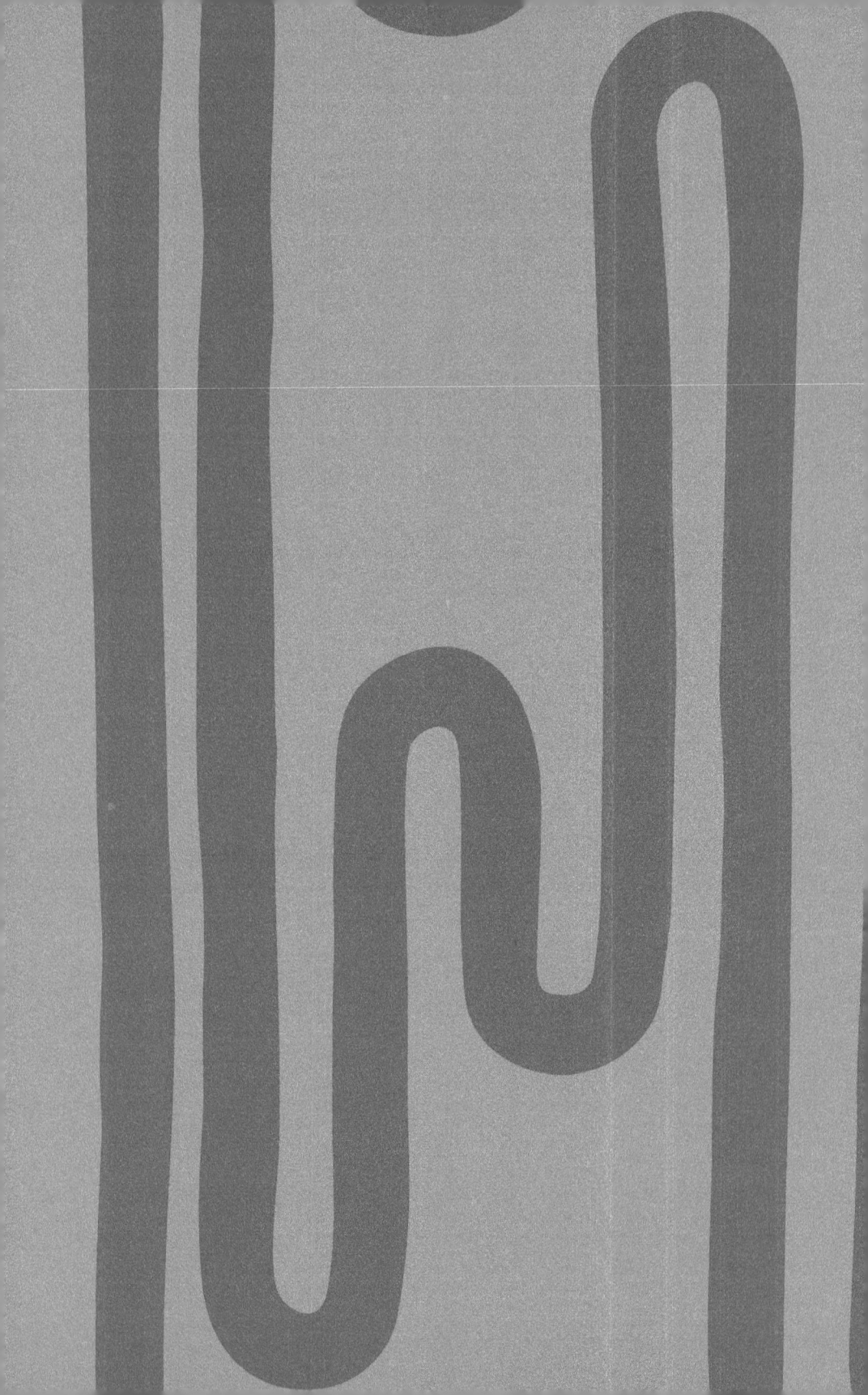

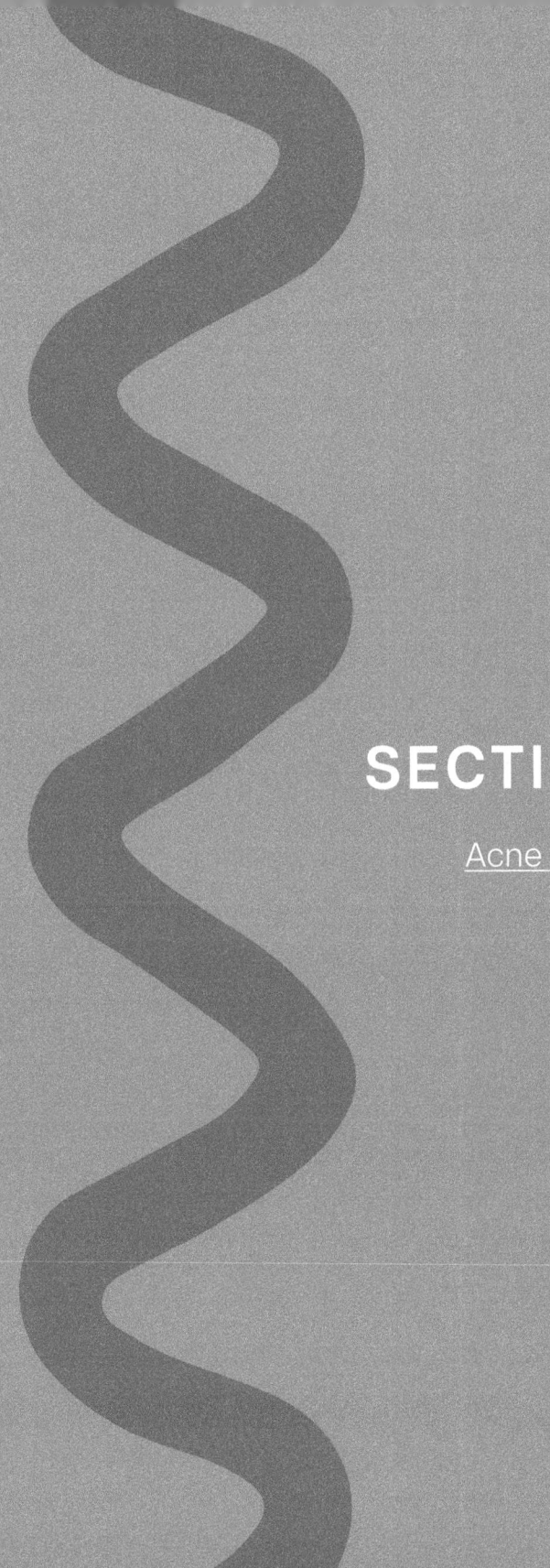

SECTION 2

Acne 101

Now that we've got the topical part of your program down, we can get to understanding acne inside and out to finally clear your skin for the long term. Your acne is a result of many factors, both topical and internal. We'll address the topically induced and more easily treatable kind first, and if after that, you're still broken out, we can take a closer look at the internally induced and more involved treatment-required ones and learn how to address those.

In about three months' time, your topical and lifestyle/internal efforts will converge, and results will be visible—you should be pretty clear at this point. By this time, all the old acne that formed before starting the program should have purged out of the skin from under its deeper layers. Using the knowledge and tools in this book will not only get you clear but also keep it that way.

Genetics and Acne

You don't need to have acne run in your family to get acne, but chances are higher you will have it if it does. Just like how we get our hair color and height, we inherit all our physical characteristics from our ancestors. The way their skin adapted and reacted is passed down to you, so if your parents had inflamed acne, you likely will, too. This also tends to be true for the age of onset and duration. People with the gene are just more sensitive and reactive than those without.

What's Actually Happening in the Pore?

Acne vulgaris is a condition that affects the skin and its follicles (or pores). It's largely a genetically inherited condition, but those without the gene—who have enough of an acne-causing aggravator—can break out, too. *Retention keratosis* occurs when pores produce too many dead skin cells that combine with excess sebum (along with comedogenic ingredients in products) that stick together and create an impaction—or an acne seed.

These seeds start out really small, forming deep in the pores as microcomedones, the tiny beginnings of acne. As they mature, these microcomedones grow in size, becoming comedones (or seeds), now visible on the skin. Each acne-filled pore has a seed stuck inside it that needs to be completely removed in order for the skin to completely clear and the acne to go away. The longer these seeds stay in the follicle (or are picked at), the more likely they are to become inflamed, infected, or even turn cystic, often leaving permanent scarring.

Section 2 - Acne 101

Typical non-acneic pores shed one dead skin cell at a time, wicked out of the pore by a hair. However, acneic pores can shed up to five cells at a time, creating a traffic jam in the tiny pore, resulting in the formation of an acne seed—often with no hair in the pore to wick it out. It typically takes between one and three months for this seed to grow in size and make its way to the skin's surface, finally becoming visible and accessible so that it can be extracted. From here, this growing seed can become either of two major types of acne: inflamed or non-inflamed.

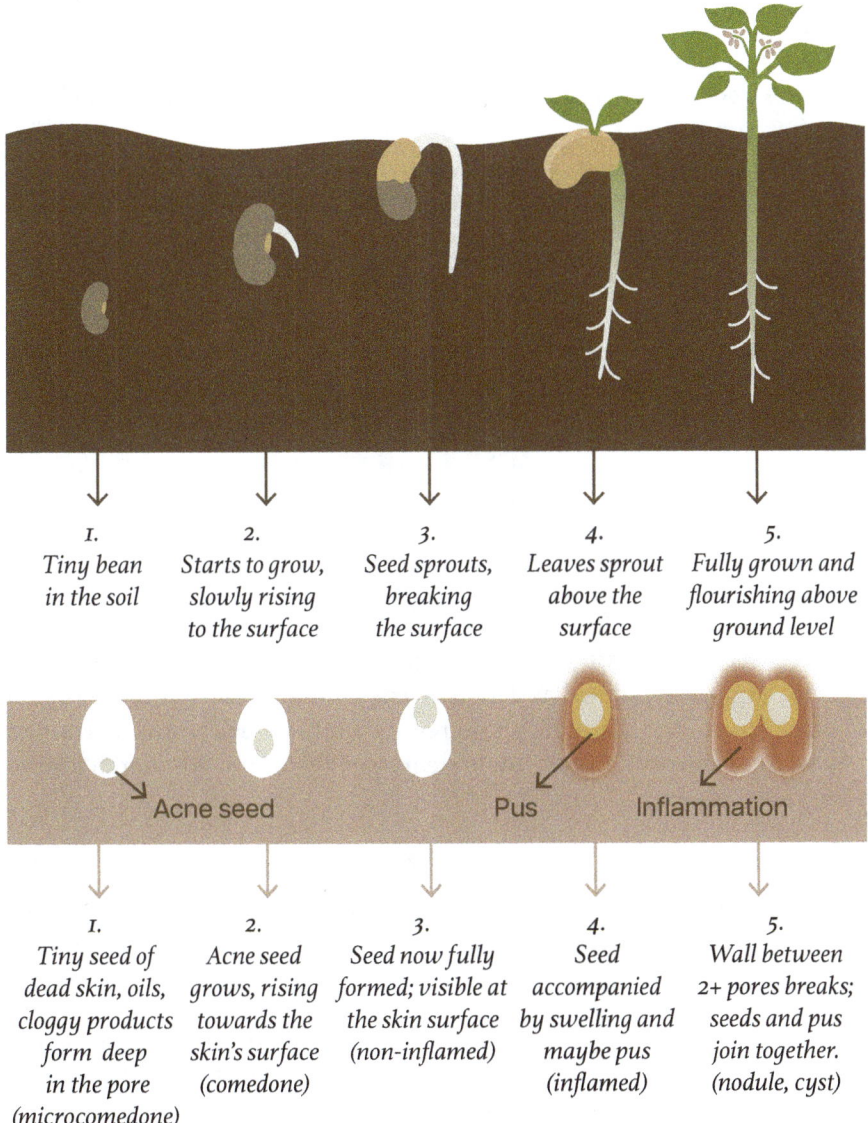

1.
Tiny bean in the soil

2.
Starts to grow, slowly rising to the surface

3.
Seed sprouts, breaking the surface

4.
Leaves sprout above the surface

5.
Fully grown and flourishing above ground level

1.
Tiny seed of dead skin, oils, cloggy products form deep in the pore (microcomedone)

2.
Acne seed grows, rising towards the skin's surface (comedone)

3.
Seed now fully formed; visible at the skin surface (non-inflamed)

4.
Seed accompanied by swelling and maybe pus (inflamed)

5.
Wall between 2+ pores breaks; seeds and pus join together. (nodule, cyst)

Removing Acne With Exfoliation

Acne seeds working their way out of your skin naturally (without the right exfoliation or extractions) is like taking the slow lane on the highway. Increasing exfoliation in your regimen is taking the fast lane; you'll get to your destination in much less time.

In nature, erosion is bad (i.e., for our forests or the shoreline). But for the skin, in the form of exfoliation, it's very beneficial in the process of purging acne, whether or not you have access to a skin therapist to do extractions. Exfoliation helps to speed up the seed's maturation and journey up to the surface so it can fall out of the pore on its own or with the help of professional extractions, sloughing the sticky skin cells away before they clump together into seeds.

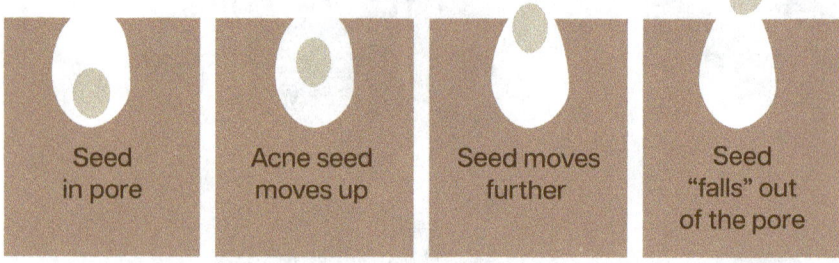

Exfoliation at the top of the epidermis "erodes" the skin surface, which "pulls" seeds out of the pore. Simultaneously, exfoliation stimulates new skin cell production at the bottom of the epidermis, "pushing" the seeds out of the pore, creating a double-pronged purging and skin rejuvenating effect.

Removing via Extractions

Extractions are the fastest way to get acne out of the skin, but only after the skin is properly exfoliated and moisturized and only with a therapist who can do this safely, thoroughly, and regularly. Their eyes must be trained to find the seeds, nails short, tools clean, and technique top-notch for the best, safest results.

Why Topical Skin Products Alone Aren't Enough

Because of how many comedogenic products are on the market, most folks' acne will improve greatly (and maybe even completely clear up) by switching to an active and acne-safe skin regimen alone. However, if there are internal acne-causing factors at play, you'll have to address them because, in due time, they'll likely show up on your skin. In these cases, changing up what's on the outside topically may help for a short while but isn't really going to fix what's going on internally for the long term.

Section 2 - Acne 101

Acne Types

Non-inflamed and Inflamed

Non-inflamed

Most breakouts start out as non-inflamed acne. The tiny "seeds," or micro-comedones, are invisible to the naked eye as they form deep in the tiny hair follicle. We can continue to exfoliate the skin in hopes that the seed will become visible, enabling us to get it out before it gets inflamed. Essentially, we just need to wait for it to grow bigger in size and move closer to the skin's surface so that we can actually see the acne and extract it.

For non-inflamed acne, the acne seeds remain in the pores without the follicle walls/skin around them swelling up. These tiny bumps that feel like Braille dots or grains of sand are generally not painful and can appear flesh-colored (closed comedones) or as dark dots (open comedones, aka blackheads). Non-inflamed comedones may not be obvious to the eye like red, inflamed acne is, but the texture is easily visible in the right light, appearing like many tiny bumps all over the face.

Non-inflamed acne can come in two forms: with the surface-level pore opening being either open or closed. An open, non-inflamed comedone is called a blackhead. The top of the acne impaction has reached the epidermis and stretched out the pore opening, exposing it to oxygen and oxidizing it, turning the exposed surface area black (it's not dirt!), hence its name.

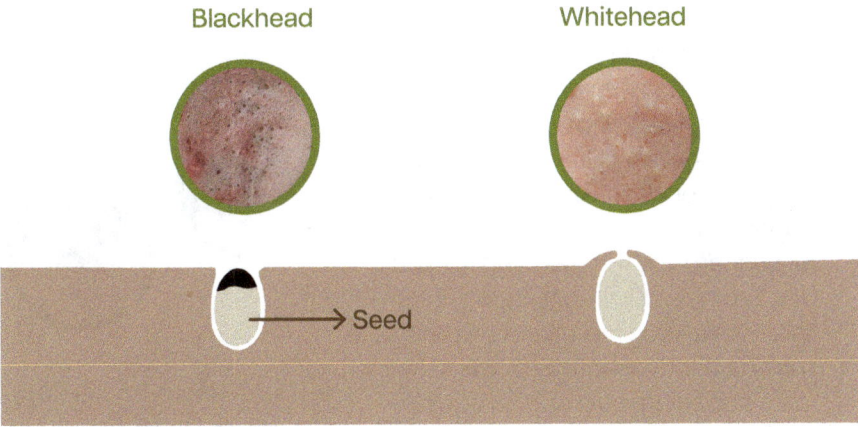

Blackheads (open comedones) are acne seeds with stretched out pore openings, allowing the exposed seed tops to oxidize, turning them black. Whiteheads (closed comedones) are acne seeds whose pore openings are sealed tight; the seed is not exposed to the air, so they remain white or flesh-colored.

Closed comedones are the flesh-colored bumps that are "sealed off" at the skin's surface, hiding the seed underneath. These require a more keen eye to locate and a precise technique to extract.

Sebaceous filaments, not blackheads

Sebaceous filaments found on the nose and chin are often incorrectly called blackheads. Though they both have oxidized "caps," the former are smaller and similar in size, don't typically turn into acne, always come back even after extraction, and often extract like toothpaste out of a tube. These protective plugs prevent bacteria from entering the body through pores.

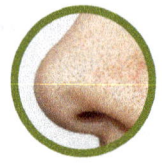

Sebaceous filaments

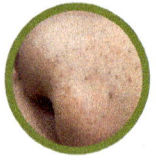

Mixed: Blackheads and sebaceous filaments

True blackheads are slightly larger, more irregular in size, may get inflamed and can appear alongside sebaceous filaments. When both are present, ensure thorough extractions to keep the skin its clearest.

Milia

Milia are a type of small, painless, non-inflamed congestion with a white, pearl-like appearance, made of dead skin cells without sebum (so they are not classified as acne, but as superficial keratin cysts). They often appear around the eyes and eyelids, and have been linked to high cholesterol or makeup ingredients. Some may be gently massaged out of the pore's opening, but usually require professional extractions to remove. They also commonly recur, so regular attention may be necessary.

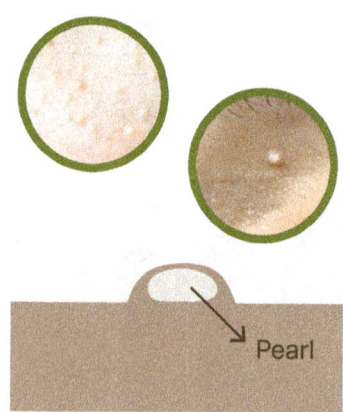

Pearl

Inflamed

As the seeds remain in the pores, the chances of inflammation setting in as the skin's first line of defense increases. The follicle walls/skin around the seed swell up, creating inflamed acne. These start off as small red or pink swollen bumps (papules) that can change color over time, turning a darker red, purple, or even blue if the blood is close to the surface of the skin and has been forming over a period of time. Pus follows inflammation as the second line of defense, turning the papule into a pustule, creating a white cap of liquid pus that's visible on the surface of the skin. From here, papules and pustules can turn nodular or cystic.

These pimples swell similar to a mosquito bite and can grow to the size of a thumbnail, sometimes larger. They can be hard or soft, are often sore, painful, itchy, or warm to the touch, and can leave post-inflammatory pigmentation and textural scarring behind. Makeup or coverup will cover up the pigment but won't hide the lumpy texture.

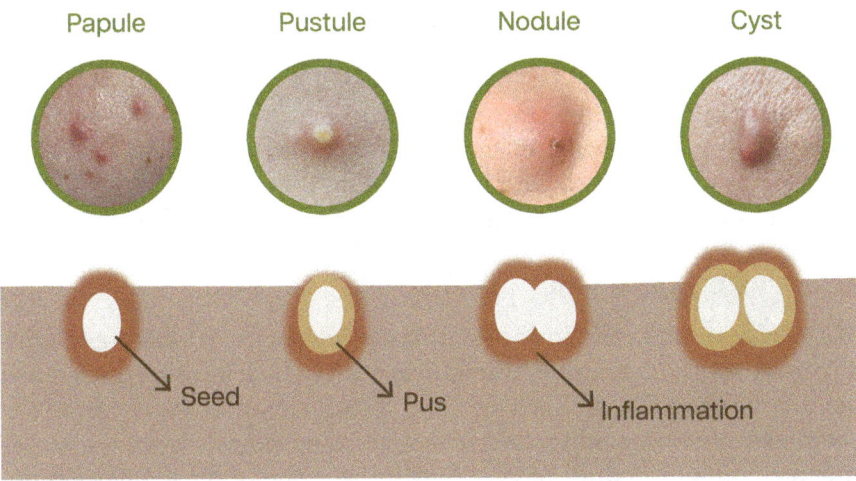

Papules are acne seeds (white oval) with inflammation (red halo). Pustules are acne seeds with both inflammation and pus (yellow halo). Nodules (firm to the touch) and cysts (soft) are the more advanced stages of both, respectively.

Some will categorize nodular or cystic acne as separate types, but I see them as more advanced types that fall under the umbrella of inflamed acne. Nodules (hard to the touch, inflamed tissue) or cysts (soft to the touch, with pus or fluid inside) may need extra help to reduce the inflammation (cortisone shots, preferably topical antibiotics versus oral), so that access to and removal of the actual acne seed is possible. The complete removal of the seed—by any safe means necessary: exfoliation, extractions, or both—is essential for the pore to clear and the acne to go away.

Bacteria, Inflammation, and the Resulting Textural Scarring

It's a common belief that bacteria is the main cause of all acne, but because bacteria of all kinds are present on everyone's skin whether they have acne or not, perhaps bacteria isn't the main instigator. Excess dead skin cells and oils, comedogenic ingredients, and inflammation are major parts of the problem, too.

Cutibacterium acnes, the bacteria most commonly believed to be responsible for acne, is actually part of the skin flora present on most healthy (non-acneic) adult human skin. However, it is present in larger, disruptive amounts when nodular/cystic acne is present, which is why acne-prescribed antibiotics have the most visibly apparent effects. The excess bacteria is killed off with these drugs, causing the inflammation to temporarily subside. But although the inflammation is reduced, the acne seeds are still left behind and need to be extracted in order for the follicles to stay clear.

Inflammation makes most everything worse, even though it's one of the body's first defense mechanisms for repair. It sees the acne seed stuck in the pore as a foreign invader. Either the skin tissue will swell in an effort to "push" or "float" the seed out or the skin sends out its white blood cell army (pus, which is indicative of a bacterial infection) to try to destroy the acne. Usually, it does both.

With the acne seed stuck inside the already tiny pore, this swelling and pus aggravate the already vulnerable follicle walls, which have been stretched out to accommodate the seed's girth. The follicle walls then rupture (on their own or with picking) and fuse with other pores, creating a larger inflamed pimple, nodule, or cyst. Becoming aware of the many ways the body's inflammatory responses are induced and managing them as best as possible while purging acne is imperative for this very reason.

When the inflamed acne isn't addressed quickly enough, permanent textural scarring can occur. Instead of digesting the acne seed, the pus starts eating away at the healthy follicle walls, creating textural pockmarks or ice pick scars. Inflammation control and proper extractions are of utmost importance when nodular and cystic acne are present to treat and prevent this from happening.

Topical Acne Types

Product-induced Acne (Acne Cosmetica)
Definitely the most common, caused by using products that have comedogenic ingredients in them, even including laundry detergent. We had several clients who broke out on the sides of their face from sleeping on their newly washed pillow cases when using a new cloggy laundry detergent.

Picking
When a seed has not been fully extracted, the tissues around the pore that just got poked at become swollen thanks to the friction and possible ruptures of the skin there. The pore will never clear up until the seed is fully extracted, and until then, inflammation may rise and fall with this particular pore. Ice your skin and let your skin-clearing regimen do the work instead.

Friction-induced Acne (Acne Mechanica)
Caused or aggravated by something external that keeps rubbing or touching the skin. This could be things like sunglasses resting on clogged pores where they touch the nose bridge or cheeks, on the sides of the face or chin if you constantly wear a helmet with a chinstrap of some kind, or hats and scarves. It's also common on shoulders from backpacks and torsos from tight sports tops or bras.

Body Acne
Similar to "regular" facial acne but it takes more time and stronger products to clear because the skin on the body is thicker than that of the face. Systemic health imbalances, prescription medications, cloggy laundry detergent, and mechanical aggravators (sweaty and heavy backpacks, dirty yoga mats) are more likely to affect these kinds.

In order to see results, you will need to use stronger products and allow them more time to work on the body when compared to the face. Check your hair and body care products and laundry detergent; wear natural fabrics and wash them often. Dry out and calm the inflamed acne with a benzoyl peroxide cleanser, and once the inflammation is under control, slowly and carefully integrate physical scrubbing of the non-inflamed seeds left behind. One can foam up the cleanser and leave it on the skin as long as possible while in the shower before rinsing it off. Adding a physical and/or chemical exfoliant on top of the benzoyl peroxide cleanser treatment can help if needed and tolerated. Benzoyl peroxide gel as a leave-on treatment may be needed for particularly inflamed or oily skin.

Use a product applicator designed for the back, much like a long-handled back scratcher with a flat pad at the end for rubbing or a long band that you hold on both ends and shimmy down your back (like the bodybuddy.com). Look for ones made of non-porous material (like silicone) so that the applicator will dispense product onto your skin instead of absorbing it, that you can clean and let dry thoroughly between uses. You'll probably want separate ones for washing and applying product. For particularly stubborn cystic areas, Dr. Fulton recommended clients apply the skin treatments and then wrap the area with plastic cling wrap to allow the product to absorb.

Recurring Acne

Some clients complain of pimples that pop up in the same exact places or pores and never seem to go away completely. They can lay dormant for months or years and randomly pop up when inflammatory responses take place. When inflammatory responses recede, so does the swelling of that still-clogged pore. Some event causing inflammation or the skin's natural exfoliation bringing those seeds up to the surface will make them reappear. Only when these are fully removed will the pores remain clear, and those recurring pimples will finally go away.

Persistent Hyperpigmentation

After inflamed acne has healed, pigmentation left behind–either red (vascular) or brown (melanin pigmentation)–usually fades away on its own or can be easily corrected with products and treatments. The longer the impaction was in the skin (or the more pigmentation-prone the skin inherently is), the longer it may take for the pigmentation to fade. More stubborn or dark marks may hang around longer than usual, though, because of a blocked pore that needs the seed to be extracted in order for the skin's pigmentation to finally brighten up.

Other Types of Topically Induced Acne Vulgaris

Medical writer Carol Turkington and Dr. Jeffrey Dover, authors of *The Encyclopedia of Skin and Skin Disorders*, also mention other types of acne: *acne detergens* (when washing the face too much, the skin gets dehydrated and oil and skin cell production increase to overcompensate); *acne excoriée* (a conscious, repetitive, and uncontrollable desire to pick, scratch, or rub acne); *acne mallorca* (mostly affects the chest, back, and sometimes face as papules and pustules; sweat causes the skin to swell and the sun increases oil production; the remedy is to stay out of the sun and humidity, avoid cloggy sun lotions); *neonatal acne* (infant acne, in which case the acne clears on its own); or *chloracne* (constant exposure to motor oil, insecticides, or cooking oils).

They also list the following as "intractable acne," types of acne that may require medical attention: *acne conglobata* (severe acne and scarring that's genetic, found in people with an extra Y chromosome), cystic acne (which we've treated successfully in clinic), *acne keloidalis nuchae* (aka *dermatitis papillaris capillitii*, which present like regular acne but with many keloids, often on the nape of the neck), and *acne fulminans* (a necrotic type of acne that causes severe scarring and is often accompanied by joint pain and fever).

Systemic and Internal Acne Types

With stubborn acne, the natural inclination would be to use stronger and stronger products to counterbalance/try to cover up/make up for/keep up with the underlying systemic imbalance. There are some things we won't be able to do much about (medical conditions or necessary medications), but along with your allopathic general doctor who can run basic lab work and test results, working with a trained and experienced holistic practitioner (like a naturopath, acupuncturist, integrative general practitioner, etc.) can run more specialized tests than a typical allopathic panel, helping to bring awareness and relief to the root causes.

The most common instances of acne cases that had a harder time clearing with the With & Within protocol alone without additional support included:

- Pregnancy, pre-natal fertility treatments, post-natal nursing and recovery
- Reproductive hormone imbalances like PCOS (polycystic ovary syndrome)
- Prescription drugs (that disrupt the digestive flora, induce acne as a side effect, or both)
- Antibiotic-resistant or recurring bacterial infections
- Hormone treatments for gender affirmation, fertility protocols, etc.
- Birth control (all kinds except condoms)
- Digestive parasites
- Fungal infections
- Chronic, long-term, high-stress lifestyle
- Too much caffeine (usually in the form of coffee or energy drinks)

- A high glycemic diet that includes many processed foods, sodas, and sugars
- Candida albicans yeast overgrowth

In these cases, it was also common for the acne to be accompanied by conditions like psoriasis or eczema, excess facial hair for women, frequent infections (vaginal yeast or urinary tract), intense sugar cravings, or irregular period cycles (both signs of hormonal imbalance), among others.

Dietary

One's diet is one of the largest lifestyle contributors to acne and can be tricky because of the many simultaneous variables, principles, and timelines that intersect. I've broken down their effects into four simple tracks: foods as both aggravator and creator of acne and its resulting immediate and delayed skin reactions. This is expanded upon in *Section 5, Digestive System, Diet and Acne*.

Aggravator: Foods that cause acne seeds already present to become inflamed.

Creator: These foods cause acne seeds to form; they don't just make existing seeds become inflamed.

Immediate reactions: Eating a certain food that causes a visible inflammatory response within hours or days of consumption.

Delayed reactions: When the acne seed has fully grown and migrated to the skin's surface and is now visible to the naked eye.

CASE STUDY: Dietary acne timeline

The first time I saw dietary acne in action was with a client who cleared up beautifully and maintained her clear complexion for almost a year, then went to Italy on vacation. She came back for a treatment a few days after her trip, bragging about how clear her skin was for having had dairy every single day she was there. She went back to living her acne-safe lifestyle as soon as she returned but had a major breakout about four weeks later. The only variable we could isolate was that for two weeks, she had dairy every day while on vacation. This is why it's so important to make sure you're all cleared up before reintroducing questionable and possible acne-causing variables, so you can see exactly what new thing is causing what reaction.

Section 2 - Acne 101

Hormones and Stress

The second most influential acne factor, hormones are not relegated only to reproductive sex hormones, as they both affect and are affected by pretty much every single bodily function that happens in the body. This acne, typically inflamed, appears on the lower half of the face and tends to come and go with various hormone cycles—menstruation, periods of heavy physical or mental stress, or disruption in sleep cycles included. Aim for a well-balanced, low-stress, and rested lifestyle.

General direct and indirect stress

All types of stress—emotional, mental, physical, digestive, and sleep—engage the endocrine system to flood the body with hormone chemicals (like cortisol) as a response, which generally increases inflammation and oil production. Both direct and indirect stressors (especially over prolonged periods) will also affect other biological processes like digestion and sleep, the very foundations of healthy living.

Hormones in the diet

Estrogen-rich foods like soy (especially the highly processed isolate kind, and/or when consumed regularly as a main protein source), cortisol-elevating foods like coffee, and oil-producing foods like peanuts can affect the endocrine system, which for the acneic person, often manifests in skin eruptions. Livestock conventionally raised in Concentrated Animal Feeding Operations (CAFO) are often given hormones to boost their yield (as well as antibiotics to treat and prevent infections), so choose organic meat and wild fish when you can. Avoiding plastics and instead using glass or stainless steel for food heating and storage also helps reduce estrogen exposure.

Reproductive hormonal acne

For a healthy person who menstruates, this monthly cycle shouldn't necessarily cause new acne seeds to form but instead can flare what seeds already exist in the pore. The body swells as a protective mechanism to protect the new, soon-to-maybe-be-fertilized egg, and these inflammatory effects affect the skin, too. Clear the pores so there are no seeds to get inflamed in the first place. Ice the skin and get extra rest, sleep, and quiet time these days.

Puberty and pregnancy, nursing

Stick to an acne-safe lifestyle as much as possible (even if it's just being consistent with your skin products) while you wait for the body to finish riding these hormonal waves. Be gentle with yourself; you're doing your best which is all you can do, and that's more than enough. Get as much rest and sleep as you can.

Synthetic hormone medications

This includes birth control, hormone replacement, and gender-affirming medications. These drugs greatly alter and even control the body's hormone balance, even if some are marketed as "non-hormonal" like the birth control copper IUD. (The copper IUD itself inherently does not contain hormones, but when inserted, alters your body's natural hormone balance, causing possible acne effects). Condoms are the only birth control that won't affect your hormones or acne.

Consistency in taking prescriptions like the pill (to the hour) and allowing enough time (three to six months on average) to acclimate onto (or off of) birth control will be necessary for the body's hormone levels to balance out before you can see skin clarity or drug-related persistent acne. Hormonal medications taken for the long term require more consideration, as discussed in Section 3, The 5 Types of Hormonal Stress Responsible for Acne.

Medication-induced (Acne Medicamentosa)

Some acne cases (or lesions that look like acne but aren't, called *acneiforms*) are inevitable when a particular medication or supplement is at play. Start by researching if the drug or supplement you are taking has acne as a reported side effect. Avoid supplements that contain iodine, soybean oil, or heavy metals, which we've all seen affect our clients in the clinic.

Some drugs that have been noted to have acne as side effects: phenytoin (Dilantin), lithium, potassium chloride (to supplement low potassium levels from heart medications); cold medicines (from the bromides and iodides within); birth control pills, injections, and implants; steroids (like prednisone); and rarely but still documented: Actinomycin D, Halothane, Thiouracil, Thiourea, Trimethadione, excessive amounts of B-complex vitamins, B12, kelp, and iodine.

Candida-induced acne

Far and away, the most common and stubborn systemic cause of acne we saw at With & Within was Candida yeast overgrowth. We found this condition to be common with clients who:

- Have a history of antibiotic or birth control use
- Have a history of frequent ear or throat infections, especially as a child
- Are highly and/or chronically stressed
- Consume a lot of caffeine (especially in the form of coffee), processed foods, and sugar
- Exhibit impaired digestive functions (chronic constipation, gas, bloating)

- Exhibit frequent and recurring yeast infections (vaginal, ear, sinus, throat, etc.)
- Needed to use very strong skincare products but they still weren't able to get or stay completely clear.

It is possible to safely and naturally rebalance the digestive flora without conventional medicine but it does take some preparation, work, dedication, and time.

Antibiotics and their lingering effects

Long-term or repeated antibiotic use has been linked to brown tooth stains, gastrointestinal disorders, breast cancer, and most commonly, contributes to digestive flora imbalances in the body, usually manifesting as a Candida yeast overgrowth imbalance. The chances of antibiotic resistance are also likely, so stronger, different, or more rounds of antibiotics may be prescribed by allopathic doctors to treat future bacterial infections, but their efficacy, even at these strengths, is still questionable.

Acne Look-alikes, aka Acneiforms

The following are often misdiagnosed for each other or for just plain old "regular" acne vulgaris, but in fact are not. However, they often coexist at the same time. These cases are typically resistant to basic acne treatments and often seem to be bacteria-, yeast-, or fungal-related.

Rosacea and Acne Rosacea

There are several types of this condition, but the skin-related kind affects people young and old and is easier to see on light or fair skin, as darker skin tones can conceal redness hiding underneath. It appears as a bright red or pink flush often on the cheeks and nose, often with visible veins or broken capillaries present. Small pustules may be present, which look like but don't act the same as acne; upon inspection, you'll see there isn't anything in those acne-looking bumps to extract. In more extreme cases, the skin can swell up, and the nose can become enlarged. Acne and rosacea can appear at the same time, so care must be taken to gently address both (exfoliate to slough off acne seeds but be gentle on the rosacea).

Topical Treatment

Topical steroids are the usual conventional medicine treatment protocol for this condition, but long-term steroid use can lower the immune system, thin the skin, and increase allergic reactions overall. In the clinic, we've found successful results from the magical yet simple and accessible combination of benzoyl peroxide and salicylic acid.

Use caution and address any skin sensitivities before using the active products. Being gentle with the skin (using products that are not too strong) and going slow with introducing active ingredients is the usual course of action. After some skin conditioning, some clients may benefit from a stronger professional chemical peel "reset" to jump-start the clearing process.

Rosacea and acne-rosacea clients can try starting slowly by using a benzoyl peroxide face wash a few times a week as the skin can tolerate, watching for dryness or irritation. Gradually increase usage, and after a few more weeks, perhaps integrate a salicylic toner or serum to boost the program as the skin can tolerate over several weeks' time. Leaving benzoyl peroxide gel on the skin may be integrated into the regimen if needed and tolerated after four to six weeks following the above suggestions. And always wear SPF!

Lifestyle

These folks may be more sensitive to extremes both in the ambient air temperature and direct exposure (like hot water from a showerhead or cold, snowy wind), spicy food, dairy, drinking alcohol, and/or stress.

The TCM (Traditional Chinese Medicine) approach for rosacea is to clear the heat from the stomach, spleen, and/or lungs that "get stuck" at the face, causing inflammation. Ayurveda says rosacea is a result of heat build-up in the body (excess pitta) from eating too much spicy food or too many unhealthy foods, overconsumption of caffeine, unmanaged stress, excessive temperature changes, sun damage, or other internal imbalances. The shared core emphasis from both philosophies is to cool the body down and clear the internal heat that's causing the redness and inflammation manifesting in the skin.

Herpes Simplex

An incredibly common virus that can affect both oral (type 1) and genital (type 2) areas of the body. Often, a tingling or itching sensation starts in the area that a lesion is beginning to appear, forming a blister that eventually scabs over and heals in one to two weeks. Clients have reported that icing the area as soon as the tingling starts has helped keep them at bay or sped up the breakout lifecycle. Take care to avoid touching, picking, or applying chemical peels and active homecare products directly on or close to the lesion if one appears, and consider skipping professional skin treatments until it has completely abated. TCM and Ayurveda recommend the same general guidelines for rosacea found here.

Keratosis Pilaris

Often called "chicken skin," these bumps, appearing on the upper arms, are not acne but dead skin cells accumulating at the surface of each pore, creating what looks like non-inflamed acne. Western naturopathic medicine says this is a vitamin A or B-12 deficiency, and both the allopathic medical and skincare professional communities simply suggest regularly exfoliating (physical scrubbing and using exfoliating lotions that are typically lactic acid-based) and moisturizing the areas affected to treat it.

Perioral Dermatitis

Note: This condition is often accompanied or caused by Candida and can also be mistaken for *Malassezia folliculitis*, below.

Who: Most common in women aged 15-45.

How it looks

Small red papules or scaly, often itchy bumps that appear around the mouth, usually in the smile lines that go from the nose to the corners of the mouth but can also show up on the upper lip on "drool" lines around the chin. This acne can be induced by:

- Sodium laureth or lauryl sulfates or fluoride found in toothpaste
- A Candida yeast overgrowth in the digestive tract
- Prescription medications like topical or oral antibiotics or birth control
- Some cosmetics and skin products, including acne-targeted products, which can make it worse
- Constant heat and humidity, like wearing PPE masks in tropical climates

How it's treated

- Try switching to sulfate and fluoride-free toothpaste and oral care products
- Avoiding acidic fruits and foods
- Trying a Candida yeast detox under the guidance of a qualified health professional
- Keeping the skin as dry and cool as possible

- Treating your skin as if you have Malassezia folliculitis (below)

Malassezia Folliculitis[9]

Note: This condition is often accompanied or caused by Candida.

How it looks

Perioral dermatitis is often a precursor of this type of acne that starts out on the face. Malassezia folliculitis presents as small, uniform, itchy papules and pustules, particularly on the upper back and chest and can include the forehead/hairline, chin, neck, and inner elbow crease. In some cases, it can spread in or around the nose, eyes, and genitals.

Red bumps and/or hypopigmentation (white spots, lack of melanin here), usually centered on or around a hair follicle; may include an ingrown hair.

Can be induced, exacerbated, or prolonged by:

- Hot and humid climates or situations where the skin is constantly damp and not allowed to air-dry (folds in the skin, after-sports hygiene)
- Excessive sebum production or sweating
- Products that don't allow the skin to breathe, like occlusive emollients and sunscreens
- Oral and topical antibiotics
- Suppressed immune systems induced by disease (like Candida or HIV) or steroid drugs (topical and oral)
- Malassezia folliculitis-aggravating and -inducing ingredients in products, some even acne-safe ones. Mostly oils, but many others as well.

This acne type can be particularly resistant and prone to recur (even after successful treatment), so maintenance, a full-body evaluation, and perhaps even treatment are vital to prevent recurrence. Many treatments and products to address "regular" acne can make this condition worse, so proper diagnosis and very careful attention to product ingredients are recommended for the best result.

How it's treated

- Topically, conventional cleansing shampoos targeted toward dandruff that contain antifungals like econazole, ketoconazole, or selenium sulfide shampoo (like a Selsun Blue brand shampoo in the US) to clear and then used regularly to prevent recurrence.

- Avoid certain ingredients in your products that are known to aggravate Malassezia folliculitis (search "fungal acne" on our lifestyle library blog for the list[10] or check *https://folliculitisscout.com*).
- Can try sparingly by applying diluted tea tree and lavender essential oils to the areas affected for itch/rash relief.
- Photodynamic therapy and, in severe cases, oral isotretinoin, have been shown to give good results.
- See a natural or integrative health practitioner to identify and treat the root cause.

Bacterial Folliculitis[11]

This condition is often accompanied or caused by Candida. It includes bacteria and staph infections within the hair follicle/pore.

How one gets it
- Damp skin that's not allowed to air-dry and/or is occluded by clothing, dressings, ointments
- Frequent shaving, waxing, or other forms of depilation
- Friction from tight clothing
- Atopic dermatitis
- Acne or other follicular skin disorder
- Using topical corticosteroids
- Previous long-term use of antibiotics
- Chronic illnesses like anemia, obesity, diabetes, HIV/AIDS, viral hepatitis, cancer
- Bathing in inadequately cleansed hot tubs or pools

How to prevent it
- Keep skin clean, cool, and if it's dry, moisturized.
- Minimize shaving and waxing. If you must, see Section 4, Practical Daily Life, Hair Removal Best Practices.
- Wear loose-fitting clothes made of natural fabrics that offer plenty of ventilation.
- Ensure adequate sterilization of hot tubs, use chlorine-free ones, or avoid altogether.
- In case of repeated episodes of staphylococcal folliculitis, allopathic medicine recommends applying Mupirocin ointment to the nostrils to eliminate *S. aureus* carrier state, the precursor to infection, in the respiratory tract.

How to treat it
- Warm compresses (or ice) to relieve itch and pain

- Medicines like analgesics and anti-inflammatories to relieve pain
- Use antiseptic cleansers
- Professionally open and drain fluid-filled lesions and abscesses
- Antibiotics
- Photodynamic therapy
- Laser hair removal

Steroid "Acne"

Steroid acne (or acneiform) most often affects adolescent or adult patients who have been taking moderate or high doses of oral steroids such as prednisone or dexamethasone for several weeks. This usually shows up on the chest but may also develop on the face, neck, back, and arms. In terms of clearing it, there's no reliable solution. For some, it can clear while continuing to take the medicine, but for others, it will persist until the steroid is discontinued. Severe cases have been successfully treated with oral isotretinoin (Accutane).[12]

Iodide Acne (or Iodide Rash, Iodide Flush)

> ## CASE STUDY: Shrimp-induced acne
>
> I've had about five cases where the clients ate shrimp as their main source of protein (two or three times a day). When they eliminated seafood from their diet and went through the clearing process, they cleared up beautifully without scarring. Some were able to eat shrimp again with no issues; some remain reactive to this day.

This looks and behaves more like a rash but is commonly accompanied by "regular" acne. It looks like a reddish or pinkish mask with a defined border around the face, is often accompanied by little non-extractable bumps (and if acne is present, extractable acne pimples, too), and can be itchy. Lines of demarcation of the rash "mask" are clear as the eyelids are not usually affected, so the skin on the perimeter of the eyes remains normal while the rash creates pink/red circles around the eyes and perimeter of the face.

From my own personal experience, using skin products or taking supplements that contain iodine-rich seaweed or kelp ingredients also caused an itchy, bumpy rash all over the face, sometimes including my earlobes and neck. Halogen drugs can also induce this reaction, particularly the ones that contain iodine and bromide. People who have this sensitivity should reduce or avoid seaweed, algae, and iodide in their skincare products (and probably their diet, too).

Pyoderma Faciale (aka Rosacea Fulminans)

Dr. Fulton describes this type of acne in his book and says that it affects people (mostly women) with a certain enzyme deficiency. This prompts the adrenal glands to dump testosterone (as opposed to hydrocortisone) into the body as a stress response, is often accompanied by super oily hair, can be verified by blood samples, and is treated by the conventional drug dexamethasone. Other studies indicate that it's a type of rosacea that is treated with oral and topical medications (antibiotics, steroids, and isotretinoin).

> **CASE STUDY: Extreme stress, extreme case**
>
> I suspect a client of mine from years ago had this condition, which she ultimately went to the doctor and took drugs for. She'd just had a major life change (she bartended into the wee hours for over a decade and abruptly switched to a daytime receptionist job) accompanied by a ton of stress. We had gotten her acne rosacea under control just a few months prior, which she successfully maintained. But when this job change happened, her face pretty much blew up. Large and intense inflamed acne literally appeared overnight, seemingly out of nowhere, and was resistant to the topical treatments I was giving her.

Other Drug-induced Acne-like Reactions

Speaking on a very general level, acute medication-related eruptions usually appear within the first two weeks of taking the medication. In the case of steroids, halogens (particularly iodine and bromine), and epidermal growth factor receptor inhibitor-induced rashes (EGFRIs), the papules and pustules often erupt over a short period of time (from days to weeks) and clear up once the medication is stopped. Chronic eruptions may appear after months or years on a medication such as lithium[13] or anticonvulsants.[14]

These drug-induced acneiforms tend to appear as red papules and pustules that have a uniform look, are typically located on the trunk, shoulders, upper arms, and face, and unlike acne vulgaris, comedones (acne impactions or seeds) are not present, so they're not extractable.

Inspiring (and Real) Acne Case Studies

Since 2008 we've successfully cleared a plethora of clients from different backgrounds with various skin types, lifestyles, and acne factors. Here is a sampling of actual case studies to help you better identify different acne types, how they may appear on different skin tones and what results have been achieved—sans prescriptions—with our philosophy and products.

Non-inflamed Acne

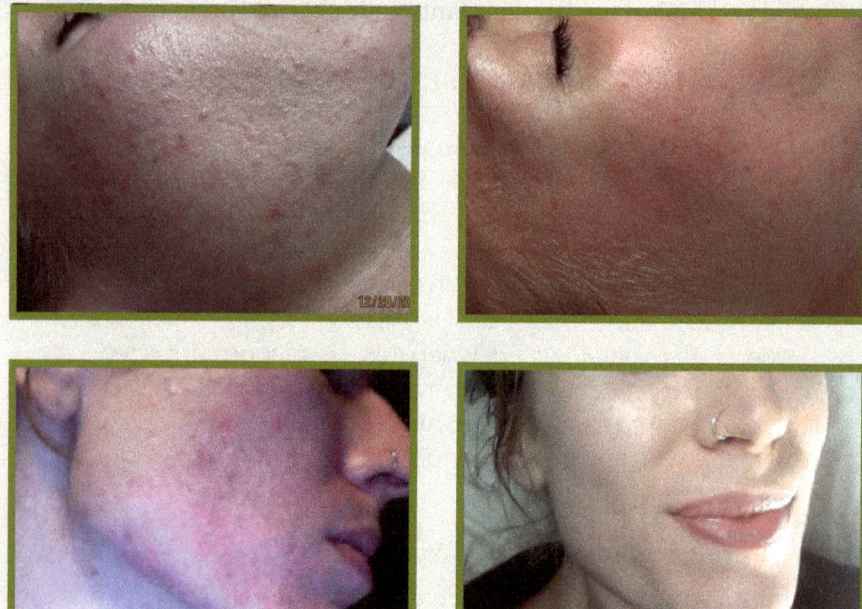

This client started with a 10% clarity rate, meaning that 90% of the pores on her face were congested. She had taken Accutane as a teen, plenty of antibiotics throughout adulthood, and when she came to us was using a lot of cloggy skin, hair and body products, and was having dairy and coffee 3-4x/day! Working together, she reached 90% clarity in 7 weeks.

Section 2 - Acne 101

Non-inflamed Acne

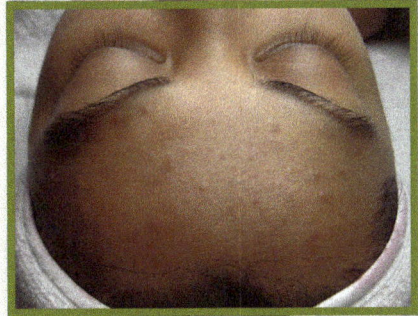 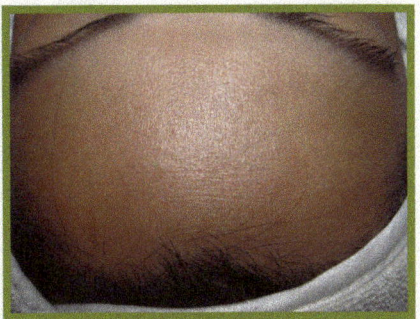

Dairy, soy milk, coffee and too much peanut butter is what initially broke out this Pacific Islander client. She cleared up but ran out of product, and broke out again. Getting back on her With & Within regimen got her clear, even after having 2 kids.

Inflamed Acne, Whole Face

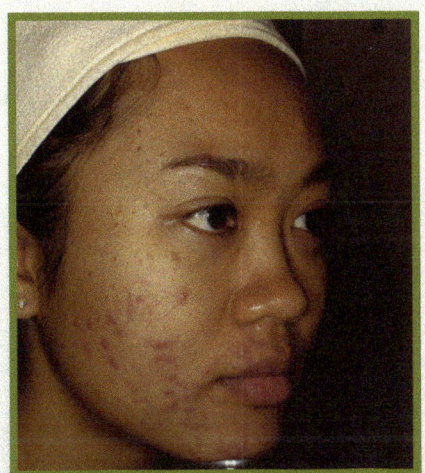 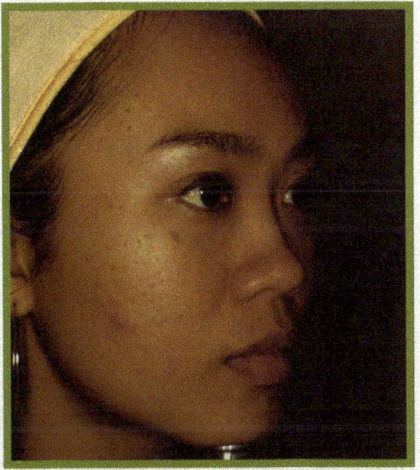

Cloggy products, birth control and diet contributed to this Southeast Asian client's acne. The breakouts were really affecting her quality of life and with a wedding coming up, she was motivated and determined to do anything to clear up. She prepped her skin by using our products for a month before coming in for treatments, and went from 50% to 85% clear in 4 weeks.

Inflamed Acne, Whole Face

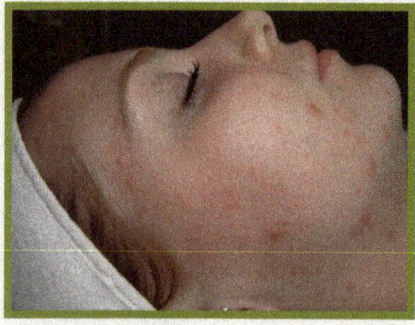 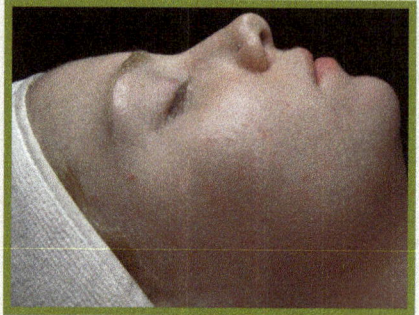

Four rounds of Accutane didn't clear this light skinned, red-headed graveyard shift NICU nurse's acne, but strict inflammatory lifestyle management, regular treatments and a strong skincare regimen got her to a 90% average clarity rate in 4 months.

Inflamed Acne, Whole Face

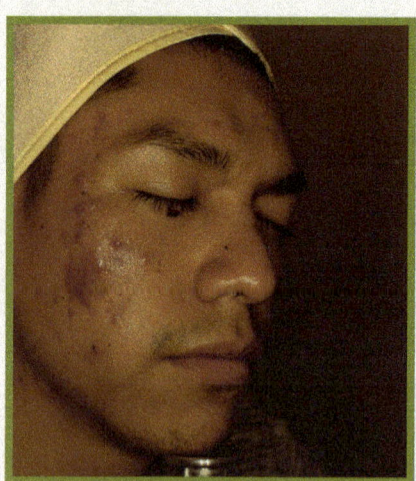 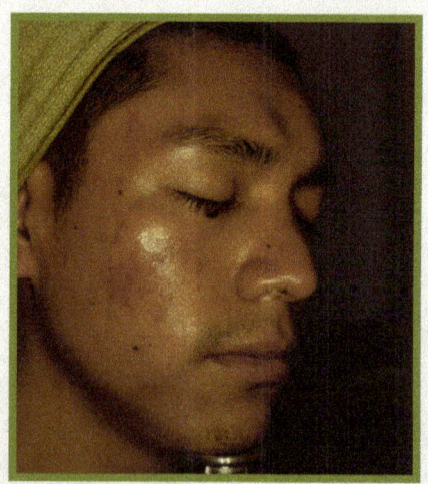

High emotional and contractor job stress, gastritis and lots of takeout food were this Hispanic client's triggers. His skin was also very dehydrated and sensitized from super strong OTC acne products, so rebalancing his skin was a must before incorporating acne-fighting active products. Choosing healthier takeout dishes, managing his stress and regular treatments cleared him up. Because he stayed clear, the resulting PIH eventually faded with time.

Section 2 - Acne 101

Inflamed Acne, Whole Face

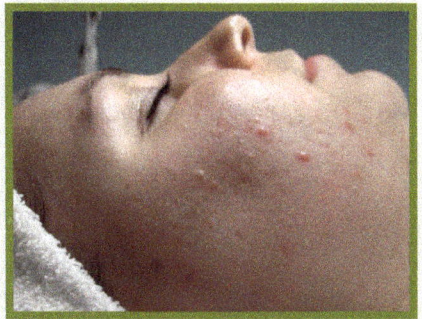 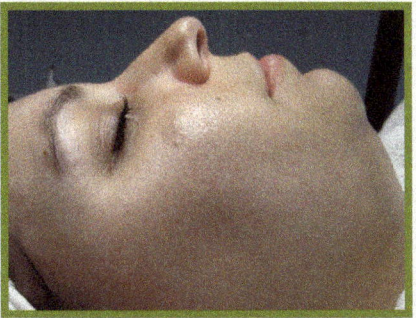

This olive skin toned client with acne in her genes couldn't clear up even after 3 rounds of Accutane, but after eliminating whey protein shakes from her diet and switching to our skin regimen, she cleared up in 3 months.

Inflamed Acne - Topical RX Induced Acne

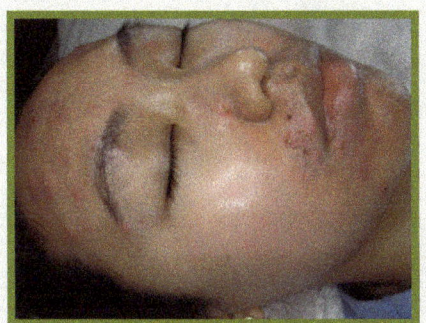 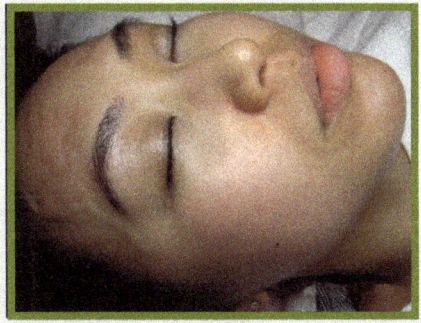

At a starting point of 55% clarity, this East Asian client came to us highly stressed and broken out from cloggy face products from another acne specialist, and terribly over-exfoliated from Retin-A and Spirnolactone. Her skin was so tight and dry that she told us it hurt to eat a banana. Balancing and desensitizing her skin before slowly incorporating active products and consistent stress management healed and cleared her very sensitive and painful acne.

Inflamed Acne, Whole Face

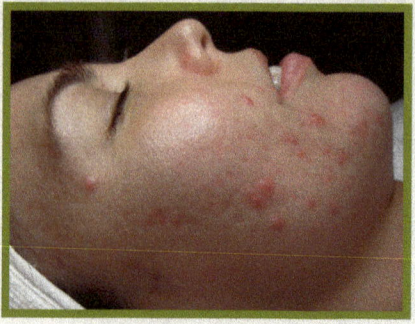 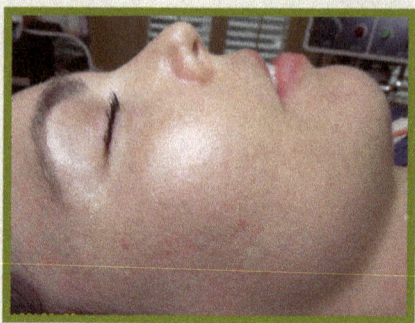

With incredibly sensitive skin and painfully inflamed acne, this client's skin turned the corner with very careful exfoliation, strict inflammation management and time. The last key to her clarity was changing her toothpaste to one that was acne-safe, ending her acne battle that started at age 14.

Inflamed Hormonal Acne

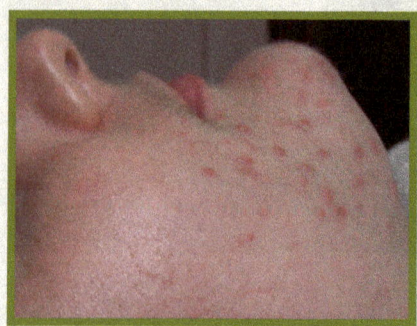 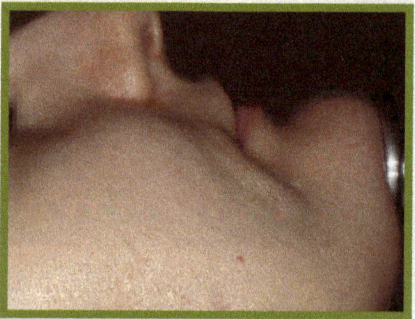

Acne in her genetic background, dairy in her diet and multiple cups of coffee a day to counterbalance lack of sleep induced hormonal chin acne in this client. Prioritizing sleep and stress management, an acne-safe lifestyle and strong skin products cleared her acne.

Inflamed Hormonal Acne

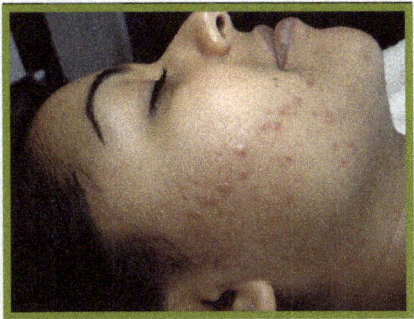 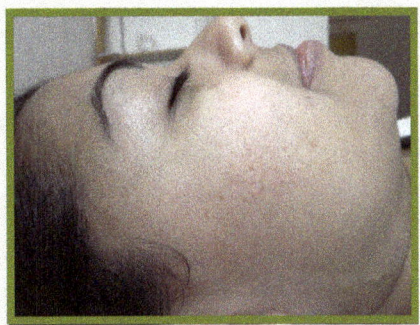

A thyroid condition, hormone therapy and an inflammatory diet caused inflamed acne for this South Asian client. To get clear, she got her hormone levels rebalanced by working with an acupuncturist and cut down on her sugar intake. In 6 months her acne cleared, and in 6 more her pigmentation naturally cleared too.

Iodide Rash

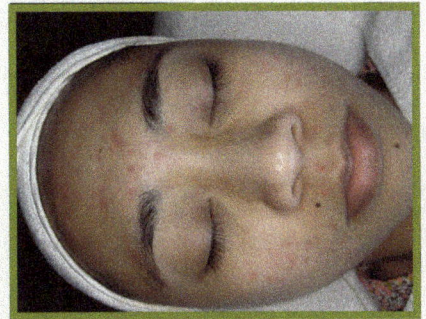 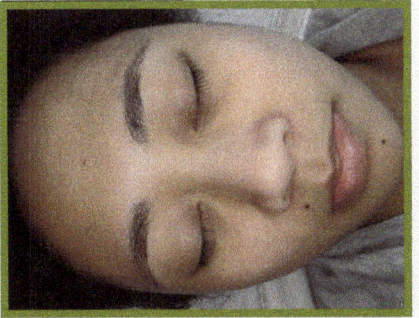

This Pacific Islander nurse came to us with extremely sensitive skin, who worked long hours under a lot of stress. She consumed iodine-rich shrimp 2-3x/day. Removing it from her diet, prioritizing self-care and discovering that the hospital PPE masks' friction worsened her skin cleared both her acne and resulting pigmentation in about 8 weeks.

Possible Rosacea & Product Reaction

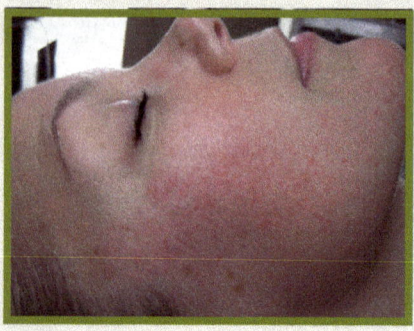 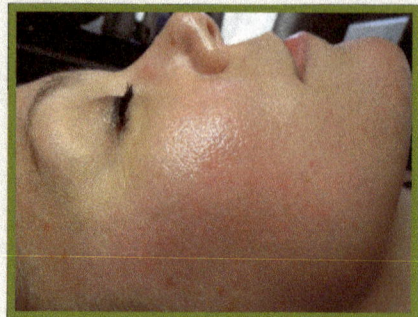

This client's case was a mixed bag: she had rosacea-like pustules with an iodide-acne-like skin texture. Her seeds extracted easily as if her skin was oily, but she complained of dryness. Birth control, comedogenic products, entrepreneur stress and RX drugs from a dermatologist were all factors. Slowly adding BP, salicylic acid and sufficient moisture along with lifestyle management cleared her up for good.

Acne Rosacea

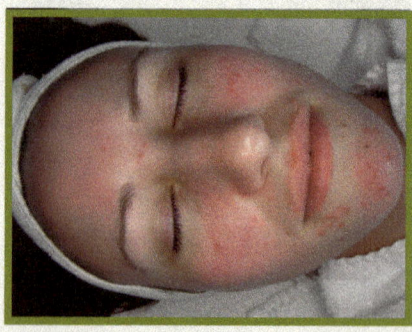 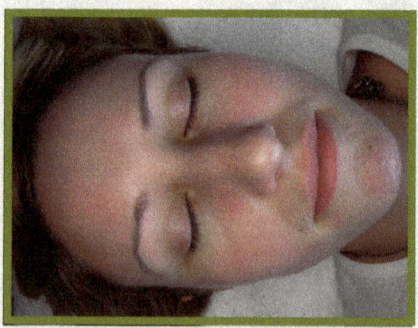

This client had acne and redness for years before finding relief and control by avoiding foods containing carrageenan which caused breakouts around their mouth, and red wine along with very hot or cold water flared their rosacea. Using Benzoyl Peroxide Gel as a nightly mask within their balanced With &Within skin regimen and using acne-safe toothpaste has kept them clear for many years, even after having children.

Other Acne Approaches

Conventional Medicine Stance on Acne

The first thing your doctor probably gave you to try was some kind of topical prescription—an exfoliant (Retin-A, Differin, Tazorac), an antibiotic (clindamycin, erythromycin), azelaic acid (which is believed to reduce Cutibacterium acnes bacteria, regulate skin cell shedding as well as brighten pigmentation left behind), or combination preparations (which usually combine benzoyl peroxide with an exfoliant or antibiotic). Prolonged use of these formulas can often result in thinning and sensitizing of the skin, discoloration, and weakening of the skin's natural protective barrier. It was very common for clients to tell me that they were never instructed to use sunscreen while using these sun-sensitizing products and were also told that daily side effects such as redness, peeling, and irritation were normal.

Dr. Fulton's protocol was largely based on treating the skin aggressively with strong topical exfoliants and non-comedogenic products. He had his patients use a BP scrub wash to exfoliate and dry the skin and apply ice, followed by a strong AHA acid toner to strip the skin of its oils, a vitamin A serum to flush out the seeds, and BP gel to further dry the skin and reduce inflammation. Dr. Terry J. Dubrow, MD, director of Acne Clinic of Newport Beach, California, and author of *The Acne Cure*, discusses a protocol that is, in my opinion, also quite aggressive. He first instructs the reader to cleanse and apply a 2% salicylic solution onto the skin before rinsing it off. Then, they perform the morning regimen (applying an 8-10% glycolic acid solution onto the skin that's rinsed off before applying a moisturizing SPF 15 sunscreen) or evening regimen (applying refrigerated BP gel on the skin with an ice pack directly on top of the face for ten minutes before wiping off the excess gel, leaving a thin film on the skin to work overnight). It's possible the aggressive peeling of Dr. Fulton's protocol would unnecessarily dehydrate and strip the skin of its natural protective barrier, as would Dr. Dubrow's protocol with multiple active products plus the cold pack on top of the BP may cause the skin to burn.

If topical approaches didn't cut it, then an oral prescription antibiotic was likely introduced, with the patient expected to use it for at least twelve weeks. Prolonged use of these oral medications created systemic imbalances for many of my clients, especially digestive disorders (like Candida yeast overgrowth).

Oral medications like antibiotics, birth control, and blood pressure and heart failure drugs are often prescribed for their "off-label" acne benefits.

They're not officially approved for the treatment of acne, but doctors have anecdotally noticed positive effects on their acne patients using these drugs. Spironolactone, a drug intended to relieve fluid build-up due to heart failure, liver scarring, or kidney disease, is the most common drug used this way and is known for its supposed effects on acne-causing and oil-producing hormone activity.

The biggest gun in the prescription medicine arsenal for acne is isotretinoin, formerly sold under the brand name Accutane, which in 2009 was pulled off the market for medical claim and lawsuit reasons. It's now back on the market with different names (Roaccutane, Claravis, Amnesteem, and others) and stricter safety use guidelines but still poses the same dangers.

The good news is that these approaches work well enough for some folks, but the bad news is that some people experience harsh side effects of these drugs (often long-term digestive problems or even hormone imbalances), temporary effects, or the drug doesn't work for their skin at all.

Drugstore/Department Store Products

These often don't work for a variety of reasons. First, they are often cloggy. For example, most face washes will contain comedogenic sodium lauryl (or laureth) sulfate in Western countries or myristic acid in Eastern ones. Second, the active ingredients often aren't strong enough to do much for the skin due to liability reasons. Also, there isn't much education out there on how to properly assess your skin's needs or what and how to properly use products. Sales representatives are really only educated on their particular brand's product, and they likely lack the hands-on clinical experience of seeing successful case studies clear up time and time again and actually knowing why.

Day-spa Facials, Medispas, Estheticians

Estheticians can be generally trained well in the school where they got licensed, but most don't get much information on how exactly to treat acne. We didn't learn what was going on in the pore when acne formed or how to safely and properly extract acne, let alone what lifestyle factors affected it. Instead, we were to refer our clients to dermatologists, who would, in turn, usually end up just prescribing drugs and not actually treating the skin. We were taught to tell the client to use acne-targeted products within the brands we were trained to use and sell at our jobs and dispense generic information like drinking lots of water, acknowledging stress as a factor (but not how to identify or manage it), and getting regular sleep (which everyone could do).

Section 2 - Acne 101

Continuing Education

The continuing education most estheticians get is sponsored by the skincare brands they are trained to use. This doesn't leave much room for unbiased information about the physiology of acne and ends up being more of a marketing infomercial on products that a skincare brand is trying to push. However, there are plenty of estheticians who are genuinely passionate about and invest in their own continuing education, and are the best ones to seek out if need be.

Treatments and Extractions

Facial treatments usually rely on the "acne line" of a skincare brand and whatever protocol that brand decides to teach the estheticians buying it. Most of these products are not truly acne-safe, as they often contain comedogenic ingredients even when they say they don't.

Professional exfoliation treatments like chemical peels, microdermabrasion, and dermaplaning can help, but when combined with comedogenic ingredients in the other products that are used during treatment or at home (or just done incorrectly) won't do much in the long term. The client will continue breaking out because they're literally putting pore-clogging ingredients back on their face.

Extractions that are commonly performed in your average facial usually address non-acneic blackheads on the nose and chin, not doing much for the active acne itself. There is also a technique for the proper, complete, and safe extractions that can only be learned through careful training and constant repetition. Extractions improperly done can leave the pimples worse off than before the treatment or even cause infection or scarring.

With & Within facials

Our signature treatment protocols combined with our truly holistic acne-safe lifestyle approach has been proven effective time and time again since we opened in 2008.

Every facial appointment includes a detailed skin analysis, our famously thorough extractions, disinfection and inflammation relief, along with whatever exfoliation and/or hydration treatment the clients' skin needs that day. For more details about our approach, see Section 8, The With & Within Standard of Treatment.

Holistic Medicine Stance on Acne

Observing thousands of clients first hand at the clinic helped me to understand that acne is more often than not a condition best addressed holistically. In TCM and Ayurveda, some of the world's oldest healing philosophies, the common theme is that you don't treat acne as an isolated issue. Instead, you evaluate and treat the entire body, at which point acne—which is seen as an imbalance side effect—should clear.

The two schools of thought are quite similar, with subtle variances. They both see the body as one: physical, mental, and spiritual. They both emphasize strengthening the immune system to prevent illness versus conventional/allopathic medicine's waiting to treat symptoms already present. They both use the elements of nature to help classify, diagnose, and treat the body. They use food as medicine, supplemented with herbs and lifestyle to assist in optimizing the body's inner workings.

The main takeaway from both philosophies is the emphasis on a well-rounded lifestyle made up of deep rest, robust digestion, low stress, and eating healthy foods to promote the best health possible, preventing disease and the need for symptom treatment in the first place.

Integrative medicine may seem more slow going compared to conventional medicine's quick and temporary fixes. However, holistic medicine's lifestyle approach works to prevent imbalance and sickness in the first place, versus simply masking symptoms already present with pills and bandages, often failing to address root causes.

The holistic work can definitely be effective, but as far as acne is concerned, clear skin results will come much faster when combined with topical treatments (like the skin regimen we describe in this book). Do the holistic *and* skin stuff in tandem, and you'll be all set up for greater long-term health sooner than you know it.

Traditional Chinese Medicine (TCM)

TCM's foundational texts were written in China between the 5th and 3rd centuries BCE and were called "Huangdi Neijing" or "Yellow Emperor's Inner Canon." It is composed of two bodies of work, the first text serving as the theoretical foundation of Chinese Medicine and its diagnostic methods, while the second text describes acupuncture in great detail. These texts were the first in the history of the Chinese to depart from the old medieval beliefs that evil spirits caused disease and instead attributed them to diet, lifestyle, emotions, environment, and aging.

In TCM, the word *shen* most closely describes the body as a whole—not just the physical body itself, but the "ensemble of functions" including both the human psyche and emotions. The five elements used in TCM, called Wu Xing, are air, water, fire, earth, and metal. Chi (also written as *qi or ki*) is the vital life force that runs throughout the body, and any stagnation or disruption of it results in disease or problems in the body.

TCM physicians believe that acupuncture helps dispel the body's internal heat and dampness that cause skin problems. They also believe that the insertion of acupuncture needles into the skin at specific points triggers the body's self-repairing mechanisms. Further, acne does not discriminate by age but by patterns or types of internal imbalance.

How Traditional Chinese Medicine (TCM) diagnoses acne

"Damp heat" (too much heat and moisture in the body, often from a damp environment, too many greasy/sweet foods, or poor hygiene, often resulting in acne, fungal infections, itching, rashes, eczema, and boils) has a tendency to trigger chronic acne. The skin is usually oily, and the acne is inflamed and pus-filled. Singapore-based registered TCM physician and acupuncturist Jun Negoro says she can confirm Eu Yan Sang's (one of Asia's largest retailers of TCM products) findings: she sees clients who have acne caused by damp heat exacerbated by late-night eating, spicy and oily food; stress, which causes liver qi stagnation, affecting spleen function and causing damp accumulation; and blood stagnation, which causes the darker red/purplish inflamed acne that takes longer to heal.

"Blood heat" (too much heat in the blood, often from poor diet, emotional stress and anger, hot environments, or spicy foods often resulting in acne, dryness, redness, inflammation, itching, and infections) may be the cause of mild to moderate acne usually on the nose, around the mouth, and between the brows. "Toxic heat" (too much heat and toxins in the body, often from poor diet, environmental toxins or infection, often resulting in acne, rashes, eczema, hives, and infections) has similar symptoms to blood heat, but the acne in this case is more serious and pus-filled, and the skin around the inflamed lesions is usually red and painful.

According to Eu Yan Sang, there are three underlying causes of acne. First, consuming too much spicy, sweet, or oily food can lead to heat and dampness accumulating in the stomach and spleen. This disrupts the normal flow of "qi," a person's life force. Second, dry heat and damp heat lingering in the organs and meridians can also cause a breakout. Careful differentiation of heat is, therefore, crucial to treat the pattern of disharmony accordingly. Third, excessive heat and wind in the lungs can also lead to a breakout (attention smokers!). In TCM, wind is believed to have a pathogenic (or disease-causing) ability, and as the skin is thought of as the third lung, it's seen as being directly interconnected to each other's health along with direct exposure to the atmosphere and air we live in.

In TCM, acne is often treated using a prescribed herbal medication, along with the advice of consuming more fruits and vegetables, drinking more water, and maintaining a balanced and healthy diet to prevent acne. Drinking cooling Chinese herbal tea like chrysanthemum tea (*Juhua*, 菊花), isatis root (*Ban Lan Gen*, 板兰根), or coix barley (*Yiyiren*, 薏苡仁) is ideal, especially in hot weather.

Face map charts
Face maps show where breakouts or issues on the face are correlated with certain organs in the body. For instance, pimples on your cheeks may indicate an imbalance in your stomach. These charts can offer some insight as to what body systems may need extra attention through the skin.

However, leading Chinese-American practitioners Sandra Lanshin Chiu MSTCM, LAc from New York, New York and Ivy Lee MSTCM, LAc from Oakland, California who are vocal in the anti-cultural appropriation movement have said that these widely circulated charts aren't always accurate and can cause harm if not used properly because you're isolating a problem to one area from one random chart versus considering the entire constitution of the person's health. These charts and practices (like gua sha) are not one-size-fits-all and thus should be used under the guidance of a licensed, qualified, and experienced TCM practitioner.

Through my years in the clinic, I've distilled the consistent acne patterns we observed into our own With & Within Holistic Acne Face Map that you can find in *Section 4, Lifestyle*.

Traditional Indian Medicine (Ayurveda)
Ayurveda (*ayur* = health, *veda* = knowledge) is the traditional holistic medicine hailing from India that first started out as oral history, eventually recorded in ancient Sanskrit texts called the Vedas from over 5,000 years ago (around 3000-1000 BCE). The Vedas taught mythology, religion, and medicine, and in terms of Ayurveda, considered all things that could affect a person's health: physiology, medicine (even surgery!), astrology, spirituality, art, and human behavior, as well as politics and government.

In Ayurveda, the five earthly elements are slightly different than the ones TCM uses (air, fire, water, earth, and space) and are called Pancha Mahabhutas, which are paired up with each other to create three basic "doshas," or body types, which influence physiological and mental characteristics. These doshas include vata, pitta, and kapha, and are present in every living thing. It is when these doshas are imbalanced that problems in the body—like acne—arise.

Figuring out which dosha is out of balance based on your symptoms helps you figure out an action plan to bring them back into balance, reducing *or pacifying* those symptoms/imbalances. Consulting a qualified Ayurvedic practitioner to determine your doshas and imbalances is recommended.

Dr. Vasant Lad, Ayurvedic physician and founder of the Ayurvedic Institute in Santa Fe, New Mexico, writes in his book *The Complete Book of Ayurveda Home Remedies* on pages 114-116 that he attributes acne to excess pitta (or fiery heat elements) to the dosha fueled by emotional stress, premenstrual syndrome, chemicals, too much sun, and sometimes, bacteria.

He suggests pitta-pacifying shifts like avoiding spicy and fermented foods, salt, fried foods, and citrus fruit and favoring blander foods such as rice, oatmeal, and applesauce. You can also use common household culinary herbs to balance pitta. Steeping a teaspoon each of cumin, coriander, and fennel seeds in a pot of hot water makes a delicious digestive support tea. Dr. Lad also recommends you drink water stored in blue (preferably glass) vessels.

Here are his topical remedies that, to me, seem acne-safe and safe to try on healed, unbroken skin:

- Chickpea flour and water as a cleanser
- Almond powder and water as a paste; leave on for 30 minutes as a skin mask.
- Sandalwood and turmeric powder with goat's milk as a paste; also leave on the skin for 30 minutes as a mask.
- Melon. Rub it on the skin at bedtime and leave the juice on overnight. Its cooling anti-pitta quality will help heal acne. It also makes the skin soft.

Here are some lifestyle tips:

- Drinking aloe vera juice to keep the colon clean
- Doing specific yoga postures for acne (Lion Pose and Moon Salutation posture sequences)
- Pranayama, or deep breathing exercises
- Breathing through the left nostril only, for 5 to 10 minutes, will help to reduce pitta. (This is called the Moon Breath and is said to be cooling; breathing through the right nostril is called the Sun

Breath and is heating.) Simply cover the right nostril with your thumb and breathe normally through the left side. If the nostril is blocked, don't force it; try again later.
- Relaxing the face by rubbing your hands together vigorously to create a bit of warmth and holding them close to your face.
- Visualization exercise: The root cause of acne is emotional stress. One effective way to relieve that stress is visualization. Close your eyes and visualize that the acne is clearing up and going away—as if you are communicating with the tissues in your skin that are bursting out in acne.

And he offers a final suggestion: Avoid frequently looking in the mirror and feeling bad about the acne.

With too much pitta being the main aggravating factor for acne, here are some general guidelines to help pacify its effects and cool the body down.

- Exercise: Swimming is cooling. Emphasize longer exercises to focus on breath.
- Detox the liver.
- Eat cooked and cooling foods like asparagus, cucumbers, sweet and white potatoes, and leafy greens. Avoid spicy foods and acid-forming foods like meat and shellfish.
- Cooling dairy and coconut oil intake are recommended in Ayurveda, but not acne-safe from a With & Within perspective. Try coconut milk and olive oil instead.

Holistic Medicine's Emphasis on Digestion

Both TCM and Ayurveda center their philosophies around good digestion (*agni* in Ayurveda, the digestive fire) in order to physiologically avoid stressing the body and instead optimize its internal operations. Eating fresh (and mostly cooked) whole foods in their natural states while living a physically active, low-stress lifestyle is the daily priority for optimal health. When needed, Panchakarma, a five-step detoxing protocol, is performed with the help of an Ayurvedic doctor, or *vaidya*, to remove excess toxins (called *ama*) left behind in the body due to disease, poor nutrition/digestion, and environmental toxins. But with healthy, clean daily living, the body should hopefully not need Panchakarma. Oja to Ayurveda is what chi is to TCM; it's the life force that keeps us going and should be kept in balance—largely by diet and lifestyle—for optimal health.

Endnotes

9   *https://dermnetnz.org/topics/malassezia-folliculitis/*

10 *https://withandwithin.co/blogs/blog*

11 *https://dermnetnz.org/topics/bacterial-folliculitis/*

12 From *https://dermnetnz.org/topics/steroid-acne/*

13 *https://dermnetnz.org/topics/lithium*

14 *https://dermnetnz.org/topics/cutaneous-adverse-effects-of-anticonvulsant-drugs*

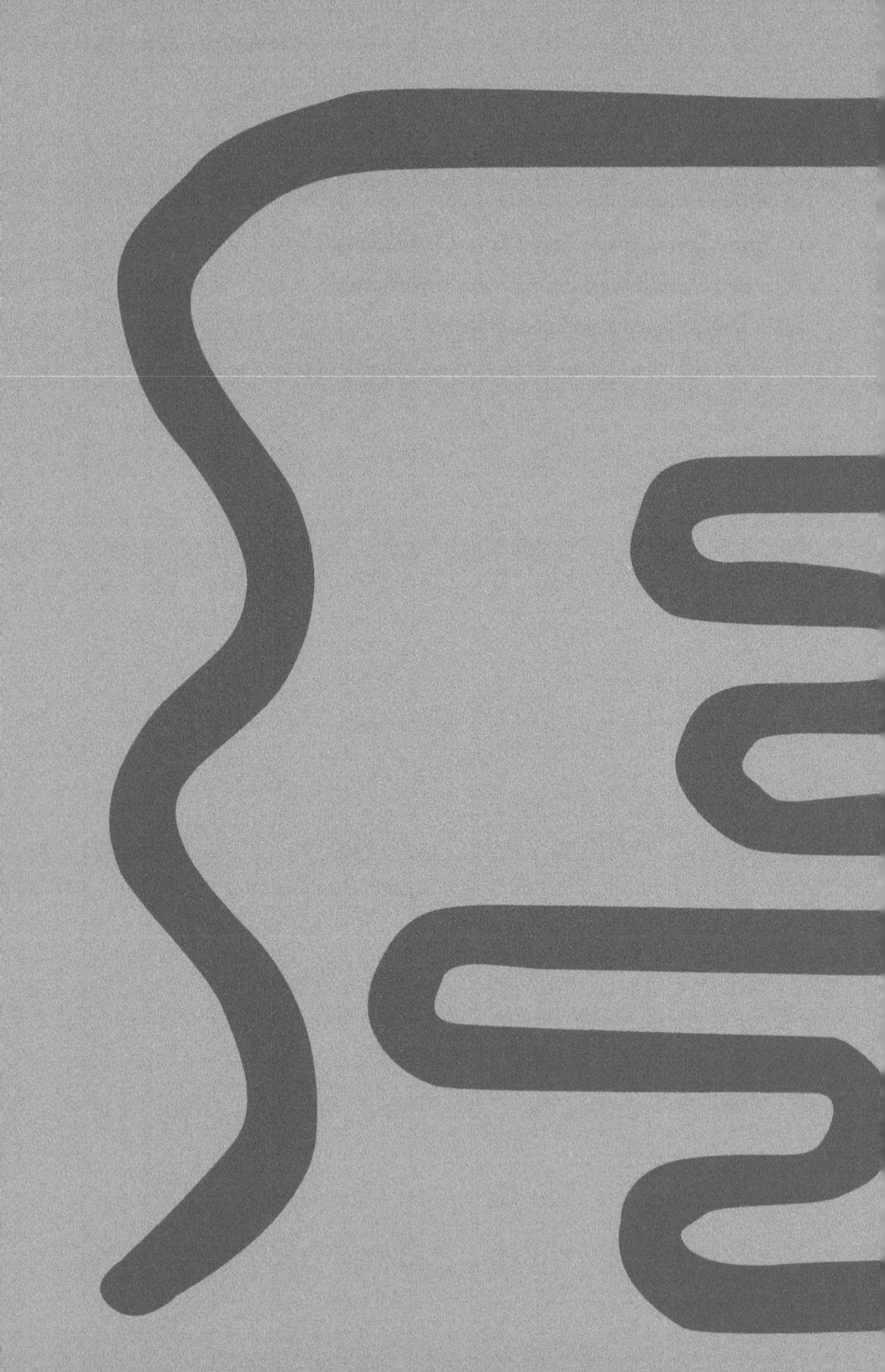

SECTION 3

The 5 Types of
Hormone Stress
Responsible for
Acne

Stress and hormones are so interlinked I'd say the easiest way to refer to them would be to talk about them like they're basically the same thing. Stress creates hormone chemical secretions, fueling the way we feel in our physical and mental bodies—usually inflamed, sluggish, unwell, sad, irritable and...stressed! Hormones are secreted as a response to stress that the physical body is experiencing. Understanding how these reactions show up in our day-to-day life will shape our awareness of how we can respond to them.

Understanding "Stress"

Stress comes in many forms—not just emotional aggravation, but also the everyday inner workings of the body, including physical, hormonal, and adrenal activity—all of which can impact your body greatly. Most people confuse stress with emotional aggravation and still do today. But Dr. Hans Selye, a Hungarian Canadian endocrinologist who in the early 1900s revolutionized conventional medicine with his concepts of stress, redefined it as any demand made on an organism to adapt, adjust, or cope, including "wear and tear within the body." Simply put, if you're doing anything other than lying down and sleeping (and even then, it's still doing stuff), your body is constantly reacting to stimuli, which requires effort, translating into stress your body has to respond to, facilitate through, and recover from. These states of alertness are produced and managed by your endocrine system where hormonal reactions originate and chemicals are secreted as a response. Start to become aware of the different stressors in your life, the physical, mental, and emotional reactions your body has in response to them, and manage them to avoid causing and exacerbating breakouts.

Stress and the hormone processes they induce create changes in the body and skin. Understanding the big picture of the human body, its fight-or-flight cortisol responses, and how they affect your stress and hormone levels will help you see the direct outcomes.

When people think of hormones or hormonal acne, they are likely thinking of their reproductive organs. These do play a big part, but the other forms of stress (and the systems affected by them) also stoke the fires of acne. While internal aggravators are more difficult to control than external ones, becoming aware of the different sources of stress and making acne-safe lifestyle choices can go a long way in managing their effects.

Section 3 - The 5 Types of Hormone Stress Responsible for Acne

Fight, Flight, or Fawn Stress Response = Cortisol Production

Humans are animals that operate largely with a fight-or-flight response—staying and fighting off danger or running away to escape it, with a large gap of relatively low activity to rest, feed, and commune. Animals are meant to forage, procreate, defend themselves from danger, and spend most of their days resting or looking for food.

The endocrine system creates and secretes hormones into the body throughout the day. At the first sign of danger, our nervous system alerts the adrenal glands to produce adrenaline and cortisol. All other body processes (digestion, healing) are deprioritized to optimize escape and survival. Adrenaline gives us the energy to run, and cortisol allows us to make quick judgments.

Once out of danger, we shake our bodies to shrug off that physical stress, allowing our minds and bodies to go back to relaxing. As humans in prehistoric times, we weren't running from cheetahs or going through that much stress all day. Life was pretty chill and spent looking for food, procreating, nurturing our offspring, and resting. Because escaping major danger like death is such a stressful production for the body to survive, adequate rest and repair are needed each time the stress state is activated to reset the body's systems, replenishing the nervous system for doing its job.

Old-school stress was rare but intense—literally running away from lions, tigers, and bears that wanted to eat us. New-school stress is not as life-threatening but more constant throughout the day. Phone, email, computer, social media app notifications! Traffic! Social, professional, self-expectations! Depressing news cycles and atrocities happening to living beings on this planet, among many, many other things. We're exposed to many constant high, medium, and low spikes of cortisol throughout the day and are never really given time to truly rest in peace and quiet without these hormone-inducing effects.

Stress + Hormones = Inflammation

It's not normal or healthy to excrete cortisol all day. In fact, it's unsustainable. Adrenaline and cortisol are precious gems and are meant to be excreted and used sparingly, not subject to constant depletion and production. Overproduction of cortisol affects us negatively in so many ways: it raises our inflammatory levels, which can result in our acne becoming more red, swollen, and painful, causing chronically painful joints to flare or digestive discomfort.

It throws off the rest of our bodies' chemical processes that affect our brain like sleep, anxiety, depression, and stress management. It's not uncommon for people who are stressed out to crave and consume a lot of caffeine, sugar, or high glycemic carbohydrates in order to make up for the lack of quantity and quality of sleep they experience. "Imbalanced dopamine neurotransmitters in the brain are connected to and may contribute to these food cravings," says Board-certified Integrative Medicine Physician Dr. Tiffany Lester (drtiffanylester.com). Eventually, our digestive system flow is disrupted, slowing down the production of enzymes needed to break down our food and metabolize nutrients.

The Five Types of Stress

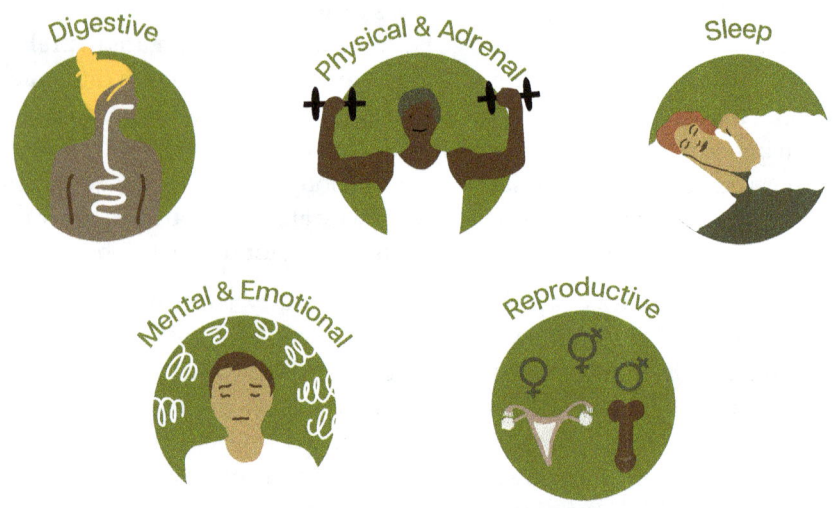

1. Psychological and Emotional

Gut and brain axis: serotonin production

Through modern research, Dr. Michael D. Gershon (author of *The Second Brain* and discoverer of the enteric nervous system) found that up to 90% of the brain's serotonin is produced in the digestive tract, emphasizing the importance of good, strong digestion.

Eating the right foods in the right way for your body will allow it to best synthesize those nutrients, powering all the body's systems to function well, and will also keep the physical health of your digestive gut optimal. Having a robust digestive system is essential to regulating the brain's emotional health chemicals. Nutrients from the food you eat are chemically transformed to greatly influence serotonin production in the gut. Brain chemical hormones like serotonin and oxytocin are instrumental to our quality of life. They help us enjoy it.

Modern-day living's stressors

We can take perfect care of our physical bodies, but true wellness rests in mind and your daily environment, especially when living in tumultuous times. Most clients I met in the San Francisco clinic (myself included) were so stressed they didn't know they were stressed. Chronic stress keeps the mind and body in defense mode, exhausting the body's cortisol processes and leading to system impairment and other bigger problems.

Managing the stress of daily life is easier said than done, of course, especially when you consider the environment in which we live has a big impact on our quality of life mentally, emotionally, and physically: the political climate, environmental decline, medical care, the increasing cost of living, and human rights being constantly attacked, all of which are constantly being spewed at us in the depressing news cycles. Things like repeated traumatic exposure, neurodivergence and intergenerational epigenetic influence can make daily living even more challenging for those affected.

2. Digestive and Nutritional

What and how you're eating

Eating food should not only be a pleasant experience for your senses but also for your digestive system. Not practicing good eating and digestive habits or regularly eating food that upsets your stomach can create chronic physical problems (stomach cramps, bloating, gas, indigestion, diarrhea, constipation, etc.), stressing the very internal organ system that fuels your body. Negative cascading effects are sure to occur, which will ultimately affect not just your skin but overall long-term body health.

Eating food that your body has a really hard time digesting (especially when coupled with stress, which reduces digestive stomach acid secretions) causes physical stress and damage to your guts, causing systemic inflammation and chemical imbalances. The entire digestive process gets worn down and works less efficiently, emitting uncomfortable symptoms like gas, bloating, diarrhea, cramps, irregular bowel movements, irritable bowel syndrome (aka IBS), or leaky gut.

Those with sensitive stomachs may want to avoid cold, icy drinks, try eating cooked vegetables over raw salads and keep fruit at least 30 minutes to an hour away from all other foods, for optimal stomach acid pH balance.

Blood sugar

Blood sugar spikes (and drops) from things like not eating at regular times or eating highly processed and sugary foods. It can affect estrogen levels, an excess of which also causes inflammation and can lead to more serious issues like cancer. If the blood sugar's extreme highs and lows persist, it can lead to insulin resistance, resulting in Type 2 diabetes, obesity, high cholesterol, heart disease, and stroke. By eating the right foods, you are supporting the health of your digestive system and its serotonin production, supplying the brain with emotional regulating hormones. In females, polycystic ovary syndrome (PCOS) is often associated with insulin imbalance, causing hirsutism (excess hair growth), irregular menses, weight gain, fertility issues, depression, and more. It's clear that there's a strong link between heightened blood sugar, insulin resistance, elevated estrogen hormone levels, long-term stress, and acne.

3. Physical Exertion, Pain, and Disability

Overexertion, overworking, and exercise

Although it's often thought of as stress-relieving for busy folks, too much high-intensity exercise, bodybuilding, hot yoga, and competitive or contact sports can be very physically stressful on the body and subconsiously anxiety-inducing for the mind, making acne worse. Moderate, daily, low-impact exercise is best for maintaining low stress levels and, by extension, clear skin. But if you have to keep on with high-intensity exercise, mix in some more calming, low-impact activities, and most importantly, know when to heal and rest. Even the best-performing athletes don't train 24/7 because they, too, need time to recover.

CASE STUDY: Forced rest

I had a client who was very active in training in mixed martial arts, and with every visit, I explained to them the effects of the intense training on their skin. Their complexion improved considerably after they started seeing us for treatments, but they still broke out and struggled with inflammation. They had to stop training for a few weeks for knee surgery, and the weeks following they wouldn't be able to train, so they were forced to rest. Lo and behold, despite the stress of the surgery, they cleared up dramatically, and the inflammation came all the way down to zero. They were dismayed to see this for themselves, but at least finally came to understand the physical exercise and stress-acne connection firsthand.

CASE STUDY: Stress from running

I had another client who was training for a marathon. He had already cleared up from being a client for years but started breaking out again once he started training. I explained to him that even though mentally he knew he wasn't in danger, his body was being forced to run long distances like it *was* running from lions, tigers, and bears. He broke out in part because of sweat that remained on his face while he ran these long distances, but the real problems were along his jawline, where hormonal acne typically presents itself. The body saw the physical exertion as stress and broke out on the skin. Once he completed the marathon, he cleared up.

Injury, pain, and disabilities—acute, chronic, and long-term

I also want to touch on bodily discomfort as a stressor because it can be majorly debilitating on the quality of one's life. Having to deal with pain—physical or mental, acute or chronic—is super stressful and thus, inflammatory. It impedes everyday functioning of life, and especially if long-term and chronic, elevates stress, which can eventually lead to depression. Pain in the body and acne are classic examples of two seemingly unrelated things that can contribute to a vicious cycle for the skin. Practice compassion for yourself and others.

4. Reproductive Sex Hormones —Teens, Adults, Female, Male, Intersex and Trans

Fluctuations in reproductive hormones affect everybody. While these fluctuations, for the most part, are expected, it's important to be aware of them. Try to reduce the other stresses on your body when you know hormonal activity is present so the body can rest and heal.

Stages of life

Puberty/teenage years

Program and dietary compliance can be a challenge for teens, especially combined with stressful teenage life. From what I've observed (and what Dr. Fulton writes), males, and those with naturally occurring higher testosterone levels, tend to experience more severe acne earlier in life (as teens) but for a shorter period of time. Females, and those with naturally occurring higher estrogen levels, tend to experience more mild acne that extends further into their adult lives.

Teenage skin can be quite sensitive and reactive, so go slowly with treatments and products. Some teens may need to get creative with their approach. For instance, they may prefer stronger chemical peels that make their skin peel aggressively for a few days over painful extractions. Raging hormones may override the most stubborn cases of acne management, but even if the desired clarity isn't fully achieved with our program, the low-inflammatory lifestyle changes introduced in this book should help reduce the severity of the acne and will benefit the teen into adulthood.

Adulthood and middle age

Arguably, the most active and potentially stressful time of our lives, where acne can be a constant. Take the time to do your skincare routine regularly and get as much rest as you can. Learning how to manage an acne-safe lifestyle as best you can with an emphasis on managing stress in healthy ways will set you up for success now and as you age.

Menopause

With these clients, the skin (and body, in general) starts to dry out; the skin isn't as oily as it used to be in its premenopausal years. Often, we find many old "tombstone" acne seeds that need to be extracted in order for the skin to clear up for good. Proper guidance, skin products, and treatments can help clear the skin and mitigate any dehydration one may experience, while acupuncture can help support the body's hormone shifts.

The Sexes

Testosterone dominant

Males, and those with naturally occurring higher testosterone levels' hormones tend to spike most at puberty, causing acne to occur in the teenage years. In most cases, by their mid-twenties, these excess hormones have stabilized, so the acne usually goes away on its own by then. Based on clinic observations, stress and diet (most often coffee, vitamins, dairy, and protein powders/shakes often made from whey or soy) seemed to be the most prevalent factor prolonging the acne into the later twenties and thirties. Acne in these folks tend to be more on the inflamed side and is more stubborn and difficult to control, perhaps because of general internalized and unexpressed stress and anxiety, too vigorous exercise, non-acne-safe protein supplements and powders, or lack of an effective skincare regimen.

Estrogen dominant

Females, and those with naturally occurring higher estrogen levels, tend to experience more and longer-standing problems with acne than do testosterone dominant folks, likely due to the daily fluctuating and delicate balance of hormones in their body around the menstrual cycle, along with the likelihood of being exposed to more comedogenic products for skin and hair.

Several kinds of hormonal changes take place throughout life like puberty, birth control, menstruation, pregnancy, nursing, and menopause. Other common hormonal imbalances and treatments can also occur, like Polycystic Ovarian Syndrome (PCOS), endometriosis, and hormone replacement therapy (HRT) to name a few.

Intersex and transgender

Because of the active fluctuation and unique management of hormones (both naturally occurring and prescription, if taking) in both intersex folks and people going through transgender-affirming therapy, the acne-safe lifestyle might simply help to improve if not completely clear one's complexion. Generally, male-affirming patients (and some intersex folks) will be more acne-prone due to the higher levels of testosterone and androgens being introduced to (or already present in) the body.

Menstruation

People who menstruate typically have a more delicate combination of different hormones that are constantly readjusting for reproductive health, which is further influenced by lifestyle and environment.

A typical menstrual cycle doesn't necessarily create new acne seeds to form, but it often inflames what's already present in the pore. Clear the pores so there is nothing to get inflamed.

Pregnancy

The acne response here is very unpredictable. The same client can have totally clear or totally broken-out skin during different trimesters of the same pregnancy or be totally clear in their first pregnancy and totally broken out in the second pregnancy, or vice versa. To make things more complicated, pregnant clients sometimes can only keep down or crave certain foods, which often are not the most acne-safe. Lack of restful sleep, physical changes, and emotional stress simply add to the mix here, further prolonged by postpartum and newborn lifestyle changes. The best bet is to give up the notion of perfect skin, know that this breakout period is temporary, and surrender to the idea that your body no longer belongs entirely to you. It is now shared by your baby for about two years (and longer if you nurse past infancy).

Thyroid and PCOS

Thyroid issues and PCOS are both common and increasingly being proven to be linked. Their chain reaction can eventually cause disruptions to the reproductive hormonal system, often resulting in acne. Acne in these cases can be more difficult to clear because rebalancing the hormones is a bit tougher to do. Watch out for kelp or iodine-rich supplements and medications often given for thyroid issues, as they can induce acne or a rash.

Hormones from our diet

Food can also affect the hormones largely in the form of coffee and soy. According to Dr. Nicholas Perricone (American board-certified dermatologist and author of *The Wrinkle Cure,* researcher of chronic inflammation's effects on the body's aging and disease), organic acids within the coffee bean (not the caffeine, so decaf won't help) directly stimulate the adrenal glands and boosts insulin, which eventually affects the hormones as well.

For some, a diet very heavy in soy, especially in the highly processed isolate form, will throw off the natural estrogen hormone balance in the body, causing acne. Soy, a legume rich with phytoestrogens that can mimic and disrupt our natural hormones, also finds its way into most processed foods under many monikers (flavoring, caramel, and soy lecithin,to name just a few), so avoid it if you can. High androgen foods like peanuts, high amounts of red meat and foods cooked in canola, corn and peanut oils can also.

Hormone medications

Birth control/fertility treatments

The synthetic manipulation of our reproductive hormones often induces acne. When starting or stopping birth control or fertility treatments, expect a three- to six-month skin breakout and clear-up acclimation period when starting, switching, or getting off birth control (even with the non-hormonal copper IUD, which still disrupts your body's natural rhythm).

Gender-affirming therapy

Because these hormones are stronger and taken for the long term, extra special attention, care, support, and maintenance will likely be required.

Be extra gentle with yourself and seek community support through this huge life-changing process (and congratulations, dearest ♥).

BIPOC/LGBTQIA+-focused esthetician Leola Davis of Pansy Esthetics in Los Angeles, California, shares that female-affirming estrogen-driven treatments result in drier skin, increased hormone-related hyperpigmentation, and possible skin thinning, whereas male-affirming testosterone-driven treatments result in oilier skin that's generally more acne-prone, accompanied by more hair growth and sweat, which may influence breakouts.

Some people going through gender-affirming therapy with particularly aggressive acne may have to resort to taking isotretinoin to get the skin under control while the body adjusts to all the other major changes happening.

5. Sleep Quality

During sleep, our bodies deep-clean and repair themselves, restoring energy reserves powered by well-digested nutritious food. Designed to follow the rising and setting of the sun to be active and to rest, our bodies ideally start the morning with their highest levels of energetic cortisol, which, over the course of the day, slowly dips down to its lowest point around bedtime. During this time, darkening skies alert the brain's pineal gland and hypothalamus to start producing melatonin, which induces relaxation and drowsiness, eventually sending us to sleep.

However, modern technology's artificial bright blue lights and electronic screens disrupt the brain's melatonin effects, tricking the brain into waking up thinking it's time to be active. If you stay off any devices for at least one to two hours prior to bedtime, it will allow your eyes, brain, and body to relax and prepare for deeper and more quality sleep.

Ideally, we all would get at least seven to nine hours of uninterrupted deep sleep AT NIGHT for the body to reset, rejuvenate, and replenish. It will be very difficult to clear someone of acne if they work nights or graveyard shifts. According to TCM, the body gets its deepest cleaning and restoration work done between 11 p.m. and 3 a.m. A popular adage in alternative healthcare is that an hour of sleep before midnight is worth two after because of the body's internal clock of routine cleansing and repairing organs.

Getting enough regular restorative sleep is crucial to supporting the skin and body's daily health and inflammation levels, along with robust digestion and effective stress management.

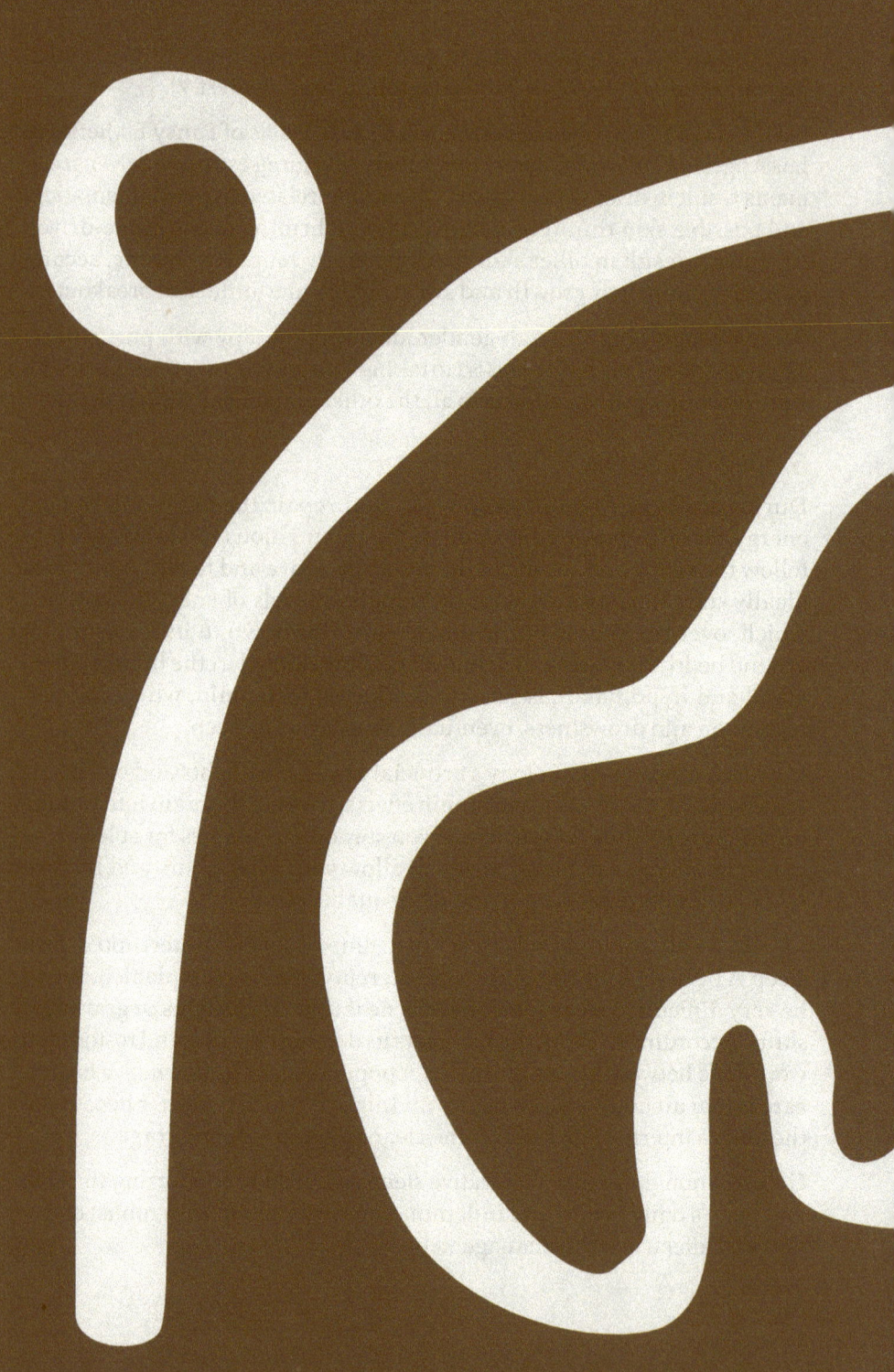

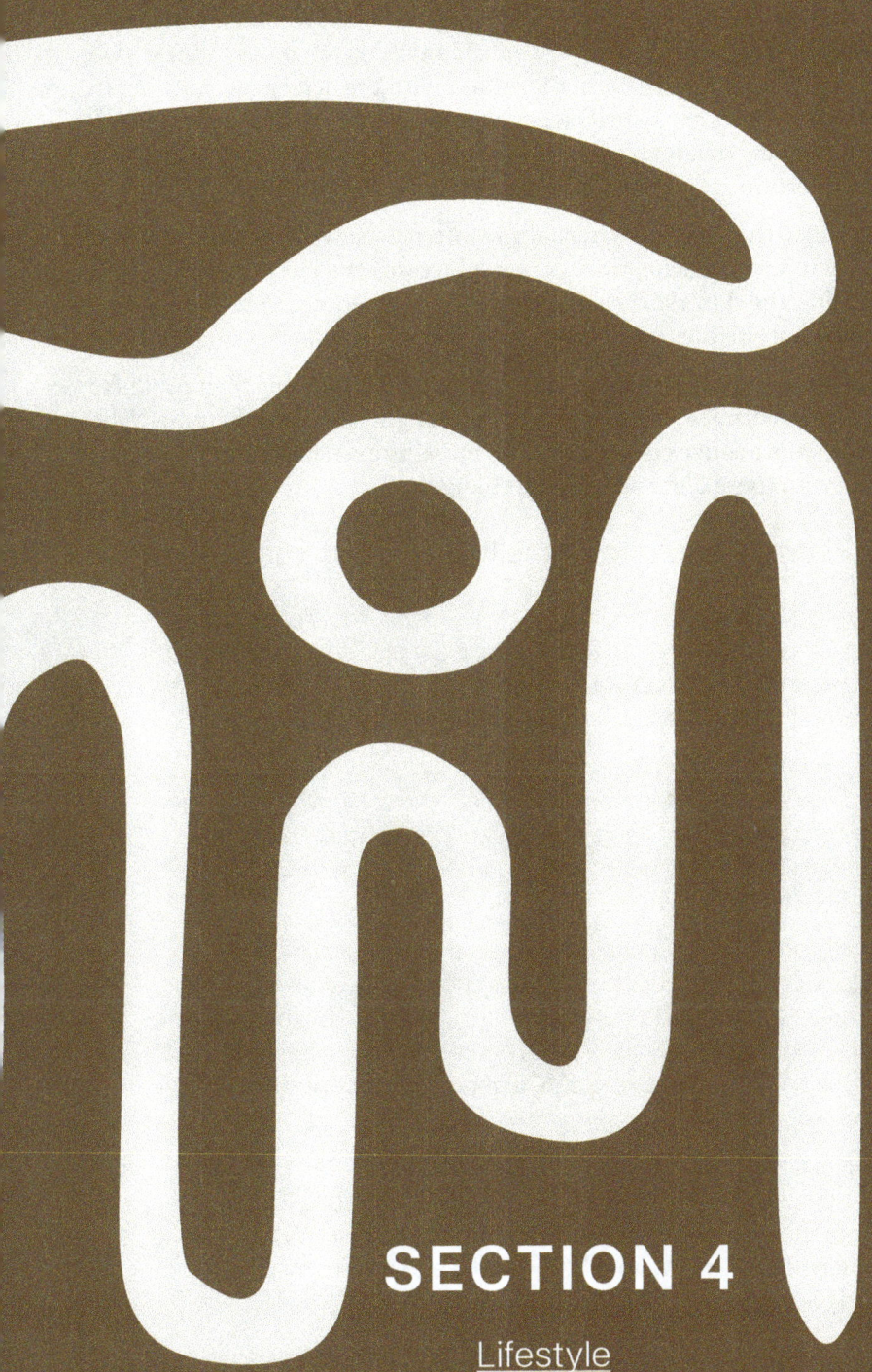

SECTION 4

Lifestyle

For the most part, most cases of acne we've seen are cases of *acne cosmetica* (acne from products with comedogenic ingredients) combined with a diet that causes acne to form from within. Though the chances of these two factors creating acne are higher for those with the acne gene running in their family history, we've had plenty of people without the genes still break out. This means that it all comes down to thresholds: your body can only handle a certain amount of *something* before acne shows up.

I've classified the factors as external and internal. Now that we've addressed the topical parts of acne, this section addresses the factors that lay skin deep, below the skin's surface. These things may require a bit more awareness and effort to integrate and become easier with time.

Most of our remote clients were able to clear up by changing their products to acne-safe With & Within ones with only slight tweaks to their diet. The ones with more active cases cleared up by being even more compliant and diligent with these diet and lifestyle changes.

TIP: Ways to make these lifestyle changes easier

It's hard to break old habits and make major lifestyle changes, but keeping your eye on the prize of clear skin with support along the way will help keep your spirits, and thus good habits, up. As you go through these changes, keep these things in mind:

It may help to set up an accountability system with a close friend or another person also looking to clear their skin who can cheer you on and support you through your challenges. The moral support can help keep you both on track for the hard things you want to tackle in life!

Try thinking of your new routine as a choice, not an obligation. Research shows that framing your choice of healthier options positively ("I get to do this") allows the brain to view the change as an optimistic preference versus depressing deprivation ("I can't have this"), helping to reinforce a generally more positive mindset and outcome.

This is about maintenance, not perfection. You aren't going to be able to have perfectly acne-safe meals or habits 100% of the time, and even if you did, you wouldn't have perfectly zit-free skin, either. Learning how your body works and how to respond to and take care of it will help heal it quickly.

Practical Daily Life

General Self-Care

Your well-being is the greatest thing you can directly influence. Doing what you can to keep your body, mind, and breath flexible, resilient, healthy, and strong will greatly influence your day-to-day quality of life. Taking care of your body, mind, and soul is truly the very best investment you can make in your life.

Sweat, stretch, and move your body regularly to maintain flexibility, mobility, and to stimulate circulation and digestion. Address injuries and pain—both chronic and acute. Eat, digest, and eliminate well and regularly. Cultivate emotional awareness, communication, relational, and conflict resolution skills for more easeful and deeper relationships with yourself and your community. Create and prioritize time for rest, leisure, and creativity. Spend time outside in quiet nature! Breathe in plenty of fresh, clean outdoor air. Be kind and gentle with yourself so you can also be the same with others.

Weekly Refresh
This could include soaking in a bath before a full-body exfoliation with a scrubbing mitt to reveal soft skin, doing your specialty hair care practices and treatments, hair epilation, or shaving, trimming nails, and moisturizing really well all over. Regularly giving your body attention and tender loving care really helps you gain self-awareness and appreciation for what it does for you every day. It also helps me discover problems and give them attention before they become more serious (like moles or pesky itchy spots).

Spas, Spa Services, and Hot Springs

Massage, Facials and Other Treatments
Sadly, most, facials and other treatments products used in these treatments are not acne-safe. I've had many accounts of clients breaking out after their treatment, and most times, they thought the momentary relaxation wasn't worth the weeks of breakouts afterward. However, I believe massages are one of life's most amazing sources of therapy and rest, so it's worth knowing the workarounds to keep from missing out!

Bring your own acne-safe oil or body lotion. I will often reach for an acne-safe oil in my kitchen, pour it into a clean, repurposed bottle with a pump, and bring it with me to the spa. Include a few drops of essential oils: eucalyptus globulus and lavender essential oils are my favorite "spa-smelling" combination. You can likely easily find some acne-safe oils (or 100% shea) at a grocery or local natural food store. One hundred percent safflower, sunflower, rice bran oils, or shea butter are safe choices.

You may opt to avoid getting your face massaged, but a scalp massage should be totally fine! If you are not inflamed and you are using your own acne-safe products, a face massage might be okay. You can also buy some massage face cradle covers to use when you're flipped over lying on your stomach. A A towel, bandana or pillowcase from home can also work in a pinch.

Steam and Dry Saunas

These include inherently inflammatory heat, but they can also do wonders to help alleviate muscle tension, stress, and to promote detoxification.

Keep your face cool by bringing some ice or a cold, wet towel into the room with you and placing it over your face to shield it from the direct heat of the hot steam or dry air. Once you exit, rinse off your face with clean water to prevent detox- or sweat-related breakouts. Be mindful of touching the surfaces within the steam/sauna rooms and then touching your face to prevent bacteria from getting onto your face, lay a towel down to act as a barrier against surfaces you sit or lay on.

Infrared Sauna

These types of saunas can be detoxifying, make you drink a lot of water, and are reputed to calm inflammation, chronic pain, and also burn fat. All this while just sitting around in a hot little room! Just wash your face and body before entering, and lay a towel down to act as a barrier against surfaces you sit or lay on and wash thoroughly afterwards.

Hot Springs

Natural springs have currents that continually cleanse and flow out into bigger bodies of water. Hot tubs (or spas) in places like Japan, Taiwan, and Korea, where communal bathing is a part of daily life wellness, have hot water that is usually not chlorinated. You're required to cleanse and scrub your body very thoroughly before dipping into the communal pools. Further, they forbid you from soaking your hair in the pools to help them stay clean, so keep it tied up.

Natural hot springs often have minerals (like sulfur) that can make the skin itchy. They supposedly have therapeutic effects when left on the skin, but you may have to deal with the itchiness. Try it, and if it gets too itchy, just rinse it off and moisturize. Monitor your skin's effects with natural springs, especially if you are acne-prone. Mineral effects may be drying on the skin but can be really therapeutic for joints and induce deep relaxation.

Hot Tubs
Conventional spa hot tubs that use chlorine and other chemicals in the water, can be irritating. See, Swimming.

Colonics
Colonics can be beneficial for jump-starting the body's digestive and elimination systems to help sluggish ones move along. Dr. Lester adds, "Our colons are one way we eliminate toxins from the body, and when that process is not happening efficiently, we can 'detox' the wrong way—through our skin." Colonics should not be relied on for regular elimination, though, and should be used more as an occasional deep-cleaning treatment. Consult an integrative therapist to see if this is right for you.

Barber Shops and Beauty Salons
If at all possible, ask your stylist to 1) omit using products altogether, especially styling stuff; 2) use only acne-safe products (bring your own or do some pre-appointment homework by using our product checker to audit the product line they carry, isolating the safe stuff, and requesting they use only those on you); or 3) let them do what they want with what they want, enjoy the amazing styling and deal with the breakouts later using what you've learned in this book. Best-case scenario is that you shower immediately after a cut or hair service.

If you are getting a service that requires product staying on the length of your hair for an extended period of time (like not washing for a few days after a chemical hair straightening appointment), wash your hair over the sink for a few days to avoid possible breakouts on your back and chest, which may happen more easily in the shower.

Bonus points if you can ask your stylist how to manage/style your hair using acne-safe products and techniques. There may be techniques they can share or a specific style or cut that might work better for you with this in mind. You may learn a thing or two, and your stylist can help others who may be concerned about this, too.

Cosmetic Tattoos
Clients have reported ink reactions resulting in months-long acne breakouts after getting their eyebrows tattooed or microbladed. Proceed with caution.

Hair Removal Best Practices

Shaving, Threading, Waxing, Tweezing, Laser, Electrolysis

Hair removal is a common, often daily grooming habit, and certain methods and products associated with it can lead to breakouts or ingrown hairs.

Regular, gentle exfoliation before and after will help keep ingrown hairs at bay, and it will also help facilitate a closer shave or more effective wax or threading experience by ridding the skin of excess dead skin cells that may be trapping or surrounding the hairs that are to be removed.

Ensure your skin is feeling strong and healthy before starting to exfoliate or epilate. Do the hair removal at the end of your day so that your newly opened hair follicles/pores aren't exposed to touching, makeup, or environmental toxins. Breaking out post-epilation is kind of inevitable, but there are precautions you can take to minimize these effects.

Shaving—fine facial hair

Use small facial razors, like the ones sold in our online shop.[15] Shave in the direction of hair growth and use on wet skin with an acne-safe cleanser to help the blade glide across the skin (although some do okay shaving dry). Try to finish the job with as few strokes as possible, as each stroke is another layer of exfoliation that can result in tender, sensitized skin and ingrown hairs. For best results, ice after shaving to help calm the skin down.

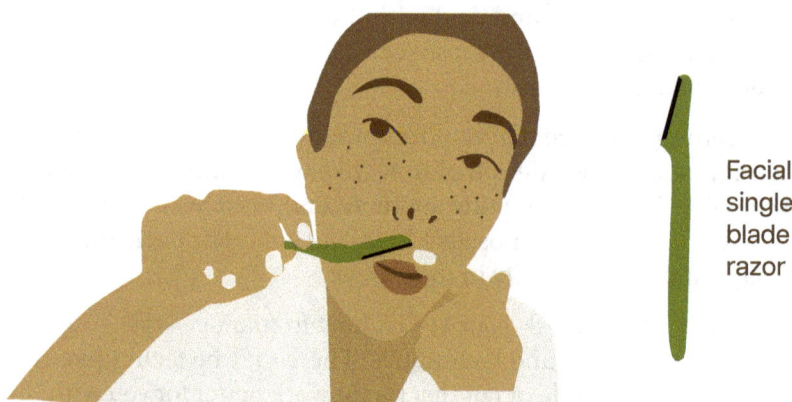

Facial single blade razor

Stretch the skin and use a small, straight edge facial razor in the direction of hair growth to carefully shave.

Shaving—thick facial hair

The closer the shave, the more chances you'll break out. The most common reason is when the hairs are cut so short, they sink underneath the surface of the skin. That hair tries to grow back, but instead of poking through the surface of the skin and out of the pore, the hair curls back into itself, burrowing deeper into the pore, creating an inflamed ingrown hair. It's best to use an adjustable electric shaver so you can better control how close a shave you get and avoid having to use shaving creams, gels, or lotions that are often comedogenic. If you must blade shave, use a light hand and choose a single straight-edge razor that has a blade guard of some kind to prevent too close a shave.

Prepare to shave by warming and softening the skin and beard beforehand, and if tolerated, a physical scrub before shaving—a steamy shower or warm compress on the beard should suffice. Applying an acne-safe oil after scrubbing but before shaving may help create a protective barrier against the razor for sensitive skin. Shave with the direction of hair growth (not against), go slowly, and try to get it done with one or two passes to prevent going over the same area several times. As always, icing helps treat and prevent inflammation, perfect for post-shaving. Avoid applying alcohol-based aftershaves and tonics, and lastly, try to shave as little as possible.

Experiment to figure out what shaving mediums (blade types, gels, oils, lotion products) will work best with your razor and skin. Many shaving foams contain comedogenic ingredients, so beware.

Play around with your regimen to see when it's best to do the more active (exfoliating toner, serum) parts of it. You may need to skip the active products at the time of day you shave (for example, in the morning) and work the active ingredients back into your regimen at a different time of day (at night). Using a benzoyl peroxide or mandelic face wash, however,

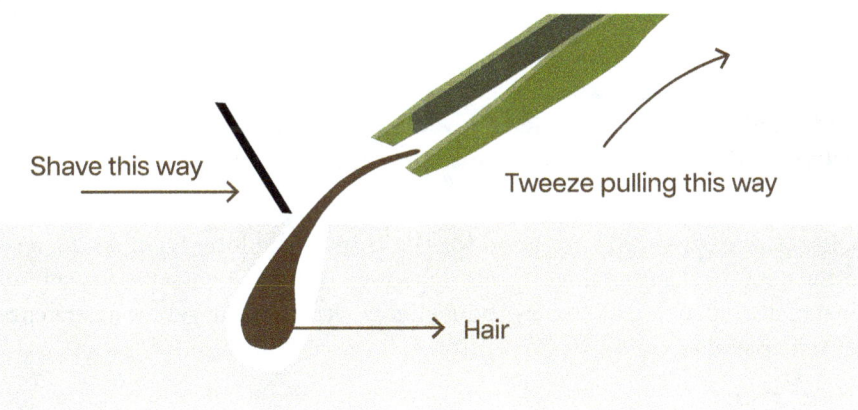

Make sure to shave or tweeze with the direction of hair growth to prevent ingrown hairs.

might be well-tolerated immediately after shaving; try and see what works best for you.

Waxing and sugaring

Most products that salons use for waxing (pre-wax or post-wax lotions, etc.) contain many cloggy ingredients. Also, if the hair is removed incorrectly (if the hair breaks at the surface or is tweezed against the grain of growth), ingrown hairs are more likely to occur. If not done properly, there is more of a chance of skin lifting, skin burns, and pigmentation issues (and in some cases, even more ingrowns). Watch how your skin responds after your wax appointment, and switch practitioners if you need to. Sugaring, similar to waxing but using more gentle products, is also an option worth looking into.

Laser hair removal

This works by first shaving the hair the day of the appointment and, in the hair removal clinic, flashing a bright light-emitting device (usually intense pulsed light therapy, or IPL) onto the skin so that the light, attracted to the root's pigment, can "zap" and kill the root below the surface. Shave with the hair growth, not against it. For small and sensitive areas, try using a small facial razor. Avoid shaving in between appointments to avoid ingrown complications. Keep laser and acne facial appointments at least a week apart to avoid scarring, and do not use exfoliants or active products post-treatment until the skin heals.

Electrolysis

This works by inserting a fine needle into the pore and using an electrical current to electrocute the hair root. This can be dangerous because of the needle aspect (it may not be inserted directly where it needs to go, causing scarring). However, this treatment has proven effective for some, especially for darker complexions that cannot safely get laser hair removal treatments. Find a qualified and experienced electrologist you trust, keep electrolysis and facial appointments at least a week apart, and do not use exfoliants or active products post-treatment until the skin is completely healed.

Hair removal creams

Chemical exposure is not good for the skin in the long term, and these often contain skin-sensitizing and comedogenic ingredients. Beauty school instructors also told us stories about clients' skin turning yellow after years of repeated use.

Threading

This is the best hair removal method because it has the least potential for skin irritation, there's little to no chance of the skin lifting (tearing upper layers of the skin off, common with depilatory waxing or exfoliants), it precisely pulls the hair out at the root without the use of any wax, gel, lotion, or cream product, and it works with just a piece of thread and baby powder.

Technique and results vary from person to person, so try different threading practitioners until you find one you like. They'll likely wipe your skin with alcohol to remove any grease, apply some baby powder or cornstarch to protect the skin, and then use thread to create a knot that precisely pulls several hairs out of the root at the same time.

There are metal spring facial hair remover tools that essentially do the same thing without the string. This may be an easier technique for at-home depilation. Just pull the spring apart and blow some air into it to remove the accumulated hairs inside, then wipe it down with rubbing alcohol and let it dry to keep it clean.

Dermaplaning (full-face shaving)

There are also many therapists who swear by dermaplaning or shaving the face (the entire face) with a straight-edge razor to encourage new skin cell growth. If you have the kind of acne where your skin texture is bumpy, the blade passing over the skin can cut those fragile pimples open. Baby hairs and peach fuzz that grow back can become ingrown. I would avoid this technique, which is basically another form of physical exfoliation.

Ingrown Hairs

Ingrown hairs happen when the hairs are cut so short that the length of the hair is actually cut below the surface of the skin. When the hair tries to grow back, instead of poking through the surface of the skin and out of the pore, the hair curls back into itself, going deeper into the pore, creating

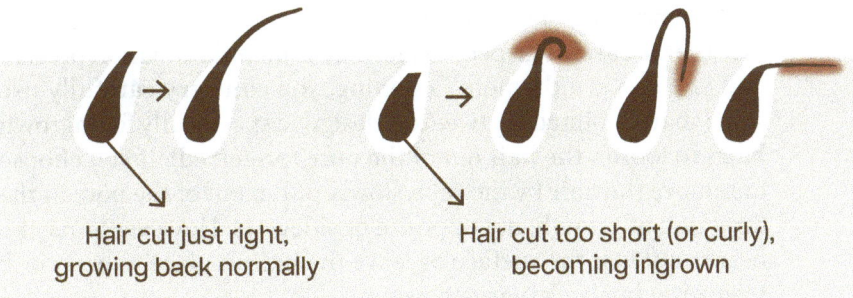

Hair cut just right, growing back normally

Hair cut too short (or curly), becoming ingrown

Hair cut just at or above the skin's surface is ideal. Once an ingrown hair is identified, carefully loosen the hair at the surface to free it from the skin. Removing this hair from the root may cause it to grow ingrown again, so proceed with caution.

an ingrown hair. This can also happen with hair that's too fine to poke through the surface, or curly hair that grows out of and back into the skin.

Preventing ingrown hairs
- Exfoliate regularly before your hair removal appointment. In most cases, days before waxing, a very gentle physical exfoliation (scrubbing) will be safer than using chemicals (toners, serums, retinols) since the combination of chemical exfoliants and certain hair removal techniques (waxing and laser in particular) can cause side effects and complications (skin tearing, scarring).
- Shave in the direction of hair growth.
- Don't shave too close to avoid trapping the ends of the hair underneath the surface of the skin.
- With methods that involve removing the hair at the root (like waxing or threading), make sure they are, indeed, thoroughly removing the hair and *taking the root along with it* instead of breaking the hair at the surface of the skin.
- After your skin has healed from the hair removal technique, continue to exfoliate the skin to prevent dead skin cell buildup. You may have to wait a few days after your hair removal appointment until the skin feels healthy, strong, and normal again before safely exfoliating.

Alleviating ingrown hairs
- Treat them like acne. Get the inflammation down with products and icing, and exfoliate with an acid (not scrub) to help coax the hair out.
- Try your best to avoid picking at it, especially if it's still inflamed.
- Ice as much as you can, let your skin warm back up from icing, and if desired, apply your chemical exfoliant. Using a cotton swab of exfoliating toner or serum will help a lot.
- With some careful inspection, if there is no inflammation present and you can see the pore's opening, you can very carefully use some sharp, pointed-tip tweezers designed specifically for ingrown hairs to loosen the hair out of the pore (preferred). If you choose to remove the hair by the root, slowly pull it out of the pore in the direction of growth, not opposite or sideways. However it may be best to cut it at the surface or leave the hair in place to prevent it from growing back ingrown again.
- If there is no inflammation present, you may try to gently squeeze *around* the pore to try to get the trapped hair to come out, much like

extracting a non-inflamed acne seed. Use clean, tissue-covered fingertips; *no fingernails directly on the skin*!
- You may need the help of a professional to perform an extraction. There will likely be some dead skin cells and oils accumulated in the pore along with the hair.
- Any and all extractions are best done when inflammation is under control.
- If worse comes to worst, seek medical attention for a cortisol injection to get the inflammation down, and then go back for a professional extraction to free the trapped hair once and for all.

Going to the Pros

Products commonly used pre- and especially post-epilation are usually super cloggy and are the last thing you want applied to the skin with open pores.

Bring your own skincare products to use before and after epilating. This can include a gentle toner, toner pad, and perhaps a gel moisturizer or SPF.

To keep your skin its clearest, protect the areas treated with the shade from a hat, covered with a clean shirt, or stay indoors to keep those open pores clean. Optimally, don't apply anything afterward (not even makeup or SPF), and make this the last thing you do for the day so you can go home, wash your face, and not expose the skin to potential environmental cloggers.

Hirsutism

Excessive hair growth in women may be a sign of a hormone imbalance like PCOS, that should be addressed on a systemic level for the best, safest and healthiest results. This hair is mostly noticeable around the mouth, chin, and torso, and is often resistant to more permanent hair removal treatments like laser or electrolysis.

Exercising and Skincare

Sweating definitely has its benefits. Sweating means that you're getting your heart rate up, which the American Heart Association recommends for thirty minutes a day, five days a week, for optimum health. Exercising regularly helps to keep your mind centered and calm and your body flexible and strong. Vigorous exercise helps increase the circulation of blood and nutrients to the joints, muscles, and organs. Sweating releases fluids;

it helps enhance our thirst for water to replenish lost moisture and electrolytes. Finally, sweating helps to detox the body's waste through its largest organ, the skin. As such, it's natural for the acne-prone to expect breakouts with this waste sitting on the skin too long.

Gym Towels

Use towels that have been washed with acne-safe laundry detergent, but this is nearly impossible to guarantee when you're not using ones you washed yourself. Bring washcloths to use while sweating during workouts at the gym and a separate one for drying your face off after showering. By bringing acne-safe toiletries, you'll cut down on a lot of exposure even if you end up having to use a gym towel.

Before Working Out

Remove your makeup and hair styling products before working out. This will prevent makeup, skin, and hair styling products from running into your eyes, avoid staining your workout clothing, and help you look your best. This also helps keep your skin its cleanest as pores open up to release detoxifying sweat. Even though you're going to sweat, you'll still need to moisturize to avoid dehydrating your skin before you start to sweat. A layer of hydrating gel, hydrating cream or a few dabs of melted shea butter or acne-safe oils should do the trick.

After Working Out

Wash your face and body with acne-safe cleansers within fifteen to twenty minutes of finishing your exercise routine. Cool down before jumping into the shower to allow your body temperature to rebalance to avoid catching a cold (according to Ayurvedic and Traditional Chinese Medicine). You'll want to moisturize your skin even if you are still sweating post-shower to avoid topical dehydration.

If you can't fully cleanse within that window, at least splash your face and chest several times with water; or even better, wet a clean hand towel and rub it all over (starting with the face, then working down your neck, chest, and body) to wick away sweat, getting as thoroughly clean as soon as you can. Moisturize to avoid drying out your skin, even if you're just five minutes away from home. Delaying topical hydration can dehydrate your skin, causing complications and sensitivities when using the active parts of your regimen or going in for a facial treatment.

Bring travel-sized bottles of your own acne-safe products to the gym to use. This is one of the main reasons I love using an acne-safe body wash; it doubles as a shampoo and allows me to bring just one product to do two jobs.

Exercise and Skincare Routines

Integrating some strategy around this will help your skin stay its clearest and healthiest. Washing a third time of day is totally fine, so long as you are only exfoliating twice a day. Depending on when you work out—as well as when it's convenient with your schedule—will determine when best to exfoliate.

Don't exfoliate or use the same active treatment cleanser (one with BP or exfoliating acid) more than twice a day. This extra "partial regimen" should consist of washing and moisturizing or applying SPF at the least; icing would be an amazing bonus. Icing a little extra doesn't hurt, but using actives too many times a day can.

On the next page are some examples of when to integrate your active products so that they stay on the skin long enough to work versus getting sweated off during your workout.

Exercise and Sports

Best Practices

- Create a clean and washable barrier between your skin and body, and the sports gear, fixtures or equipment.
- Create a sense of ventilation so that sweaty fabrics can dry out quickly
- Reduce points of friction to prevent *acne mechanica*
- Avoid touching your face with dirty hands to prevent infection
- Thoroughly wash your face and body as soon as possible after your activities

Create an acne-safe barrier between you and the surface with clean hand or face towels. If you are going to lay your face on a surface (say, a face-down-directly-on-the-mat yoga pose), place a clean hand towel to lay your face on to avoid rubbing up on a dirty yoga mat. With practice, this towel placement will become second nature.

If you are going to lay back on a lifting bench, wear a T-shirt that covers the areas that touch your body or lay a towel down to form a safe barrier between your skin and the sweaty communal bench. Using the alcohol

Clear Skin for Everyone

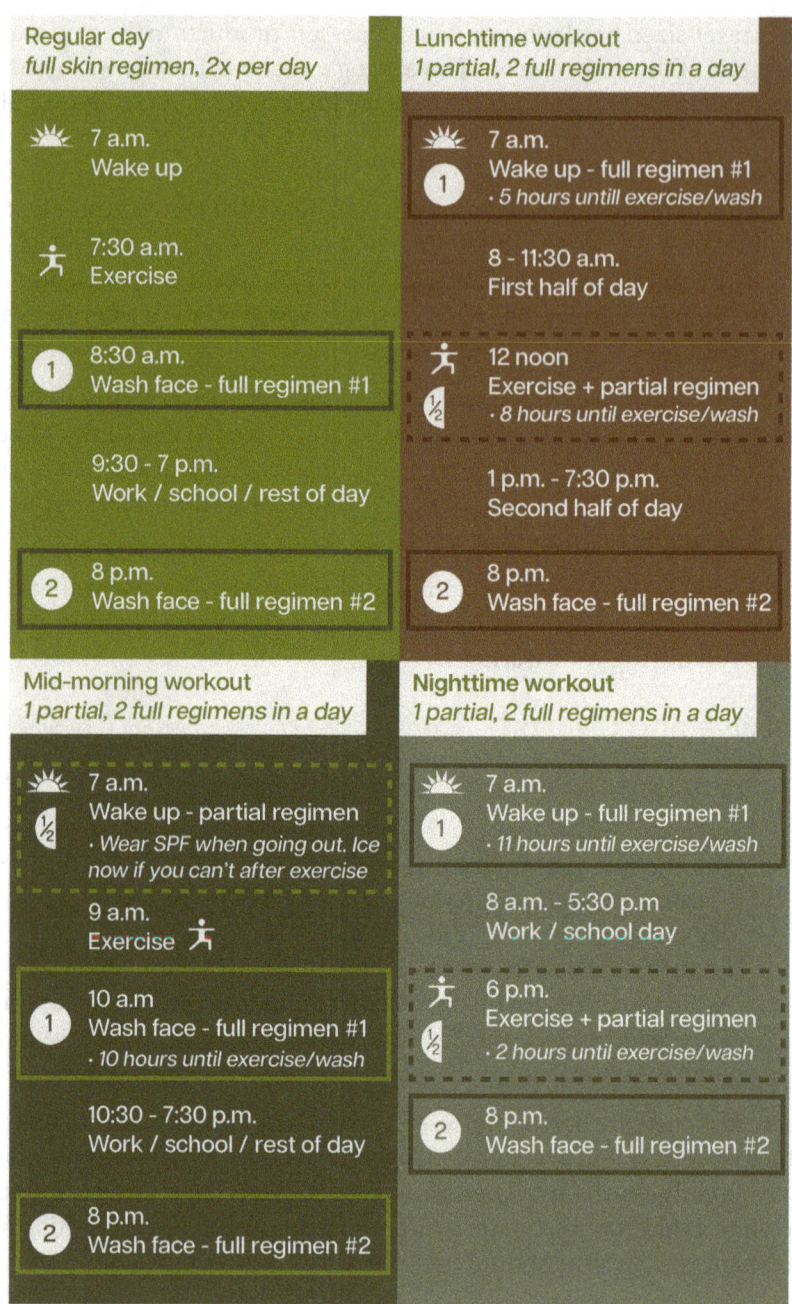

Here are four skin regimen and exercise schedule ideas aimed at keeping the active products on the skin as long as possible. Ice as much as you can and always wear SPF.

wipes and sprays at the gym is a good idea and highly recommended, but laying down a clean barrier even after spraying things down is the best bet.

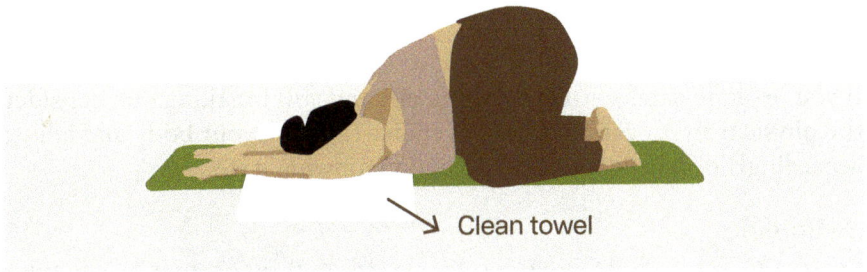

Lay your face onto a clean towel, versus directly on the yoga mat.

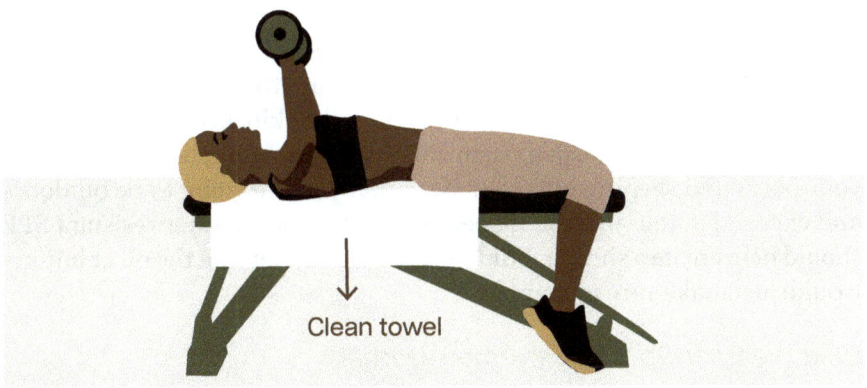

A towel, t-shirts or long pants will protect exposed skin when laying on exercise equipment.

Keep your hair tied back (for the face touchers)
Tie your hair tightly back and wear a headband that will keep those wisps out of the way so you don't touch your face with dirty hands during your workout. If you *must* touch your face or wipe off face sweat, use a clean hand towel and try to designate one side for your face only and the other side for your (dirty) hands or surfaces you lay it down on.

Everything in moderation
Too much of a good thing can become a bad thing. Overexercising puts extra physical stress on the body, fueling inflammation just the same as other types of stress. To find out if you are exercising too much or not enough, check out the *Physical Activity Guidelines for Americans*.[16] Also, research has shown a link between weightlifting and acne.[17]

Rest!

Exercise that's too physically or mentally vigorous can count against the nervous system, especially if you already have a very mentally or physically stressful day job. Lower impact exercise can better support your nervous system.

If you're "acne-safe" with everything else but still breaking out, consider the physical stress your exercise of choice takes on your body and adjust accordingly or accept your skin's reaction for what it is.

Swimming

Most swimming pools and hot tubs contain chlorine, which has iodides and bromides that can break you out. They can also be very dehydrating and smelly. Ocean water is very salty and can make your skin itchy and dry as well. If you are a swimmer or a hot-tubber, apply a thin layer of shea butter, sunflower, or safflower oil onto your skin before getting into the water and washing it clean as soon as you can afterward. Applying the butter or oil will create a protective layer on the skin, keeping the drying, damaging, and acne-causing chemicals, minerals, and salts from clogging your pores and seeping into your system. If you are going to be outdoors and exposed to the sun, you'll need sun protection. A water-resistant SPF should help create a similar iodide-protective barrier that the oil or butters would; just make sure to reapply.

Cold Weather Sports, Extreme Weather

Do your best to avoid getting sunburned, wind-chapped, or very dry, sensitive skin. Applying extra layers of moisturizers and sunscreens (perhaps shea butter on easily chapped areas) can help create a protective barrier against the harsh elements. Avoid active ingredients and foaming cleansers in your regimen until your skin is healed. Thicker sunscreens that really stay put (like our Safeguard SPF 40 or Tizo) are highly recommended. Watch for dryness and try to occlude the skin from the harsh weather elements as much as you can.

Mental Stress of Exercise/Competition

Your endocrine system still engages the body's defense mode by producing cortisol, the stress hormone in the body that fuels physical activity. This can be true if you are in a competitive or super-active sport like high-intensity interval training, marathon running, or weightlifting; although your life isn't in danger, the body's nervous system reads it as stress and reacts as such.

Breaking up more active or competitive sports with lower-impact ones like yoga, walking, tai-chi, or chi-gong will be beneficial for your mind, body, and endocrine system.

> ### CASE STUDY: Pillowcase acne
>
> I've seen clients mysteriously break out on the sides of their faces when they hadn't changed anything else in their routine or diet, only to find out they ended up using a new type of laundry detergent and upon closer inspection when they got home, found it had pore-clogging ingredients in it. It got only to the sides of their faces because they used that detergent to wash their pillowcases!

Laundry

Pillowcases, Bedding

Clean pillowcases are a must for those who are acne-prone. Residue from your hair, whether from natural oils or styling products, transfers onto your pillowcase and then to your face. Washing your hair thoroughly before sleeping is best, but the next best option would be to wrap your hair with a clean, new natural fabric wrap or cap each night and change your pillowcases every other night. Sleep on one side of your pillowcase one night, flip the pillow over to use the next night, then switch to a new one the third night to avoid congestion.

It's a good idea to change your pillowcases regularly because your face products inevitably rub off onto your pillowcase. This is particularly important for those who use BP, and especially if you sweat. The sweat and products also rub off onto your pillowcase and into your eyes, irritating them. Apply just enough BP onto your skin to work.

> ### CASE STUDY: Exercise and commuting stress
>
> I had a yoga teacher client who would travel from studio to studio several times a day throughout San Francisco's highly trafficked streets on a scooter. We had a really tough time clearing her up even though, in her mind, she was used to the hustle and didn't regard her zipping around town as a big factor. When she started her own practice in a stationary studio, her skin cleared up dramatically, though she didn't change anything else in her lifestyle.

She finally realized that scooting around all day in a busy city put her nervous system in "defense mode," and stopping that really lowered her stress levels. Her mood vastly improved, allowing her to be more engaged with her clients and loved ones, and she became calmer and more relaxed with her life overall.

Pajamas

If you sweat and break out on the body, keep your room cool and blanket thin. Maybe try a pillow chilling pad or keep a fan running in your room while you sleep. Frequently wash your bed linens and wear new clean PJs to bed every night for sweat reasons, but also for product residue buildup. Wear white and use white linens if you use BP to avoid unwanted bleaching.

Clothing

Along with washing with acne-safe laundry detergent, try to choose clothing made from natural fabric to avoid excess irritation, perspiration, or potential skin allergies. Hang exercise clothing turned inside out to dry after sweaty activities, then wash after each wear.

Wash new clothing before wearing it. Many chemicals, including formaldehyde, are sprayed onto them to prevent things like mold and wrinkling when being transported from the overseas production plant to your hands.

Laundry Detergent

Pick laundry detergents that are not only fragrance-free but also use acne-safe ingredients. Softeners leave a residue on fabric that rubs off on the skin, so try wool dryer balls or pinning a metal safety pin onto an article of laundry going into the dryer to capture static.

Dry cleaning is actually just dipping your clothes into chemical solutions that are terrible for our health and the environment. It's called "dry clean" because a bath of chemicals is used instead of water. Try using a garment steamer or handwashing to maintain your clothes.

Eyewear

To prevent breakouts along the eyeglass-affected areas (ear, temple, nose, and cheeks), keep your glasses clean and wash them occasionally, using acne-safe soap and warm water. Try to keep them off your head and hair, as any hair styling products will transfer from the glasses to your face. Hang them on the neck of your shirt, in a chest pocket, on a chain, on top of your hat or headwrap, or keep them in a case. Remember that nose pads, frames,

Section 4 - Lifestyle

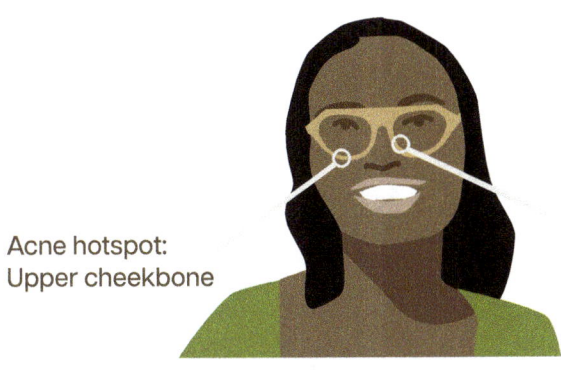

Common eyewear acne hotspots include the upper cheekbones and nosebridge, where they commonly rub against the skin.

and temples—the parts of the eyeglasses that touch your skin—can create enough friction for your skin to break out even if everything else is acne-safe. Clear nail polish or clear acrylic spray paint can be applied onto metal parts if you have a metal allergy, as I do. This works for metal buttons (like on jeans) and earrings.

If you're actively breaking out on the eyeglass-affected areas, refrain from wearing this particular eyewear until the acne clears up. Those bumps will never purge and heal if they constantly have something rubbing up against the already irritated pores. Give it a rest, exfoliate it a bit, and keep inflammation down to purge the seed.

If breakouts here are a persistent problem no matter how good you are with your skin routine and keeping your frames clean, you may need to switch eyeglass frames for the sake of your skin (or at least until you clear up). Larger frames with dark polarized lenses can help offer physical protection for the skin around the eyes against the sun and squinting, which leads to wrinkling.

CASE STUDY: Eyewear acne

We had a client with a face full of acne that we cleared up nicely. She just had one pesky pimple on her upper cheekbones (that sat directly under her glasses) to deal with. We extracted that pore, and post-treatment, she wore contacts while using her acne-clearing regimen. As her skin was allowed to heal without the constant pressure/friction of the frames, she cleared up nicely and was able to go back to wearing her glasses without any problems thereafter. Because she was darker-skinned, the dark brown pigmentation left behind from the acne finally lifted and disappeared without the seed in the way.

TIP: Sunglasses and anti-aging

Larger frames with dark polarized lenses can help offer physical protection for the skin around the eyes against the sun and squinting, which leads to wrinkling.

Hats, Helmets, Sports Gear

There's only so much you can do about gear like this. Protecting your head during transportation and sports is definitely more important than avoiding acne. The focus here is to protect the skin, reduce friction, and keep it clean.

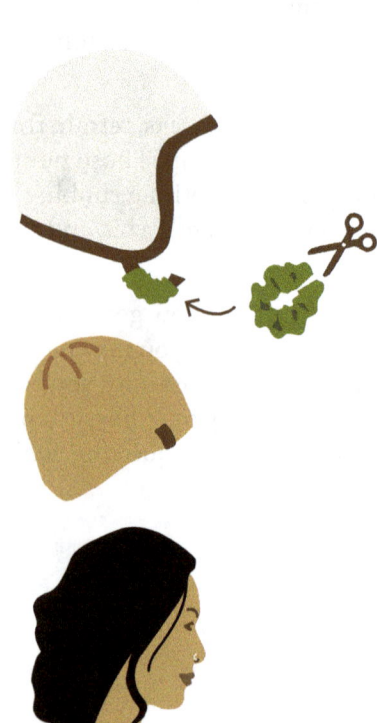

Create washable barriers between your body and the item causing the acne. For example, wear a headscarf, beanie, shower cap, bandana, or natural cloth bonnet to create a barrier between your skin and your hat or helmet. Sweat, hair/skin products, and makeup can rub into the hard-to-clean fabrics that line a helmet, so this barrier will help keep you clearer and also extend the life of your gear.

Regularly deep-clean everything that touches your skin. Give your hats, helmets, and makeshift barriers (beanies, bandanas, or chin strap covers) several regular good, hot, soapy water scrubs and rinses, letting them completely air dry after

Washable barriers like a beanie between your head and helmet, or a chin strap sheath can help keep you clear.

To make the sheath, cut open a fabric hair scrunchie, remove the elastic and pull it around the helmet chin strap.

washing and between uses. Generous sprays and swipes of alcohol in between deep washes can help.

No matter how much you wash or clean, sometimes the repeated friction alone may be enough to make someone break out.

PPE Masks

If you can, aim for the types that form a cup around your nose and mouth versus the pleated rectangular surgical ones (or use a mask frame underneath) to minimize friction between the mask and your nose and lips. Cup-shaped masks create space to allow air flow, hopefully making for a less humid environment there.

Keeping your body cool and the affected areas as dry and air ventilated as possible will speed the recovery and prevent it from recurring. Rotating different mask styles will change the pressure points on your face, hopefully reducing acne formation.

> ### TIP: PPE mask heat rash
>
> If an itchy rash develops on your upper lip due to the heat and humidity, try applying a mix of hydrating gel (or hyaluronic acid serum) and tea tree/lavender essential oils sparingly as much as possible, avoiding creams, lotions, or oils until the rash subsides. The key to this trick is to use as little hydrating gel/serum as possible (over-moisturizing will prolong the rash) but just enough to dilute the essential oils to prevent burning your skin and help them spread around better.

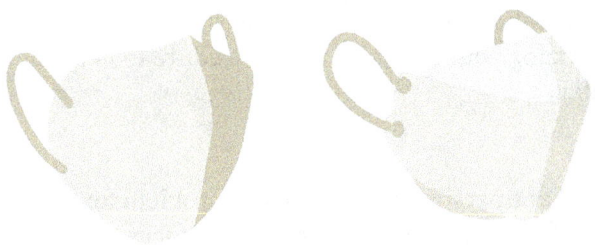

Look for cup shaped PPE masks like these, versus pleated surgical masks.

Other Skin and Body Products

Body Lotions and Moisturizers

Be sure to use an acne-safe body lotion or hand cream to keep clear, especially if you are a frequent face toucher. Treatment moisturizers that have active ingredients, such as exfoliating acids, can be helpful in smoothing out your skin. Exercise caution and wear sun protection if you are exposed to the sun, and monitor your skin to address any irritations before they go too far and become more serious complications or reactions.

> ### TIP: Hand massage as meditation
>
> I love using the time to apply hand cream as a meditation. A few minutes of thoroughly massaging it into every single finger and knuckle, squeezing various points on my palm and giving my hands and arms a good stretch helps to reset my mind and attitude. Plus, if you're using something like shea butter that takes a few minutes to absorb into the skin, you're sort of forced to stay off your devices and be with yourself until your hands are no longer greasy.

Self-tanners

Make sure it's acne-safe prior to using both at-home and salon formulas. Any reputable tanning salon should be able to show you the ingredient listing of the tanning solutions they use. Avoid using a professional spray tan on your face if the solutions at the salon are comedogenic, and consider using an acne-safe one at home to match the bronze glow on your body to your face.

I recommend exfoliating your skin prior to the tanning solution and regularly moisturizing your skin after the procedure to help your tan last as long as possible.

Deodorant

Deodorant and antiperspirants may pose a problem for your acne if they somehow transfer from your underarms to surfaces that touch your face, like a pillowcase or sheets. If you struggle with ingrown hairs here, look at the ingredients of the deodorant you are using and switch it out to something that has acne-safe ingredients. You can apply ice and your skincare regimen products to these areas to help those congested pores clear, but the help of a professional who can actually see the pores and try to extract what's stuck may be best.

When your skin is healed, scrub your underarms prior to hair removal, and use proper post-epilation care to avoid the recurrence of ingrowns in these areas.

Gua Sha and Jade Rolling

If you are clear-skinned and a fan of Gua Sha or jade rolling, enlist the guidance of a professional either in person with an actual TCM practitioner (not an esthetician) or via instructional videos. *Sandra Lanshin Chiu,* MSTCM, LAc is a good resource with many instructional videos.[18] Use an acne-safe serum, cream, or 100% shea butter to provide the slip needed for the tools to slide across the skin easily.

Both Gua Sha and jade rolling are forms of Traditional Chinese Medicine, performed to enhance lymphatic flow, relieve muscle tension, and encourage detoxification by oxygenating blood flow to the areas that are "scraped." Traditional Gua Sha is actually really intense and painful and is usually performed on the body (not on the face) via a blunt-edged wood, jade, or stone tool used in a scraping motion. When done correctly (and if there are toxins present), the skin will be left bruised and red with a blood clot-like appearance. However, the gentler approaches on the face popularized in the late 2010s are generally marketed to enhance lymphatic flow, which gently sculpts the face, making it appear slimmer with a more "lifted" appearance, thanks to the lymphatic drainage effects of the physical upward and outward sweeping motion.

Depending on how much moisturizer or shea butter you use during this step, you may skip moisturizing an additional time as part of your normal regimen unless you are going out into the sun, during which sun protection should be applied. Blot off excess moisturizer used during this step if you are going to apply your SPF or makeup on top.

Dating and Acne

Dating can be a healthy and nourishing part of life—it provides necessary intimate social connection and physical touch, which has been shown to increase serotonin levels while lowering cortisol, great news for those with acne-prone skin. Here are some tips to keep in mind.

Making Out

Cloggy lip balm and toothpaste can transfer from face to face and break you out. Saliva and other bodily fluids are best washed or rinsed off or at the least wiped off with a warm, wet hand towel. Your skin may dry out after being splashed with water, so a quick application of moisturizer would be ideal before dozing off.

Making out with scruffy faces

Beard burn is a common incidence among folks who make out with bearded people, where the skin around the mouth may feel chapped or sore. Treat it with care as if tending to a sunburn.

Avoid using exfoliants (mandelic toner, salicylic or glycolic acid, or vitamin A, to name a few) around the mouth, and treat the lower half of the face like you are recovering from a treatment. Gently cleanse, lightly ice, avoid toner and any exfoliating serums, and moisturize extra. You can do the clearing regimen on the rest of your face and resume applying those active products on the sensitive areas, but only after they have healed. Treat these tender areas gently and avoid touching them to allow them to heal, as overzealous toner application can make it worse.

Navigating sleepovers

At the least, bring face wash and moisturizer. Icing and toning would be awesome, but at least these two basics will be okay for a night. If you've got nothing, splash your face with water and moisturize with acne-safe lip balm (scrape off a ¼" chunk, melt in your fingers and press onto the skin), or wait till you get home and do your regimen.

A clean pillowcase washed with acne-safe detergent is ideal, but a clean t-shirt can work in a pinch if the borrowed pillowcases are questionable.

Change your sheets regularly, once every week or two, depending on your home climate and your body (if you sweat a lot at night, change them more frequently).

Long nights with no sleep can wreak havoc on your energy levels the next day, making you want to drink coffee to compensate for lost sleep. Get plenty of good night's rest in between late nights.

Sexy time

These are best practice suggestions; do the best you can while enjoying yourself!

Clean face: Wash your face before sex so you don't get your makeup all over your partner and the sheets and again afterward to get all the sweat and fluids off your face.

Clean body: Showering (or at least quickly rinsing) before and after sex can prevent sweat breakouts (and infections). Or use a clean towel soaked in hot water, then wrung out to wipe your face and body clean. Rubbing your body down with the same technique is also highly recommended and feels great post-coitus.

Use water-based, fragrance-free lubricant. It's non-toxic and is usually free from potentially cloggy and irritating silicones.

Birth control and the Plan B pill
Plan B is basically a supercharged birth control pill designed to delay or prevent ovulation wherever one is on their menstrual cycle in order to prevent pregnancy. Expect a similar response to daily birth control pills, disruption in the period cycle resulting afterward, and for it to take a few months for the body to readjust back to normal hormone levels. See an acupuncturist to normalize hormone levels as soon as possible.

Pets and Acne

We love them! But they can definitely complicate skin issues. Try to keep them from snuggling into your scarves, towels, bed, and pillows—where you'll eventually be laying your face at night. Pet dander, pet fur, flea care products, and all else leave residue everywhere they lay. Cover your bed with a tightly tucked large flat sheet or duvet, and leave a small pet blanket on top for them to snuggle. Check out your pet's shampoo and treatment lotions, and try to go for formulas that are acne-safe and fragrance-free. And if you can bear it, the less kissing and snuggling on your face, the better it may be for your skin.

Travel

Skincare While on the Go

No matter what, stick to your regimen! Even though you are traveling and as long as your skin is healthy for it, you should still be cleansing, icing, exfoliating, and moisturizing twice a day.

Pack and Prepare Your Products

Having a travel-sized (3.4oz or 100ml max per piece, to meet most airline regulations) set of all your homecare skin, oral, and body products always ready to go (to the gym, an overnight bag, or on a trip) can be a real time- and skin-saver!

Your skin may be fine with a foaming cleanser in your home climate but could really use a more moisturizing one in the new climate. The same goes for active exfoliants and moisturizers. Bring a bit of everything to have a more comprehensive toolkit in your travels, should you need to address the gamut from healing and calming the skin from sunburn, giving yourself a mini-facial to keep travel acne at bay, or soaking up extra oiliness from a particularly humid climate.

An exfoliant (either toner or serum) keeps your acne at bay and purges existing zits. For practical efficiency, taking your serum along might be easier than toner. The serum will be helpful if you need to spot treat or if your toner spills.

Spill-proof containers like silicone *Gotoobs*[19] are especially good for liquid products like toner and cleanser. Their wide necks also make for easy cleaning and refilling. You can reuse plastic zip bags (*Sea to Summit* makes mine, which I love[20]) or use reusable bags like silicone *Stashers*[21] or *Full Circle bags*[22]. You can also try placing a piece of plastic film between the bottle and the cap when screwing it shut.

Pack your toner or exfoliating serums into a resealable plastic bag and put it into your carry-on, as there are fewer chances of it being squeezed, jostled, and thus leaking. Make sure the toners or serums are within the size limits of carry-on liquids per TSA regulations.

Eat fresh foods and try to avoid eating too much salt, which bloats you and makes you thirsty. Eating light would be best because you don't want your body to have a hard time digesting heavy food while in flight.

Digestive teas, probiotics, and digestive enzymes can also be helpful in keeping your digestion healthy. Drinking plain hot water can help tons.

Topically, Especially During Plane Travel

The less you touch your skin (and the more you keep your PPE mask on for safety reasons), the better. Preventing topical dehydration is key.

Wash your hands and apply a layer of moisturizer as needed, preferably before takeoff. You can also try layering two to three drops of acne-safe oil under your moisturizer and using shea butter (in a pinch, try acne-safe lip balm) in areas prone to extreme dryness, like the nostrils.

If the insides of your nose get really dry, try cutting some cotton swab sticks in half and keep them in a little pouch along with a small jar of shea butter. Just before takeoff, balm your lips with it and then gently swab some shea butter into the nostrils to help keep them moisturized. Saline rinsing can also help.

Have a small spray bottle of hydrating toner or rosewater with you to keep your skin hydrated. This, along with essential oils, can also help calm nerves.

Climate considerations

Be prepared for any climate by bringing both regimen types, healing and clearing. You don't really know how your skin is going to react once you get to your destination, so having a comprehensive care kit will help remedy any situation.

Your healing regimen is generally the more moisturizing products commonly used in cold or dry air climates or in case of sunburn. Your clearing regimen is typically comprised of the more drying products, which are likely to have active ingredients in them, too. These are commonly more tolerated in warmer climates, but watch for sun sensitivity and adjust your skin routine accordingly.

Hot and humid: Some breakouts may be inevitable no matter what you do. Foaming cleansers will probably do better for your skin here. Showering at least twice a day is pretty much mandatory. Make sure your towels and clothing dry thoroughly to avoid bacteria growth, rashes, and infections.

Hot and dry: If you feel dry, use extra moisturizers, especially under SPF. Drinking water with electrolytes, eating fresh fruits and vegetables, and having chia seeds can help retain water in the digestive system, preventing constipation that's common with overall dehydration.

Cold and dry: Cold, gusty winds and central heating can wreak havoc on skin and an cause chapped skin. This is where acne-safe oils (safflower, sunflower) and shea butter/acne-safe lip balm could really come in handy to treat and occlude those areas (nostrils, nose, or cheekbones). Hydrating and non-foaming cleansers will probably be better for your skin, which will likely be on the drier side with cold, dry weather. Showers and baths can also be used as warming agents to help induce a better night's sleep, but take care not to use too hot water that can be dehydrating and itch inducing.

Lifestyle While on the Go

Travel is physically rough on the body; being catapulted several hundreds of miles per hour (i.e., on a plane) is stressful, unnatural, and dehydrating. Here are some things you can do to minimize the effects of travel on your skin.

Digestion

The focus here is adequate hydration and smooth digestion. Drink plenty of water to avoid dehydration, which can lead to constipation and other digestion problems. Try to drink more than you typically would. Taking electrolytes with you may be helpful to keep your body hydrated. (Pink Himalayan or Celtic gray salt have plenty of minerals; a pinch of either in a glass of water should do.)

Sleep

When traveling, new time zones, different beds, and rooms will inevitably affect your sleep somehow. Washable eye masks, ear plugs, essential oils, and spa music/meditation playlists are part of my sleep-well toolkit. You can also try supplements like chamomile tea, valerian, and melatonin.

This may not be accessible to all, but padding a few extra days before and after international trips to acclimate and recover from jet lag going and coming back can be a huge help. This way, you're not pressed to show up feeling miserable for work the very next day after a long-haul flight.

Try to start acclimating to your destination time zone as soon as possible. For example, stay up the entire flight going there so that when you land in your destination's evening time, you can go straight to the hotel and crash (or vice versa). Use eye covers and blackout curtains. This can help reset your sleep clock a bit faster with minimal adjustment pain.

Managing Inflammation

Stay icy. Most hotels have ice, so get it from the ice machine, convenience store, or room service, and continue icing your face. This is one of the easiest and cheapest ways to prevent and keep inflammatory acne down while traveling. If a pimple opens up while washing your face and you *must* do something about it, go to Section 1 (Picking) to learn how to take care of it properly.

New foods, wonky sleep schedules, and the general disorientation stress that comes with travel raise inflammation, so making good choices and integrating routine, low-inflammatory lifestyle practices like deep breathing, meditation, and calming exercises will help a lot.

Supplements can also help lower inflammation. Consider 50-100mg of OptiZinc (zinc methionine is combined with copper, which apparently makes for better absorption) each day with meals. Several research trials found this particular zinc and copper combo to be helpful in calming down inflammation from the inside out. New Chapter's Zyflamend is another powerful anti-inflammatory that's herb-based, so it can be easier on the digestive system. They also have a nighttime formula that can aid sleep. Turmeric and black pepper, when combined, are a powerful duo available in pill form or powdered to make a drink or sprinkled onto foods.

Managing Food While on the Go

The closer to an acne-safe diet you can stay, the clearer you'll be. Do some research on common local dishes and their ingredients. Asking questions about what is in your food, opting for the acne-safer option whenever possible, and advocating for your dietary choices are the best things you can do. However, it may also be less stressful to enjoy your trip as is and deal with the acne when you return than trying to stick to all the rules during it.

While traveling, carrying a card or screenshot of some translated phrases like "I cannot eat milk, cheese or soy products" to show local restaurants can be helpful.

Traveling around in regions like the Mediterranean, Southeast Asia and Latin America, you may be surprised to find that most local indigenous foods are actually naturally acne-safe. You may have to make do with some coconut oil here and there or ask to omit cheese, but these are relatively small and common adjustments to make.

Research

Learn about local dishes, seasonal foods, restaurants, and cooking schools run by local people in the area you will be traveling to. Seeking vegetarian and vegan options will usually guide you toward healthier choices. Food from small local outlets will be much more delicious and lovingly made than what you'd find at any chain restaurant. "However, chain restaurants consistently source the same ingredients in their dishes, and usually publish information on them online, making it easy for you to see what's potentially safe to consume." Cooking classes help you get an in-depth understanding of what goes into your favorite recipes.

Taking a cooking class early on in your trip can be a relaxing and enjoyable activity to help you settle into your new destination, and you will get an in-depth understanding of what (potentially non-acne-safe) ingredients go into the local dishes.

Pack Your Food Favorites

Learn about the acne-safe lifestyle choices you can control and what you cannot. Mapping these points out will help you plan ahead and make acne-safe decisions as much as possible ahead of time. It may be helpful to pack some items with you so that you have some safe food choices at hand, like your favorite matcha or collagen protein powder or a chia and flax seed mix for a protein and fiber boost easily added to any smoothie, juice, soup or oatmeal.

Dinner Parties

If you are traveling for the holidays or going to other people's homes for meals, here are a few suggestions:

- Bring a dish that's acne-safe so you know you've got at least one safe option to eat.
- Submit your dietary requests to your host. They are (hopefully) happy to accommodate you with food that won't make you feel ill.
- Eat before you go to the event so you can get away with grazing at the actual meal.
- Just eat the food, enjoy the love, and relish the moments. Deal with the acne later, now that you know exactly what to do to help it heal.

Kitchen/Mini Fridge

It's a great idea to go to a local grocery store to stock up on even just a few pantry staples and to have healthy, acne-safe things for quick breakfasts, snacks, and/or meals on the go. Consider a travel smoothie blender. Fill it with your favorite fruit, veggies, and smoothie ingredients from the local farmer's market, grocery store, or hotel buffet. Adding chia or flax seed and psyllium husk is super helpful and adds protein and fiber that regulates the digestive system.

Canned sardines or smoked salmon, avocado, and tomato toast fixings, salads with the dressing on the side, proteins (like roast chicken, boiled eggs, and falafel), trail mix, fruit, and dark chocolate are favorites. Dinner leftovers that can be eaten at room temperature work, too.

Section 4 - Lifestyle

Extra Digestive Support

In addition to all I write about in Section 5, you may need to pay extra attention to your digestive powerhouse while traveling due to all the changes travel inherently brings. Bring along your digestive supplements of choice, keep hydrated, put herbal digestive tea bags into your water bottle to calm the nerves, and nourish digestion all day.

Stomach upset might happen, so consider bringing supplements like charcoal pills, pre- and probiotics, digestive teas, fiber supplements, and anti-bacterials/-virals like oregano, peppermint, and/or fennel oil capsules for travelers' food poisoning and diarrhea.

Hotels

Hotels can be tricky because you never really know how clean the mattresses and pillows are or what detergents they use for their linens. But there are workarounds.

Consider bringing your own pillowcase to cover the pillow, or at least use a clean scarf, shirt, or towel so that you can rest your face easily on a clean surface. Avoid using decorative pillows and blankets, as they are less likely to be washed regularly (if at all) than sheets and towels.

Ice

Hopefully, your room will come with a mini fridge to store your acne-safe foods and ice. Look out for the hotel's ice machine so you can easily keep icing a part of your travel skincare routine. Asking for a cup of ice for takeaway when you're out at a restaurant is a good solution, too.

Laundry

Bring your own pillowcases, small washcloths for drying your face, and clean T-shirts or clean fabric like camping towels or sarongs to lay, sit, or sleep on.

Forever New Granular Unscented Detergent can help with your laundry needs while traveling.[23] It's lightweight to travel with and works wonders for everyday use, whether washing by machine or by hand. Try to bring clothes that you can easily hand wash and dry overnight by hanging them in your hotel room (or in the sun).

Camping

Camping acne-safe is possible with some planning, even with limited resources, and will help put you at ease, allowing you to further enjoy the great outdoors.

Keeping Clean

Try using a water dispenser with a spigot to have running water to use for drinking, cooking, and also brushing teeth, hand washing, and wetting towels. It's helpful to have a couple of these at base camp. You can buy the one-time disposable ones anywhere you buy bottled water or get a reusable and refillable one. Treat and cover up any scabs, cuts, or scratches on your skin to keep it clean and safe, avoiding infection.

Face

Because exfoliation is inherently sensitizing and who knows what weather elements you'll experience while camping, your regular skin routine may irritate it. Focus on keeping clean, moisturized, and sun protected, and then worry about exfoliating later when you're back home.

Disposable wipes make things easy but often contain irritating chemicals (and are environmentally not great). Instead, consider a washcloth wrung out of water (preferably warm) and use that to wipe down your face, neck, chest, and body, then moisturize (with warm, clean hands). The manual wiping down with the towel will provide a bit of physical exfoliation, so be gentle. If your skin can tolerate it (and the weather isn't too hot or cold), you can try using your active products.

If inflammation is an issue for you, definitely try your best to ice, even if only for a few seconds.

In every case, make sure to properly apply SPF often to avoid sunburn.

Body

After a few days of not being able to take a proper shower, it's inevitable that gunk is going to build up on your skin—sweat, dirt, sunscreen, and bug spray. Therefore, when you get home, take a really thorough shower—a bath would be optimal—and scrub yourself down thoroughly but gently with a soft mitt and acne-safe body cleanser to scrub and wash off all the dirt, skin, and SPF. If you're taking a bath, you'll be surprised at how dirty the water is when you're done.

Eating

As always, enjoy yourself and just do the best you can! A good cooler and a mix of prepped fresh and shelf-stable items work best. You can eat dehydrated foods so long as you drink a lot of water and watch your sodium intake, but of course, fresh foods are the best option. Research ways to pack healthy camping eats for inspiration and ideas.

Digestion

It's very important to use the bathroom and have regular bowel movements. Holding it all in and purposely constipating yourself is not healthy and can lead to more complications in the future, including acne. Drink lots of water, eat healthy food, and get physical activity in to keep your digestion moving. Digestive beverages like ginger tea, herbal fruit cider, or a turmeric latte by the fire would be great!

Sleeping

Try to keep your tent or cabin area clean. Remove dusty clothing and change into clean ones before climbing into your sleeping bag to keep everything as tidy as possible.

SPF

Sunscreens that come in tubes or bottles require you to massage them into the skin thoroughly, which is exactly what's needed to ensure good coverage for sun protection. It also allows you to get as much product out of the package as possible. You can cut tubes open and get several uses out of the remaining product or store bottles upside-down to get the product to drain out through the neck to get every last bit out.

When using spray sunscreens, you'll still need to rub the product onto your skin to really make sure it stays on. Sprayed-on sunscreen actually just floats on the hair or peach fuzz where you apply it, so it actually needs to be pressed down onto and spread across the skin. The spray function can be misleading in this way because the liquid should still be rubbed into the skin for best results and staying power.

A nice trick is to keep your SPF in your cooler. This helps keep your SPF cool and preserves the SPF in it, which can degrade in the heat. It'll also feel really good putting it on, and chances are you'll reach for drinks more than the SPF, so this will help remind you to reapply before indulging in another cold drink.

SPF types

Gels, lotions, creams, powders, oils...so many SPF types. You can layer them throughout the day's sun exposure.

Definitely always use SPF, big glasses, a big hat, and cover up exposed skin. The sun can be unexpectedly strong in seemingly cool climates, so always have protection at your disposal.

Start with a thorough base application of SPF lotion/cream all over the face and body before putting your swimsuit or clothes on. Doing this well will serve as a good foundation for reapplications the rest of the day (and keep your clothing tidy).

Powder SPF for the face may be easier to apply because the brush will be touching your skin, not your dirty, sandy fingers. Start with an all-over application of your lotion SPF, and be very thorough with applying the powder on top.

Mineral-based SPF lotions and creams are usually in a thicker formulation that can take some getting used to, but ultimately, the thorough rubbing helps ensure better SPF coverage and staying power.

Other Skin Conditions

Mosquito Bites

Natural versus chemical bug sprays

Try to stick with non-toxic products at least on the upper half of the body (in case of accidental ingestion or inhalation) and the stronger chemical/DEET-type products on the lower half (especially helpful for hiking through bushes or dinnertime at restaurants, where mosquitoes hide under tables). In every case, constant reapplication is always needed to ensure a better chance of protection, especially if you are hot and sweating it off—whether you go natural or chemical.

Prevention

Mosquitoes are mostly active at dawn and dusk and in swampy, humid, forested nature areas or bodies of still water. Diligently applying and reapplying your anti-mosquito treatments, sitting in front of a fan, and staying inside with your doors and windows closed during dawn and dusk are preventive measures you can take.

Spray products may be more convenient, but lotions adhere those protective ingredients to the skin better. Bug and sun protective products should always be applied liberally, rubbed into the skin thoroughly, and used repeatedly for maximum effectiveness.

If you're spraying, spray onto your hand, then rub onto the skin (or at least spray onto the skin and rub into the skin thoroughly), so it actually coats and protects the skin.

For the lower body, try the *Sawyer brand Picaridin Insect Repellent Lotion*.[24] Picaridin is synthesized in a lab (as most skincare ingredients are) that is modeled after an extract from the chrysanthemum flower and also has been shown to be just as effective as DEET without the toxicity or fragrance (check out the EWG's stance on bug repellents[25]).

For the upper body, try making your own acne-safe mosquito spray: 2 oz. filtered water in a spray bottle with anywhere from 20-50 drops of either or both citronella or lemongrass, and it would be optional to add a few drops of the following: lavender, tea tree, eucalyptus, or rosemary. You can also find mosquito-focused blends from essential oil companies at your local health food store in lieu of the single oils above.

Treatment—after you get bitten

Don't scratch or pick at it. Relieve the itching without scratching by:

- Applying ice. Ice will numb nerve endings and reduce inflammation. You can do this anywhere, including at a restaurant, by taking out a piece from your drink.
- Slap it or rub the skin around the actual bite. It's better than scratching if icing isn't an option.
- Apply something minty. TCM recommends warming muscle rubs like Tiger Balm or White Flower Oil. Consider an essential oil roller you can refill with peppermint and lavender essential oil. Other oils like camphor, eucalyptus, spearmint, or even lemongrass or rose can help.

Lifting the pigmentation left behind

Hopefully, you were able to manage the itching to avoid tearing the skin via scratching. Once the skin is healed and back to normal, you can use your skin-brightening products to help brighten the dark spots (the same as post-acne pigmentation scars). You can also get professional chemical peels to even out the skin tone, but time, an effective brightening product, and regular moisturization will help a lot in any direction you choose.

Polymorphous Light Eruption (PMLE, or heat rash)

PMLE, sometimes considered a sun allergy, is a condition where the skin develops a pink or red, itchy, and bumpy rash when exposed to the sun—either too much of it or at all. It can affect the entire skin or only in certain areas like in the folds of the skin: neck, inside the elbow, underarms, or behind the knees. Cool, dry temperatures, avoiding physical scratching, and treating the skin by either drying out or moisturizing it will bring relief.

Treating Heat Rash

Scratching at and opening the skin will make the rash worsen, persist, and spread. To treat the itch and prevent scratching, apply ice directly to the skin to numb the nerves causing the itching sensation and relieve inflammation. "Minty" essential oils like peppermint or camphor, which are commonly found in analgesic products for topical muscle pain relief, can quell the itch and simultaneously induce a cooling effect on the skin. Consider muscle oil roll-ons, BioFreeze gel, or wet clay like Thanaka (Thanaka tree bark that's finely ground into a powder, found in central Myanmar).

I find using essential oils to prevent itching and allowing the rash to dry out helps the most. I foam up an unscented antibacterial soap, apply it to the affected areas, leaving it on for several minutes before rinsing off with cool water, ice, air dry (preferably with a fan), and then apply a drying body powder. Some people find relief by doing the exact opposite by moisturizing the rash generously, slathering light moisturizers like our Hydrating Gel or aloe vera gel onto their skin to soothe the itch and heal the skin. Experiment to see what approach works best for you, and remember to avoid breaking the skin by scratching.

Preventing Heat Rash

Keep covered up with loose long sleeves and long pants made of silk or thin cotton, both of which are natural, very lightweight, and dry quickly. Synthetic fabrics trap heat and moisture.

Protect your skin. Thoroughly applying SPF *before* you're exposed to the sun can help immensely versus applying when you're already in it.

Keep cool. Avoid direct sun exposure onto the skin (especially sunbathing—but applying physical SPF beforehand may help) and other things that generate internal heat like smoking and alcohol, along with TCM and Ayurveda heating foods like spicy chili, alcohol, fried and barbecued foods, and lamb. Emphasize eating hydrating foods that also cool the body and lower inflammation.

Keep your skin dry. Using unscented body powder in the creased areas of the skin and body is really helpful to keep those areas dry, as moisture helps itchy rashes form and persist. Thailand's Snake Brand Prickly Heat Powder works well, but any baby powder should work too.

Stay hydrated. Sip lots of water and cooling drinks (cucumber slices, peppermint, chrysanthemum, or chamomile tea) throughout the day rather than taking big glugs a few times.

With & Within Acne Face Map

Seeing thousands of clients in our clinic over the years allowed us to notice patterns in our clients' acne: how they looked, where they showed up on the face and what seemed to consistently cause them to occur. On the following pages you find a guideline of the most common findings and placements we observed in our clients.

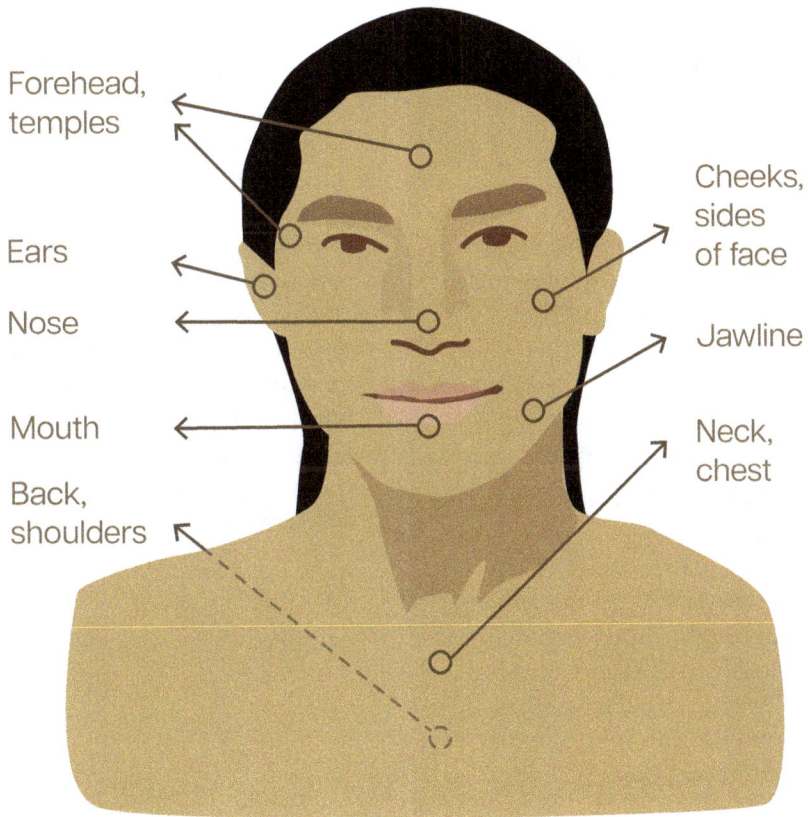

Clear Skin for Everyone

Mouth

Topical
- Cloggy lip products like lipstick, lip liner, lip balm, toothpaste, cold sore medication
- Petrolatum-based products can create dark sebaceous filaments along the lip line
- Upper lip hair removal like waxing
- Cooking oils, oil pulling
- Kissing partner with beard or who's using cloggy lip products
- PPE face mask

Internal
- Soy, coffee
- Perioral dermatitis
- Candida yeast imbalance

Nose

Topical
- Overmoisturizing
- Eyeglasses, PPE face mask
- Friction from noseblowing, rubbing, tissues, allergies

Ears

Topical
- Not washing or cleaning inner, outer or behind ears, piercings regularly
- Residue from hair or skin products, cloggy, not rinsing thoroughly and/or applied closely to areas breaking out
- Earrings, head coverings, headphones, telephone, ear buds

Forehead, Temples

Topical
- Head coverings like hats, beanies, hijab, headscarves, helmets, bonnets, cloth wraps from friction, dirty or washed with cloggy laundry detergent
- Cloggy hair products especially shampoo, styling products on bangs, skin products
- Sweating and not washing off soon enough

Internal
- Dairy
- Candida yeast imbalance

Cheeks, Sides of face

Topical
- Sleeping on pillowcases washed with cloggy laundry detergent
- Cloggy makeup like blush, bronzer, highlighters, contour
- Hair products that transfer via sweating, pillowcases, head coverings
- Leaning face on hands, unconscious picking, phone headsets, dirty yoga mats
- PPE face masks
- Upper cheeks could be eyeglasses if touching here

Internal
- Dietary, digestive
- Rosacea or acne rosace

Jawline

Topical
- Cloggy hair products
- Repetitive touching, leaning face on hands or unconscious picking
- Turtlenecks, scarves, yoga mats (unclean or friction)
- Straps from bike helmets

Internal
- Soy, soybean oil, coffee, high androgen foods
- Reproductive hormones imbalance, hormonal stress

Neck, Chest

Topical
- Necklaces, shirts and turtleneck collars dry cleaned, starched or washed with cloggy laundry detergent
- Cloggy hair or body products
- Perfume residue
- Clothing manufacturer chemical sprays on unwashed new clothing used to protect clothing in transit
- Residue from skin, body or haircare products, not rinsing thoroughly after cleansing, sweating, swimming, sex
- Dirty yoga mats

Internal
- Candida yeast or hormone imbalance, iodide rash
- Medication side effect

Back, Shoulders

Topical
- Constant friction or pressure from things like sweaty backpacks or sports gear
- Laying on surfaces such as dirty yoga mats, exercise equipment
- Cloggy shampoo, hair, body products, laundry detergent
- Not rinsing quickly or thoroughly after cleansing or sweating
- Massage with cloggy oils, products
- Unwashed new or used clothing

Internal
- Excess sugar
- Candida yeast imbalance, hormone imbalance
- Medication side effect

Endnotes

15 https://withandwithin.co/products/facial-single-blade-razor
16 https://www.cdc.gov/physicalactivity/basics/adults/
17 https://healthfully.com/332766-why-is-lifting-weights-causing-acne.html
18 https://lanshin.com/
19 https://www.humangear.com/shop/p/gotoob
20 https://seatosummit.com/collections/toiletry-bags
21 https://www.stasherbag.com/
22 https://fullcirclehome.com/products/ziptuck
23 https://forevernew.com/products/forever-new-granular-unscented-detergent
24 https://www.sawyer.com/products/picaridin-insect-repellent
25 https://www.ewg.org/consumer-guides/ewgs-2018-guide-bug-repellents

"On behalf of all of your clients,
thank you so much for all you've done for us
over the years. You've certainly improved my life
in immeasurable ways - from my skin
to my health, to my perspective and way of life.

I'm traveling the world now pursuing
my wildest dreams and would never
have found myself in this position
without With & Within.

As you know, I'm still very loyal to W&W
products and have friends bring me
refills along the way."

- KS, client since 2016

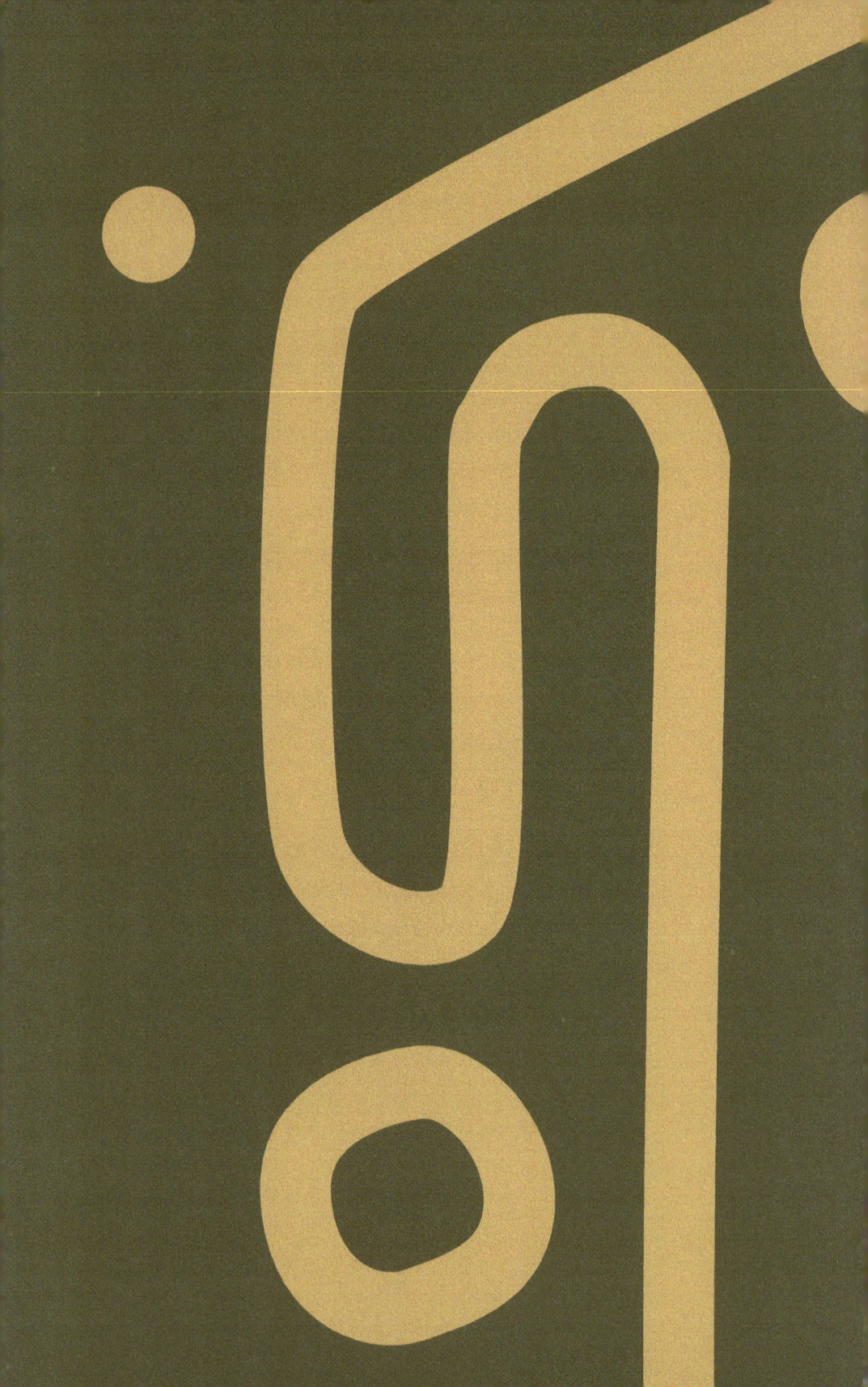

SECTION 5

The
Digestive
System,
Diet and
Acne

"You are not what you eat, but what you digest and assimilate."

– Tony Robbins

Learning exactly what foods will aggravate or cause acne is great, but without regular and robust digestion, assimilation, and elimination systems, you can be missing out on a lot of the long-term anti-inflammatory, body-fortifying qualities your foods have to offer.

Food can be a very emotional thing, and changes with it can be challenging to navigate, adjust to, and stick with. Many of our clients report that they generally feel better with the acne-safe diet, so once you get over the acclimation hump, trust that it gets easier to stick with (considering the benefits) and will soon feel natural.

Certain things you ingest (like medications) are necessary, so you may have to deal with the side effects of acne if you aren't able to switch to another type.

There's a lot to learn about here, so slow and steady wins the race. Read along and, at your own pace, try implementing one new thing at a time. See if you can notice the effects before, during, and after you try them on your body and on your skin.

How to Eat

Digestion

First lesson: digestion starts in the mouth. Food's first mechanical process is through our chewing, stimulating the first chemical pass via saliva (amylase enzymes), before making its way down to the rest of the organs to further mechanically and chemically break down the food. Chewing very thoroughly relieves stress on the rest of your organs to more fully and efficiently concentrate on assimilating the nutrients needed for feeding the body's processes (versus mechanically breaking down what could have been done in the mouth), preventing issues like gas, indigestion, and bloating. If chronic, these symptoms can lead to more complicated conditions like food intolerances, ulcers, infections, bleeding, and gastroesophageal reflux disease (GERD), which can develop into even more serious health issues like gastric cancer. A compromised digestive system puts unnecessary physical stress on your organs, which in turn makes your body more

Section 5 - The Digestive System, Diet and Acne

vulnerable to the effects of external stress. Controlling what and how you eat is a lot easier to manage than stress, so do what you can to crush these points of vulnerability.

Physiologically, your body will exert more energy to digest these foods than to push blood flow to your brain, where you'll need it more if you're going back to work after lunch. Mentally and emotionally, let's also not forget the brain and gut connection mentioned in the last section, as a two-way highway. If you are stressed in the brain, your guts won't digest so well. If your guts don't digest so well, the 90% of serotonin production that happens in the gut is disrupted.

If you really can't chew your food thoroughly, aside from seeking medical care to examine your teeth, consider consuming protein smoothies, blended soups, or soft foods that are easy to chew like avocado or eggs instead. Foods that are broken up in this way are already predigested (chewed up), so there is a lot less chewing needed. All you have to do is swallow.

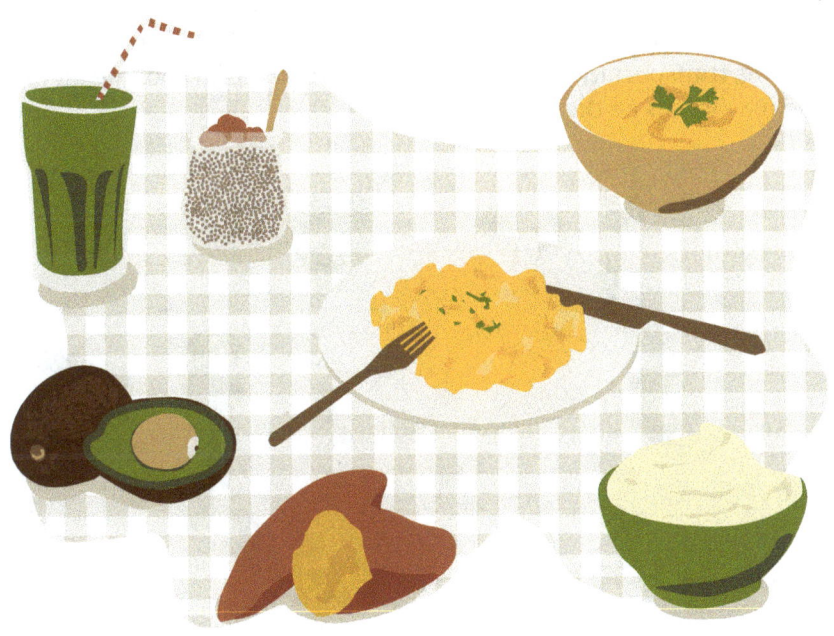

Soft and easy to eat-and-digest foods like green smoothies, chia seed pudding, blended vegetable soups, whole grain sweet or savory porridges, kitchari, avocado, sweet potato, mashed potatoes and eggs are good choices for quick meals.

Mindful Eating

Take it easy. Don't eat too fast, or when you're on the go. Eat intentionally and in a relaxed fashion. This will optimize and make most efficient the very first part of the digestive process that begins in your mouth: the saliva production and mechanical breakdown of those foods powered by chewing.

Eat in peace. This also counts as the time you can spend undisturbed, in a relaxed fashion. Ayurveda says that it's best for you to eat alone, or to eat with little to no talking, and certainly not under emotional distress, to maximize the body's digestive processes. Air is inhaled while talking, which can make for gas and improperly digested food.

Get out. While at work, get up and away from your desk, eat outside in fresh air and natural light, if you can. Your mind needs a mental and environmental break so that your organs can relax and do their job. The digestive process won't be as efficient if you—and your body + organs—are tense.

Savor your meal. Put your fork down between bites, really taste your food and think of mindful eating as a time to really enjoy and honor all the efforts of the supply chain that got the food to your plate. The hardworking farmers, the abundance of nature's soil, water, and sun, the harvesting, cleaning, transportation, recipe planning, and careful cooking all had a hand in what sits on the plate before you.

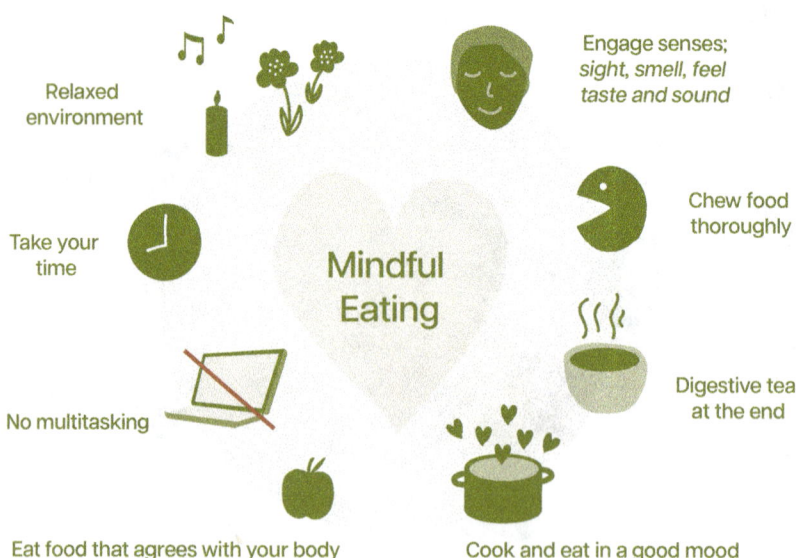

Practical Eating

Eating at regular times is a cornerstone of holistic wellness, to maintain a healthy blood sugar balance (which can affect blood sugar spikes and dips), and to avoid your digestive system from acting up in between meals. The body runs on timed cycles, so variations in what should be regular occurrences stresses the body and thus the mind.

Try not to drink too much water before or during your meal, as this can water down the digestive acids and enzymes. Hot herbal teas after meals are encouraged to enhance digestion.

Avoid cold drinks, especially ice, as this also slows down digestion; the digestive system generates heat to digest food, and drinking ice cold liquids halts the digestive process, forcing the body to work twice as hard to warm up again to produce more acids. You may notice extra bloating or indigestion the next time you simultaneously consume an iced drink and eat, now that you're privy to this school of thought. (Both TCM and Ayurveda advise warm or hot beverages instead, and tepid in hot weather.)

A tip I learned from California-based herbalist Kami McBride is to incorporate carminatives into your diet. Warming herbs like cinnamon, chili, fennel, and ginger enhance the digestive system. She likes to make herb sprinkles you can easily add to any dish, soup, or salad. Herbal teas made by boiling these spices in filtered water also works.

Take your probiotics first thing in the morning, on an empty stomach. You can take them in supplement form, or from food sources like fermented veggies (kimchi, sauerkraut) with every meal, acne-safe yogurts, and enzyme-rich foods like apple cider vinegar, papaya, or pineapple first thing in the morning.

Consider digestive reset days. Every month, try a day or so of consuming only raw fruits and vegetables, smoothies or blended soups (while drinking plenty of water) to help give your digestive system a break, allowing it to rejuvenate and reset.

Reflection

Pay attention to how your physical body, mind and emotions feel after eating certain foods. Do you experience brain fog, thirst, fatigue, or bloating in your belly? Keeping a food journal may help you track down what foods make you feel a certain type of way.

In today's world, people have gotten used to feeling terrible in their bodies because they're too busy to notice or care about the details, or just chalk it up to getting old. Imagine how much better your quality of life can be if you optimized your body's operational systems. You'd have more energy, be more alert and clear-headed, healthier, and happier all around.

Digestive Support

Constipation is a common problem with acne sufferers but luckily, there are a plethora of ways to naturally enhance your digestive system, as our ancient active lifestyles and holistic medicine have done for centuries. With modern-day sedentary and stressed lifestyles, extra help in this department is likely needed. Consult a qualified natural health practitioner or nutritionist to learn what types of supplements are right for you, and how best to take them. Paying attention and taking care of your digestion will in turn lower systemic inflammation, including the skin. Here are some ideas to get you started.

Physical Stimulation and Activity

Physically stimulating your organs can help physically move things along, and there are many ways to do this. Yoga poses like Ananda Balasana (aka happy baby), Malasana (yogi squat), and Ardha Pawamuktasana (one leg wind-removing pose) can be quite effective. *The Squatty Potty*, a foot stool that elevates your knees above your hips while sitting on the toilet claims to move your colon into an ideal position to easily eliminate.[26] TCM's Chi Nei Tsang, a type of abdominal massage, focuses on pressure points to stimulate the internal organs.

Gentle belly massage

A simple self-massage technique to encourage bowel movements: Use a gentle clockwise motion starting from the right side of your belly (looking down, this serves as 3 o'clock), working your way to the middle top just under your ribcage (6 o'clock), left belly (9 o'clock), and just above the pelvis (12 o'clock). You can enhance the effects with some acne-safe massage oil, essential oils, or minty muscle balms.

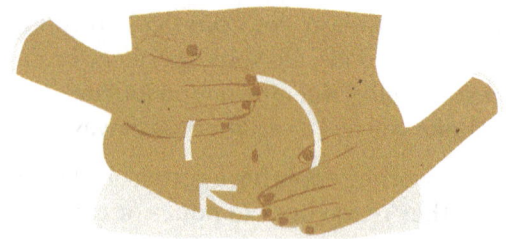

Section 5 - The Digestive System, Diet and Acne

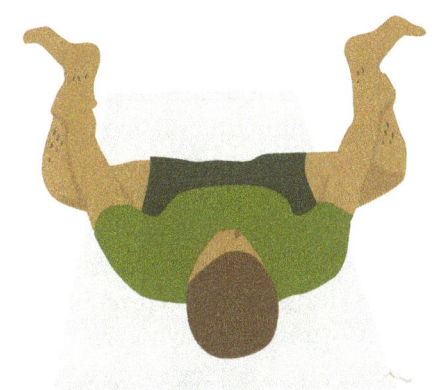

Ananda Balasana, or happy baby. Lay on your back, grab your knees, ankles or feet, bending your knees, aiming them towards your shoulders. Breathe deep.

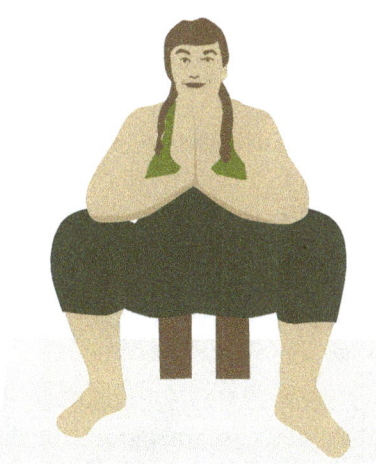

Malasana, or yoga squat. With your feet slightly wider than hip distance apart, squat down as low as you can. Touch your palms and use your elbows to push your knees apart and back. Sit on yoga blocks or a cushion as needed for additional support. Breathe deep.

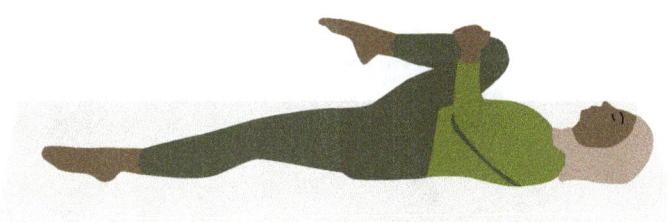

Ardha Pawamuktasana, or wind removing pose. Lay on your back, hug one knee to your chest, aiming it towards your shoulder for a deep stretch, all while keeping your back and neck flat on the mat. Repeat with the other leg, and again with both knees. Breathe deep.

Herbs

Before conventional over-the-counter symptom-targeted drugs like Tylenol and Nyquil came along, herbs (and food) were the medicine people used to promote health and cure ailments. These modern drugs do a good job of alleviating symptoms, but don't do much to actually heal the body and come with side effects that herbal medicines typically do not. It's common to experience bowel movement changes (especially constipation) while starting any new diet or cleanse, as your body acclimates to the new foods you are eating and protocols you are implementing. Additional herbal remedies may be utilized to help promote good and thorough elimination and luckily they're quite easy to incorporate.

Herbs can be taken in several forms in order of most to least potent: tinctures (herbs distilled into grain alcohol or glycerin concentrates), pills (dried herbs in capsule or tablet form), infusions (herbs steeped into liquid such as teas, soups or syrups), and in my favorite way, eating them (herbs added to recipes).

Ginger is an example of a centuries-old effective herbal remedy. It is taken to help alleviate motion sickness (in tablet form), settle the stomach while promoting digestion and elimination (eating it or drinking a tea of it), and even soothe a toothache (by placing a piece of ginger directly over the tooth). In fact, ginger ale was first made as a fiery medicinal tonic to cure all these ailments before the big soda industry turned it into the mainstream, high fructose corn syrup, ginger-flavored beverage it is today.

Herbal teas to try include senna, peppermint, ginger, dandelion, licorice root, marshmallow root, chamomile, parsley, cascara sagrada, buckthorn, rhubarb, and triphala. Most any spice, herb or root you find in the kitchen (like cinnamon, fennel and coriander seeds; mint, thyme and rosemary

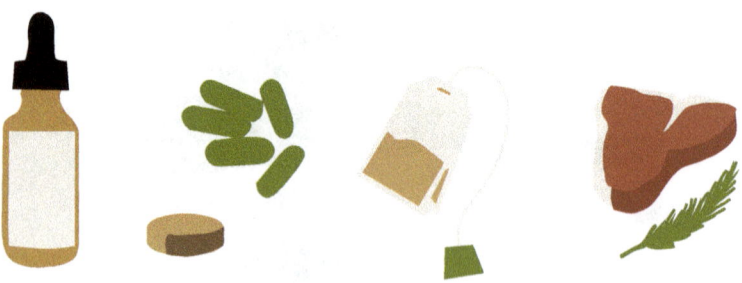

Herbs can be taken in forms such as concentrated tinctures, capsules or pills, infusions like tea or eaten in its most natural state with food.

leaves; fresh or dried ginger or turmeric) can be steeped to make soothing, caffeine-free teas. Magnesium and probiotics can also help facilitate bowel movements, along with soluble and insoluble fiber. With any and all remedies, sufficient water intake is vital! There's a plethora of ways to improve digestion. Do some research, try out a few ideas to see what works best for you, and build your digestion toolbox.

Fiber

Acne sufferers often also have digestive issues, so consider supplementing your diet with some digestive support to literally scrub your guts, to produce regular, long and formed bowel movements. Insoluble fiber scrubs your digestive tract, and soluble fiber aids in easier, smoother, elimination.

Insoluble fiber
(Psyllium husk, oat bran, chia and flax seeds.)

Recommended brands: no brands, just find raw and organic at your local health food store (for flax seeds, grind it yourself and store in the freezer to maintain freshness, as they go rancid quickly).

Oat bran, chia, and flax seeds add protein, anti-inflammatory omega-3s, insoluble fiber and antioxidants.

Sprinkle ground flax seeds or whole chia seeds onto salads, into soups, stews, or cooked into meatloafs, meatballs, or casseroles (they help make these foods moist, and also work great as vegan and shelf stable egg replacers).

Chia pudding is easy to make when you combine it with acne-safe milk, topped with nuts or fruit for a quick breakfast or simple dessert.

For more intensive cleaning, psyllium husk can help bulk up bowel movements, but caution must be exercised. Mix small amounts of psyllium with water and drink, blend into a smoothie or take one to two capsules to start, and drink liberal amounts of water afterward, as psyllium is very absorbent. Not enough water can cause constipation, among other possible complications.

Soluble fiber
(Prunes, cooked vegetables, apples, dried beans, oats, the skins and peels of most fruits and vegetables, potatoes, whole grains, cereals, and seeds.)

These can help ease the elimination of those bulked-up, insoluble fiber-filled movements while providing some anti-inflammatory, healing, and moisturizing properties to the lining, as well as provide food for the digestive flora.

Supplements

Probiotics

Probiotics help to digest food and assimilate nutrients that acne-prone people are often deficient in, thanks to this day and age of processed food, constant stress, and prescription drug consumption (especially antibiotics, antidepressants, and birth control). All these factors eventually disrupt the delicate balance of good bacteria that exist within the gut, necessary for strong digestion. When the biome of the gut is out of balance, other organisms in the gut—like Candida yeast—are given the chance to overgrow and cause bigger problems like brain fog, fatigue, depression, digestive issues, and treatment resistant acne.

Probiotics come in the form of supplements like pills and powders (look for shelf-stable ones that don't need refrigeration), and in fermented foods. Acne-safe choices include pickles, sauerkraut, kimchee, sugar- and carageenan-free non-dairy yogurts, soy-free miso (chickpea is a common one), and koji (fermented rice). Non-acne safe choices include soy-based miso, natto, tempeh, animal dairy based kefirs and yogurts. I think kombucha and miso can be eaten in moderation, but it's best to get your probiotics from acne-safe food sources. Important to note that true probiotic-rich foods are made sour *without* the use of vinegar but by natural fermentation. You can ferment your own pickles naturally at home, or buy them at your local health food store.

It's generally suggested to take probiotics first thing in the morning on an empty stomach, so long as it doesn't make you nauseous. Kyolic and Jarrowdophilus are good brands to try.

Enzymes

Enzymes like papaya or pineapple found in natural fruit or supplement form can help further the breakdown of heavier proteins, relieving gas and bloating. They can be really helpful while you rebuild your digestive system while restoring the natural digestive fire's ability to create its own enzymes.

Hydrochloric acid (HCl)

Naturally occurring in the stomach, stress and other factors reduce HCl's production, essential for protein breakdown and keeping the digestive tract strong. Supplementation can reduce bloating and other digestive woes associated with heartburn-like symptoms. Natural medicine theorizes that heartburn is a sign of *not enough* stomach acids, versus the conventional medicine's diagnosis of *too much* acid in the gut. There are simple tests that you can do at home to try and determine if you have too much or too little stomach acid, like the baking soda, lemon juice, or apple cider vinegar tests.

Imbalanced acid levels in the gut can result in bad breath, gas, indigestion and eventually constipation.

Oils and healthy fats

Increasing your intake of omega-3 and flaxseed oils not only help boost hydration from the inside out, but also help regulate elimination of the body's toxins. Good quality fish oil supplements do triple duty: they keep inflammation down, raise your vitamin A + D levels, and are essential to repair and regenerate organs such as your brain and eyes. Eating wild oily fish, nuts, seeds, and incorporating more healthy fats like nut butters and avocados can help too. Nordic Naturals is a brand we trust.

Eliminate

The goal is to get your digestive tract to eliminate as much as possible, so that the toxins don't start looking for alternate exit pathways out of the body (like the skin—it's all gotta come out somehow!). The concept of digestive constipation is also true for acne in the skin; we need just enough hydration in our pores/intestines so that the impactions/waste within can easily glide out of the body, with minimal effort and fuss.

Starting the day with a big glass of warm water, perhaps with some lemon or mineral salt added or an ounce of aloe vera juice, can help clear the digestive tract.

If you have the urge to poop, do so as soon as you can. Delaying the evacuation will cause dehydration and likely more long-term constipation, as the water within fecal matter gets reabsorbed by the colon, drying it out as it sits. It also makes the intestinal muscles weak, further compromising the system in the long term. Exercising, strengthening, and massaging the abdominal muscles help stimulate the digestive organs that lay underneath to work well.

Get Regular

The body's main pathway of detoxing is through regular bowel movements. If you are chronically constipated, your body is more likely to rid its toxins through your skin, triggering breakouts. Optimally we should have one movement per meal, two to three times per day, preferably long and formed—just like babies or dogs do—that evacuate quickly and easily without any effort or exertion. Regularity is different for everyone; for some, a few times a week is their norm.

If you have chronic constipation, even after making dietary and lifestyle changes, a Candida imbalance or some other systemic issue may be present as a result of a sluggish/overtaxed liver, so check with a doctor.

In order to facilitate healthy and regular bowel movements, there are several things that need to be in place. As mentioned earlier, eating mindfully and carefully with adequate hydration and physical stimulation are good starting baseline habits to build.

Hydration

Making sure your body is properly hydrated helps things move smoothly, ensuring a properly moisturized digestive tract is operating at its best. Your small intestine absorbs 90% of your body's water intake, and the large intestine (aka colon) is responsible for absorbing the balance of what is left over, along with producing electrolytes, and eliminating the body's waste. (Electrolytes are the chemicals and minerals that allow water to hydrate the body, maintain the blood's pH and pressure, regulate nerve and muscle function, and rebuild damaged tissue.).

Drinking Water

The general rule for how much water we should consume is half our body weight in ounces, and more if you live in a dry climate, are taking supplements, medications, or drinks (like coffee) that induce dehydration, or work out (and sweat) a lot. For example, if you weigh 150 pounds, divide that into two which equals 75, and convert that to ounces. This means you should be drinking at least 75 ounces of water throughout the day—not chugged all at once or twice a day. The body works best with regular amounts of hydration throughout the day. Your urine should come out pale yellow gold or clear, indicating that you are consuming enough water. However if you are experiencing intense thirst, consult your doctor.

You can also try adding electrolytes to your regimen: either sprinkling them into your drinking water or taking them in capsule form, as well as a magnesium supplement nightly.

Eating Water

Eating foods that are rich in fiber and water help to do two jobs in one to scrub your digestive tract clean, while replenishing lost moisture. Water you retain from eating these foods also counts toward your daily consumption of water.

Section 5 - The Digestive System, Diet and Acne

Water-rich foods to emphasize include:

- Cucumbers
- Lettuces, especially Iceberg lettuce
- Celery
- Radishes
- Zucchini
- Grapes
- Sweet peppers
- Green cabbage
- Cauliflower
- Spinach
- Strawberries
- Watermelon
- Grapefruit
- Bean sprouts
- Zucchini
- Tomato
- Watercress
- Cantaloupe
- Peaches
- Pineapple
- Raspberries
- Cranberries
- Oranges
- Apricots
- Carrots
- Kiwi
- Broccoli
- Eggplant
- Jicama
- Soups and broths
- Apples
- Brussel sprouts
- Hydrated chia and basil seeds

Electrolytes

Most all sea salts, especially pink Himalayan and gray sea salts, are suggested because of the high levels of mineral + electrolytes they contain, which help the body retain more water, promoting good digestion. I personally like a pinch of pink Himalayan salt and a squeeze of lemon first thing in the morning. Magnesium is another supplement that helps to calm the nervous system and relax the digestive organs, promoting good elimination the next day.

Clean filtered water is best, but be careful of drinking distilled water for too long; it's great for detoxing the body due to its lack of minerals but over time may cause problems, since the very minerals that have been distilled out of it are necessary for healthy body function. Processed or low-fat foods can be dehydrating, especially if they have a lot of iodized salt in them, so drink lots of water when eating them, and emphasize whole natural foods.

Eating Acne-safe

As we've alluded to earlier in the book, there are certain foods that we've seen aggravate or cause acne to form in our clients. As such, there are likely some dietary changes that can be made for optimal results. However, these dietary changes are not necessarily permanent; they are in place at the beginning of the clearing process to lower any inflammatory reactions your body will have as your skin starts to purge acne. Ingesting these foods may not necessarily create new acne for you, but they will almost certainly make whatever existing acne you have worse. Once you are clear, you can try reintroducing these foods to your diet to see if and how they affect your skin.

Some clients cleared up very quickly when they followed the acne-safe diet precisely, and then later, once they were clear, found what they could and couldn't get away with. Perhaps coffee wasn't a trigger for them, but dairy was. Or that tofu once a week was okay, but any more than that caused painful acne to erupt around the mouth. Or they could eventually eat anything they wanted because it really was just the products they were using that were breaking them out. Or their bodies are just sensitive, and the closer to the acne-safe lifestyle they live, the better—until they grow out of their acne.

Each person's reactions are very different, and it's hard to tell what your specific triggers are in the beginning stages of the purge when one can be broken out from so many different mystery factors.

Being Vegetarian Isn't Necessary for Clear Skin

We often have to dispel the rumor that you need to become a vegetarian to clear acne. Diets and bodies are very personal and bespoke things. Some have definitely cleared up going vegetarian or vegan, while others cleared up after reincorporating animal products into their diets. Some broke out while on the Candida cleanse and got better when they stopped the cleanse early because the mental stress of adhering to all the restrictions was too stressful.

Acne only really becomes a problem when the body reaches a threshold of how much of any particular substance (be it a food, cloggy skin product, or lifestyle stressor) it can tolerate before acne manifests as a visible sign of imbalance.

Acne-specific Food Reactions

Understanding how foods directly affect the skin and body will likely make it easier to make the changes needed to clear up. From an acne standpoint, there are three general reactions that I've noticed occur with certain foods. They are:

- Inflammatory (aggravating): most immediate effect, can be seen within hours or days
- Acne-producing: takes longer for the seeds to become visible; about one month
- Candida-yeast feeding: can cause immediate reactions for those with this condition

The reactions you'll notice will depend on your baseline on that particular day. A person with a healthy and balanced digestive system who consumes a little too much sugar one afternoon might experience a sugar rush and crash but no new acne. But if another person with a Candida yeast imbalance consumes just a tiny amount of sugar, intense reactions can occur. An inflammatory reaction occurs, and existing acne on the skin flares up. New acne seed formation in Candida-related cases happens much faster than typical acne and can be seen within days, and other symptoms appear or worsen, like recurring yeast or sinus infections.

Foods like dairy, soy, and coffee are inflammatory *and* acne-producing. Some sugar can be okay with those with balanced digestive systems but can wreak havoc on someone with a compromised system. Nightshades and grains don't necessarily cause acne formation but can certainly severely inflame those who have a very, very sensitive inflammatory reaction.

How to Shop

Quality of foods and dietary philosophy

The acne-safe diet is generally good for everyone, regardless of whether or not acne (or Candida imbalance) is present, thanks to its low-glycemic nature. It closely resembles what's popularly known today as the paleo diet: natural and fresh nutrient-rich foods and whole grains while minimizing dairy, sugars, refined grains, and processed foods. Ideally, the food is grown locally and organically before being simply prepared.

Dr. Weston A. Price, a Canadian dentist who traveled the world studying the diets and lifestyles of several indigenous communities in the 1920s, found that their traditional, whole, and natural food diets provided these folks with very strong and healthy minds and bodies that were resistant to disease, accompanied by straight teeth and clear, acne-free skin. People in places where highly processed foods prevailed had poorer health, more disease, and dental and skin problems. Turns out the secret to a healthy life is following the simple ways of our indigenous ancestors.

Moreover, many foods are now pumped with things like pesticides and growth hormones to encourage bigger crop and livestock harvests. Pesticides, antibiotics, and GMOs are used to treat or keep them from disease, making their way into us when we consume them. Food researcher and writer Michael Pollan's book *The Omnivore's Dilemma* explains more of how this affects us personally and globally. Choose local, organic, and sustainably raised whenever possible.

Acne-causing Foods – Primary Triggers

Dairy

Dairy has induced acne in many of our clients; there are countless cases. It's also a food that's difficult to cut out, especially when clients realize how much of it they consume in their daily lives. Even regular but small amounts of dairy (like a splash of milk or cream in your tea) can cause breakouts, so at least in the beginning of your clearing process, try eliminating *all* animal dairy products, including cow's, goat's and sheep's milk (whole, low fat, lactose free), cream, yogurt, ice cream, cheeses, sauces, frozen yogurt, kefir, and whey protein. Whey or soy isolates are often in protein drinks, smoothies, and bars, so check the ingredients.

There are a few "official" medical studies as to why dairy is problematic for so many, but many of them are marked inconclusive, contrary to what I've personally seen in my practice over the years. If it breaks you out, makes your stomach hurt, or clogs up your sinuses with extra mucus, then it's very likely that it's just not good for you.

Hormones: Milk is sourced from pregnant animals, and pregnant animals have a lot of hormones on their own, not including the artificial ones that are injected into them to boost growth and production. Naturally occurring hormones are in milk to help baby cows grow big and strong.

Unnatural: No other mammals in the animal kingdom consume milk after infancy, let alone that of other animals. We are an anomaly in nature. It's no mystery why most humans are lactose intolerant.

Antibiotics: Notoriously and widely used in commercial livestock and food production, cows are often fed antibiotics as both medicines and within their food to cure but also to prevent disease. There are often so many animals packed into a small space that it's easy for them to get sick from each other. Animal rights groups claim that cows that are commercially milked often contract a form of mastitis, or udder infection, from the rough machinery that injures them. Because all the milk collected from individual cows is combined into large tanks, virtually all milk has some pus contamination. This may be a big reason why milk sold commercially is pasteurized; the heat kills bacteria like this.

Iodine: Dr. Fulton believed that the salt licks that cows graze on to promote milk production are so rich in iodides that they make their way from the lick past the cow's digestive system and into the milk, passively passing the iodides into the finished product that humans will consume. Seafood, sea vegetables and supplements derived from them can also induce a negative reaction.

Traditional medicine: In Traditional Chinese Medicine, dairy is considered a food that creates dampness and stagnation in the body, an imbalance that causes acne. In Ayurveda, dairy products can be cooling for the body's overall temperature, but they are also a factor in phlegm creation, which creates a kind of congestion in the body on a systemic level.

Clinical evidence: In the clinic, I have seen time and time again over the years the effects of dairy causing acne in my clients. Sometimes, a scientific explanation isn't needed so much as the evidence of what I see my clients experience in my practice every day.

Instead of dairy:
Dairy- and soy-free milk made of almond, oat, hemp, cashew, coconut, and rice are just a few of the many good substitutes available. Beware of carrageenan in mass-produced nut milk; it's a common thickening, stabilizing, and texturizing additive that is derived from (acne- and rash-causing) seaweed. Studies on carageenan, like this one found on Dr. Andrew Weils' website have linked it to autoimmune, inflammatory bowel disease

and others.[27] Dr. Weil is an American medical doctor, author, teacher and advocate of integrative medicine for over thirty years.

> ### TIP: Make your own acne-safe milk
>
> Make your own homemade nut milk. With a blender, some nuts (or nut butter) and water, you can easily make your own milks at home. Try one part nuts soaked overnight and drained with 3-4 cups fresh filtered water (or 2 tablespoons nut butter and 1.5 cups water); add a pinch of salt, some vanilla and/or a date to add some sweetness, and strain if you like.

Beware of soy-based dairy alternative products—soy milk is not an acceptable substitute, as that will likely break you out.

Cheese-flavored nutritional yeast comes in powder form that can be used in recipes or on top of salads to impart a cheesy flavor while providing vitamins, minerals, and antioxidants.

There are lots of vegan cheese substitutes on the market. Look for soy- and coconut oil-free ones. As these are largely oil-based, consume occasionally.

Possible exceptions:
Butter, in moderation, should be okay, but those with extreme dairy sensitivity may wish to do without.

Ghee, or clarified butter, is a better option than plain butter because the milk solids have been removed, possibly making it a lower-inflammatory option to cook with.

Some allopathic doctors say that aged dairy products like hard cheeses are okay, but drinking fresh milk is not. Abstain until you are clear enough to see their direct reactions.

Dairy can also be found hidden in foods like breads and sauces, so make sure to read your ingredient labels. In shelf-stable products, it will often show up as powdered milk, milk solids, or whey isolate.

Acne-safe sources of calcium include almonds and almond milk, oranges and orange juice, sardines, dark leafy greens like kale, collards, and chard, herbs, chickpeas, and chia seeds. Remember, vitamins from eating whole, natural foods are more easily processed and better assimilated by your body than synthetic or processed ones.

Dairy-caused acne often first shows up as very small, non-inflamed acne, almost like grains of sand. It often starts across the forehead, slowly moving to the temples and the rest of the face. With enough time (or depending on the person's inflammatory response), it can also get inflamed and make existing inflamed acne worse.

Soy

Soy products contain phytoestrogens that mimic estrogen in the body, and in high enough amounts, can throw off our own naturally balanced hormones, affecting the skin. Too much of any one hormone will cause an imbalance, causing a trickle effect of symptoms. Soy seems to take longer than other foods to purge out of the skin and body, as evidenced by our in-clinic clients.

Commonly listed as an allergen on processed and packaged food ingredient lists, soy shows up as a main protein source (commonly listed as isolated soy protein or textured vegetable protein, tofu, or tempeh) in commercially baked breads such as soy flour and soybean oil, and are the bases of ingredients like vegetable oil, soy sauce, caramel colorings, and flavorings. Fermented condiments like soy-based miso and soy sauce in moderation should be okay for most. Pretty much all other beans, whole grains, seeds, and nuts (aside from peanuts, which in moderation should be okay) are acne-safe protein sources.

Soy-caused breakouts often show up as inflamed acne in the lower half of the face, around the mouth and jawline. They can inflame existing acne, making it much worse. Soy-induced acne also seemed to take longer to clear as compared to dairy within my practice.

CASE STUDY: Soy lattés and acne

I had a client who had cleared up and maintained her clarity on her own for about two and a half years but started coming back in for treatments because of some really inflamed acne she started getting around her mouth. After quizzing her during the treatment, we discovered that she had developed an affection for soy matcha lattes, and that after several weeks of habitually drinking them, she started breaking out with painful, inflamed acne concentrated mostly around her mouth. Soy seems to take longer than other foods to purge out of the skin and body, so she took a full three months of active purging to clear, going from a 50% clarity rate to 90%.

Coffee

According to Dr. Perricone, it's not the caffeine but the organic acids in coffee beans that raise cortisol (the stress hormone) levels for twelve to fourteen hours after you drink it, boosting oil production and inflammation. Drinking coffee is basically like drinking liquid stress and inflammation—both to be avoided when you have acne. Even decaffeinated coffee will raise your cortisol levels because it's these natural acids—not the caffeine—that ramp up your stress hormones.

With the elevated cortisol response, anxiety levels are raised and the energy-crashing effects are induced, potentially encouraging one to pick at their acne and destroy their face, prolonging the clearing process and increasing the chances of permanent scarring. The inflammatory and excess oil production effects just make existing acne worse, not to mention the nerve-racking increased heart rate and adrenaline production.

Because it spikes cortisol that comes from your endocrine system (hormones), this acne often shows up as inflamed along the jawline and around the mouth—much in the same way as soy, because they're both inflammatory and have direct effects on the hormones.

Instead of Coffee

<u>Water.</u> Start your day with a glass of clean, filtered, and preferably warm water (bonus for a squeeze of lemon and a pinch of pink salt) to hydrate your body and flush out toxins that accumulated while you were sleeping. Doing this first thing in the morning on an empty stomach allows your body to optimize its cleansing and repair processes. A drop of organic citrus essential oil in cold sparkling water is delightful.

<u>Caffeinated teas are fine but are still dehydrating</u> and in high enough amounts, and can result in a cortisol spike. Make sure to drink enough water to make up for the caffeine you are drinking, at least 1:1. Drink green, matcha, and black teas; yerba mate is a very powerful one that energizes without the jitters or the afternoon crash. Chai (an Indian black tea with spices) is delicious; try it with acne-safe milk or plain.

<u>Caffeine-free herbal teas:</u> All of them. Your standard peppermint, mint, rose, and chamomile are fine. I love making them from fresh herbs like rosemary, thyme, mint, and lemongrass to make a lovely digestive-supporting tisane. Slices of fresh turmeric and ginger in hot water are great (add ground black pepper to boost turmeric's anti-inflammatory properties). In Sri Lanka, roasted coriander seeds and fresh ginger tea are commonly taken as a traditional digestive remedy.

Herbal teas that are dark and roasted like Dandyblend, Celestial Seasonings' Roastaroma and chicory "coffee" may help curb the flavor craving of coffee. Dandyblend's roasted dandelion root, chicory, beets, barley, and rye blend offer a full-bodied flavor very similar to coffee without the adrenalizing inflammatory effects.

Mushroom coffee from brands like Four Sigmatic sound funky but they just might be your new jam. Mushrooms are known for their plethora of healing and antioxidant properties. Many people swear by how focused and alert they are when taking this, without the coffee crash.

Hot cacao. Yep, similar to hot chocolate but with cacao (unroasted cacao beans) instead of cocoa (roasted cacao beans). Combine pure cacao powder, acne-safe nut milk, and a bit of sweetener if desired. High quality cacao offers high levels of antioxidants and caffeine, which may surprise you. Some people drink it as a sweet pick-me-up treat during the day or at night to help relax their adrenals, promoting good sleep. Try it out and see how best you can fit it into your regime.

Haldi Doodh, as it's known in India (referencing where the drink originates), popularly known in the West as golden milk or turmeric lattes, are made up of the very same spices that may be in your pantry. Blending powdered turmeric, ginger, cinnamon, clove, and black pepper with some honey, acne-safe milk, and hot water is delightful. Diasporaco.com is a good, ethical source of Indian spices.

"Bulletproof" (fill in the blank). You can technically "bulletproof" anything, even if the traditional Bulletproof is made with coffee. Introduced to the mass US market by entrepreneur Dave Asprey, who traveled to Tibet and was inspired by their yak butter tea drinks, the idea is to blend up your nut milk and beverage of choice (matcha, turmeric, cacao) with grass-fed butter (or ghee) and MCT oil to create a satisfying, relatively high-protein drink that will keep you satiated, focused, and caffeinated without the crash, thanks to the brain-loving butter/ghee and MCT fats.

Many clients were able to successfully reintegrate coffee back into their diets without breaking out (but only after clearing up completely). In order to reintroduce it, start slowly with plain black coffee with perhaps acne-safe milk to begin with. See how your skin does with a new variation over a month's time. If you jump right back into drinking lattes with cow's milk and start breaking out—you won't know if it was the coffee or that milk that did it.

Acne-causing Foods – Secondary Triggers

These foods may not be the primary foods that break people out per se, but they can certainly make existing acne worse. You may be able to get away with a little bit of these foods, but too much of them may pose a problem.

For some folks who are super sensitive by nature or have compromised immune/digestive systems (like Candida yeast or eczema and psoriasis), these foods can flare symptoms because of their inherent inflammatory nature and/or how they are processed.

Most folks are able to clear up from just abstaining from the above, but if you have a very high inflammatory response or just aren't seeing results (inflammation isn't getting better or clarity isn't coming) from abstaining from the above primary offenders (and doing all the topical things like your regimen and icing), consider cutting out the following foods for one to three months to see what happens. If it doesn't help, your acne case may be indicative of a more serious underlying health condition that should be assessed by a proper medical doctor or practitioner.

Sugars and Other High Glycemic Foods

High glycemic foods are closely linked to acne in several cases I had in the clinic as they increase the body's inflammatory response—so whenever possible, eat as low glycemic as you can. Sugars include not only the sweet stuff, both natural (sugar cane, fruit) and the highly processed fake stuff (artificial sweeteners, high fructose corn syrup) but also simple, quick-to-digest carbohydrates like white rice and pasta.

All sugar is inflammatory. Refined white cane sugar is one of the worst as it robs minerals like copper, magnesium, and calcium from your bones to process through the liver. Many agave brands have been proven to be mislabeled and sold as such but are actually corn syrup (which is just as high glycemic as white sugar). Other healthier sugars derived from alternative sources like beets, yacon, honey, coconut, and dates are much better because they contain beneficial enzymes and minerals but should still be consumed in moderation. All sugars—refined or not—elevate blood glucose and inflammatory levels.

Some sugar should be tolerated just fine by healthy bodies; however, if you feel your sensitivity is very high, then you may have a digestive flora imbalance that you'll want to investigate further. We have seen extreme reactions in those with a Candida yeast imbalance.

Choose organic whole grains like barley, quinoa, brown rice, buckwheat, and pasta made from these grains. Try dried stevia leaf (it ideally should be green, not bleached white) or other lower glycemic sweeteners like yacon, monk fruit, coconut, or date sugars instead of cane or fake sugars. Try eating fruit as the main or only sugar in your diet. Keep in mind that whole, unprocessed grains are digested by the body more slowly than pasta (which is already ground up and broken down for you—learn more about refined and processed grains coming up next). Look at labels and choose ones with no added sugar.

Artificial sweeteners

We recommend completely avoiding artificial sweeteners; they are nothing more than chemically synthesized chemicals that disrupt the body's endocrine receptors. To date, there have been no long-term studies to confirm the safety of these newly developed sweeteners, but many have reported negative symptoms associated with these products, including migraines, digestive issues, and skin irritation.

Fake sweeteners like saccharin, aspartame, sucralose, xylitol, and erythritol all have many negative side effects and can disrupt the natural flora of the digestive system, resulting in more serious digestive and skin sensitivity issues (along with scandalous political backstories—look them up! Search: Donald Rumsfeld, Dr. Arthur Hull Hayes Jr. and FDA approval, Monsanto, GD Searle[28]).

Natural sugars in fruit

Fruit is an important part of a balanced diet, but fresh or dried, can also be a major source of inflammatory sugar. Dried fruit can and often does have the same amount of sugar as candy bars. Consider combining dried fruit with a healthy fat like nuts to help balance the sugar rush. Our blog post[29] and informational website *The Paleo Diet*[30] has helpful articles on fruit sugar content.

Most healthy digestive systems should be able to tolerate refined/processed grains and nightshades, but some with really difficult-to-control inflamed acne cut these out, and they saw positive results. Once they were clear, they were able to reintroduce these foods safely because they had little to no seeds in their pores to get inflamed.

Clear Skin for Everyone

Fresh Fruits	total sugar (g)
apples	13.3
apricots	9.3
avocado	0.9
banana	15.6
blackberries	8.1
blueberries	7.3
cantaloupe	8.7
casaba melon	4.7
cherries, sweet	14.6
cherries, sour	8.1
elderberries	7,0
figs	6.9
grapefruit, pink	6.2
grapefruit, white	6.2
grapes	18.1
guava	6,0
guava, strawberry	6,0
honeydew melon	8.2
jackfruit	8.4
kiwi fruit	10.5
lemon	2.5
lime	0.4
marney apple	6.5
mango	14.8
nectarine	8.5
orange	9.2
papaya	5.9
peach	8.7
pear	10.5
pineapple	11.9
plum	7.5
pomegranate	10.1
purple passion fruit	11.2
raspberries	9.5
starfruit	7.1
strawberries	5.8
tangerine	7.7
tomato	2.8
watermelon	9,0

Dried Fruits	total sugar (g)
dates	64.2
dried apricots	38.9
dried figs	62.3
dried mango	73
dried papaya	53.5
dried peaches	44.6
dried pears	49
dried prunes	44
raisins	65
raisins, golden	70.6
zante currants	70.6

Pure Sugars	total sugar (g)
brown sugar	89.7
high fructose corn syrup (42)	71
high fructose corn syrup (55)	77
high fructose corn syrup (90)	80
honey	81.9
maple sugar	85.2
molasses	60
sorghum syrup	65.7
sucrose (table sugar)	97

Candy	total sugar (g)
almond joy	44.9
baby ruth	42
bit o honey	42.4
butterfinger	48.8
caramello candy bar	54.2
hard candy	62.3
hershey's kisses	50
junior mints	82.2
lifesavers	66.5
m & m chocolate candy	64.7
milk duds	50
nestle 100 grand candy bar	63.5
nestle crunch candy bar	52.4
nestle plain milk chocolate can	51
nestle raisinets	62.5
reese's pieces	50
skittles	76.4

Grams of sugar per 100 grams. Source: https://thepaleodiet.com/fruits-and-sugars/

Refined and Processed Grains

Extruded grains are grains that have been highly processed with heat and pressure to form a paste that is easily formed in shapes like flakes and "o's," so commonly found in breakfast cereals and pasta. This long, high-heat processing strips the originally nutritious whole grain of fiber and nutrients, which is why manufacturers 'enrich' these products with synthetic vitamins and minerals that are unrecognizable to the body. Furthermore, the body digests these very finely ground grains extremely quickly, effectively treating them like sugars—raising inflammation.

Instead, choose low-sugar granola or whole grain porridges, batches of which can be prepared at the beginning of the week. Porridge can be slow-cooked or soaked in the refrigerator overnight and be ready for morning consumption. Any whole grain will work—steel-cut oats, barley, quinoa, brown rice, amaranth, teff, buckwheat, etc. Choose whole-grain pasta when you can.

Nightshade Vegetables and Fruit

If you're having a particularly hard time fighting inflammation, looking into removing more inflammatory foods could be an option. While not triggers for most people, research has shown that a low-glycemic diet that avoids nightshades (tomatoes, potatoes, peppers, eggplant, goji berries) and has little to no gluten or grains can combat inflammation. Paleo AIP (auto-immune protocol) is an easy guideline to follow that avoids foods that trigger inflammatory responses in those with auto-immune disorders.

High-Androgen Foods

Dr. Fulton says that foods high in androgen (similar to peanuts) increase oil production, and eating enough of these foods will lead to more oil, translating to more acne.

The following foods might not only increase androgen and testosterone levels in the skin (that induce oiliness) but have been known to also trigger hormonal diagnoses like PCOS. Try reducing your consumption of these foods (along with sugars and refined grains), especially if you have other hormonal imbalance symptoms present (PCOS, very oily skin, hirsutism): peanuts, peanut butter and foods cooked in peanut oil; high amounts of red meat, turkey and organ meats; vegetable, soybean, corn, canola, wheat germ, and cottonseed cooking oils.

Iodides

If your diet contains too many iodides, these will often flush out of the body through the skin in the form of an inflamed and itchy rash. Although this sensitivity and reaction to iodides are not a problem for most, I saw it often enough in the clinic that I think it is worth mentioning.

Do your best to keep to a minimum (or avoid) all obviously high-iodine foods, including seaweeds (kelp, spirulina, algae, carrageenan), iodized salt, and "green" protein powders, drinks, or supplements. Less obvious sources include molasses, sports and energy drinks, meal replacement bars, multivitamins (listed as potassium iodide or iodine), shellfish (shrimp, clams, crab, mussels, etc.), saltwater fish (tuna, cod, mackerel, sardines, etc.), and cured deli meats.

Bromine and other bromides can behave similarly to iodides and can be found in many pesticides used on strawberries and other fruits (another reason to buy local and organic and to wash your produce before eating), dough conditioners in mass-produced and shelf-stable bread and pastries, and in cold medicines.

Topically, hot-tub detergents and chemicals in swimming pools contain iodides as a disinfecting agent. Applying a layer of shea butter or petroleum jelly as a barrier onto the skin prior to swimming and then washing thoroughly afterward is a good approach.

Protein Powders

Eating whole natural foods is always the best choice, but we understand some need extra supplementation that's easy and shelf stable. Green powders that contain ocean algaes and seaweeds can cause iodide acne, and the protein itself can cause digestive issues and inflammatory acne, as seen in one of our case study clients.

CASE STUDY: Protein powder-induced acne

We had a very active vegan client with a complicated case. About 40% of his face was broken out, 90% of which were very stubbornly inflamed (and impossible to extract), accompanied by a case of candida yeast imbalance. As his gluten-free protein options decreased after cutting out soy, he leaned heavily on protein powders to fuel his vigorous workouts. As his exercise activity decreased, he eventually replaced the powders with whole natural foods. With these diet and lifestyle changes, some candida-control implementation and regular treatments, we were able to clear his skin dramatically.

He successfully maintained his clarity after moving away, but months later started breaking out again. The only lifestyle change he made was taking those seemingly acne-safe protein powders again. He then discovered a third-party research study showing the particular brand he used was found to have very high levels of toxic heavy metals. After sharing his success story of working with us on social media, many others came forward with similar protein powder and acne-related stories.

Instead of prepared protein powders, try making your own. Mixing simple, non-processed ingredients such as psyllium husk, acne-safe nuts, seeds (chia, flax, sunflower, etc.), cacao and/or freeze dried berries work well. Prepping other ingredients (preferably cooked for easier digestion) like whole grains (brown rice, buckwheat, quinoa, etc.), nutrient-dense greens, peas, beans or winter squashes then combined with fruit will make whole food smoothies that are easier for your body to digest, assimilate nutrients from while keeping your skin its clearest.

If you must consume protein powders, find a soy-, sea vegetable-, dairy-, and whey-free one. Sea vegetables include things like seaweed, algae, spirulina, and many others with many different names. Be diligent with checking ingredients, especially if your powders are green. There are many seemingly acne-safe protein powders on the market; however, we strongly suggest you avoid these powders as best you can, and stick to whole, natural foods.

Sweets

There are *so many* new nut-based ice creams on the market worth trying; just watch out for coconut oil, soy, carrageenan, and high amounts of sugar. Try to find something that's made locally and in small batches. Chances are that the ingredients smaller bakeries use are of higher quality with fewer additives and fillers used.

Look for paleo style, dairy-, soy- and carrageenan-free frozen desserts in the freezer aisle of your natural health food store. Fruit sorbets and "nice cream" (blended frozen bananas) are a good choice instead of traditional dairy ice cream, but again, watch the sugar.

Chocolate is fine so long as it's dark and milk-free. It's the milk chocolate's dairy (and higher amounts of sugar than in the dark chocolate) that you want to avoid. The higher the percentage, the darker the chocolate, and the less inflammatory sugar is present. Cacao is more nutritious than cocoa.

Most baked goods contain dairy, and if commercially produced, they likely contain soy as well. Try to find ones made from whole grains like sourdough, whole wheat, buckwheat, quinoa, almond, or coconut flour.

How to Eat Out

Eating out is inevitable, and by knowing how to navigate menus and getting comfortable advocating for yourself, you'll have the best chances of eating acne-safe. By cooking at home, you have more control over the ingredients you are using and will gain an awareness of how dishes at restaurants are prepared. Although dairy and soy are more easily visible (and avoided) on restaurant menus, the cooking oils are harder to navigate around. With acne, aggravators accumulate and become a culmination of all factors adding up to the acne equation. Treating acne-causing foods like allergies can be helpful as your server guides you through the menu. To make it easy, just ask to avoid the two biggest aggravators (and food allergens): dairy and soy.

General guidelines for acne-safe eating include:

- Minimizing fried foods (because of the often acne-causing oil used; share this dish as an appetizer versus having it on your own as your entree)
- Ask for sauces and dressings on the side.
- Vegetable oil (composed of various, usually inflammatory and acne-causing sources) is probably the most commonly used oil in restaurants, so choose foods that are not super greasy or ask for little to no oil.
- Asian cuisines tend to use a lot of soy sauce, soy products, prepared sauces and sugar.
- Italian, French, and American cuisines use a lot of dairy and refined white flour.
- Fresh, local, natural foods simply prepared are best—seasonal vegetables, salads, local meats and catches of the day. Mediterranean cuisine, avoiding dairy, is a good choice.
- Aim for grilled, roasted, poached, steamed, or braised dishes or sauteed in acne-safe oil.

~ Eat local and organic at small, locally owned restaurants, avoiding chain restaurants (and their frozen, processed, genetically modified foods) as much as possible.

Medications and Nutritional Supplements

Many prescription medications and supplements are known acne aggravators and creators. We have seen clients break out from drugs, medications, and supplements, both prescription and over-the-counter.

They don't necessarily appear as extractable acne but are often mistakenly referred to as such nonetheless. In conventional medical terms, this acne-like reaction is called *acneiform drug eruptions* or papulopustular eruptions, drug-induced folliculitis, and drug-induced acne. The treatment recommended for these types of reactions is to stop the drug if possible and treat the skin the same as you would regular acne, with or without the typical, conventional acne prescriptions (benzoyl peroxide, antibiotics, retinoids, oral antibiotics, or oral isotretinoin).

Here is a list of types we've seen affect our clients' acne as a side effect of taking a drug or supplement. Drug-related cases that we have personally seen in clinic are notated with a double asterisk (**). A more comprehensive list of drugs known to induce these reactions from *dermnetnz.org* follows.[31]

Prescription Medications

Birth Control**

Regardless of the type, effects on the skin over the three- to six-month acclimation period (both getting on or off a medication) are to be expected and observed. Some, like the birth control pill (BCP), require precise dosage for best results; methods like the hormone shot or implants don't require daily attention. Avoiding prescription birth control and using condoms is the most acne-safe way to go.

If you're traveling for the short term (less than one month), keep taking the medications according to your home time zone if you can. Disruptions in manually manipulated hormone levels (as with the Pill) can drastically affect the skin, so take it at the same exact time daily on a twenty-four-hour basis to prevent breakouts as much as possible.

Oral Contraceptives**

In terms of acne, pills seem to have a higher margin of error that results in fluctuating hormone levels because taking the pills even an hour off the regularly scheduled time would be enough to see the skin change. Even worse is when a pill is entirely missed and then is (often) doubled up the next dose.

There are so many different types of pills, but the common thought process among professionals is that drugs high in testosterone or androgens are more likely to cause more oil production and thus acne reactions, whereas estrogen-heavy ones dry out the skin (theoretically resulting in less acne).

Choose one that has the lowest number of hormones possible, being very good about taking the pill at the exact same time each day, and hope for the best. Expect some changes to happen to the body and hope that acne isn't one that persists past the three- to six-month acclimation period.

Hormone Shots**

Some of our clients have gotten hormone shots, and though it does require less day-to-day maintenance, there are some acne-related effects. These clients noticed an immediate uptick in acne the week or two following the shot, which eventually tapered off a week or two after the hormone levels reset from that spike.

IUD**

Once inserted, there is no daily precise management to manage. If given a choice, the copper Paragard IUD is preferable over the Mirena one, which contains hormones. The Paragard lasts for ten years and inherently has no hormones in it. The Mirena lasts for five years and has hormones that are slowly secreted into the body over time. Although the Paragard is "hormone-free," it's still shifting your body's own "normal" hormone balance, so expect some acclimation symptoms, of which acne may be one.

Hormone Replacement Therapy and Gender Affirming Drug Treatment

See *Section 3, The 5 Types of Hormone Stress Responsible for Acne.*

Antidepressants**

These medications can have some skin side effects. Some can dry you out, so you'll need to stay hydrated internally and externally. Some can increase your energy, which can affect getting enough quality sleep, inducing

Section 5 - The Digestive System, Diet and Acne

inflammation and breakouts. Some can cause sweating, which can be stressful, and thus are inflammatory and breakout-inducing. There's a fine balance between getting what chemical help your brain needs and seeing how it'll affect your skin. If your medications are affecting your skin, talk with your doctor to discuss options.

Halogens (Iodides and Bromides, Often Found in Thyroid Medications and Kelp Supplements)**

Too much iodine in the body flushes out of the skin, resulting in a red and often itchy mask-like rash on the face. This can be accompanied by acne. Going through the acne-clearing protocol and abstaining from eating iodide-rich supplements and foods can help them clear up.

Allergy and Cold Medicines**

These often contain potassium iodide, which helps to thin the mucus and loosen congestion in the throat and chest, acting as an expectorant or a sedative to get a better night's sleep. Allergy medicines, in a quest to dry up excess mucus in the body, can also dry out the skin.

Other Medications

(See *Section 2, Acne Look-alikes and Acneiforms*)

- Immunosuppressants (specifically Prednisone**, azathioprine, cyclosporin, and sirolimus)
- Anticonvulsants
- Lithium** taken in high amounts has been found in the skin, suggesting that it can accumulate there and result in the occurrence of follicular and cystic acne eruptions.
- Epidermal growth factor receptor inhibitors (EGFRIs) like sirolimus. The mechanical cause is unclear, but it appears that the effects of these drugs cause the skin to undergo apoptosis, a kind of self-destruction of the cell, which causes blisters and inflamed pustules to form.

Vitamins and Supplements**

Vitamins

Check the ingredients for acne-causing ingredients like iodides, especially softgel vitamin capsules, as these are often made of or filled with soybean oil.

CASE STUDY: Soybean-oil based supplements

I had a male client who we were able to get almost all clear, but his jawline kept breaking out. I was concerned about his stress levels (as stress acne often occurs here), but he assured me he was a pretty chill guy and wasn't at all stressed out. After much questioning, I found out that he was taking supplements, and when I looked up the ingredients, I saw that they were filled with soybean oil! Once he stopped taking those, he cleared up and didn't need to come back for treatment.

*Vitamin B***

Vitamin B complex supplements are often marketed as hair, skin, and nail growth boosters and can also be great for supporting the stress response in the body. However, some people will break out from taking too much. Stopping the supplement, allowing the body to detox the excess, and then slowly working it back into their regimen at a more reasonable amount can be a way to take care of this type of vitamin-induced acne. *Dermnetnz.org* specifically cites B1, B6, and B12.

*Steroids***

These are not birth control but can contain and affect hormones like birth control pills do. Often taken long-term as a prescription for auto-immune disease (like eczema, allergies, or organ transplant maintenance) or for athletes looking to gain more muscle, these are definitely to be avoided as much as possible not only for their acne-causing tendencies but also for the plethora of very dangerous side effects. Dermnetnz.org cites that they may specifically affect the sebaceous glands and specifically mention adrenocorticotropic hormone (ACTH), androgens, and systemic corticosteroids.

Caffeine, Drugs, Alcohol, Smoking, and Chemicals

Take care. We want your body to prioritize healing versus detoxing. But if you must indulge in some partying, prepare your body by resting, eating, and hydrating well before, during, and after, and enjoy the highest quality libations you can find.

Your immune system can only take so much, so too many things piled up (changing seasons, poor diet, emotional stress, lack of sleep, travel) on top of an intense acne treatment, especially while hung over, may send your immune system over the edge, resulting in a cold, making your skin worse, or other complications.

Smoking

All kinds, but especially cigarettes, cause the skin to thin and blood vessels to dilate, making it more difficult for the skin to heal and clear. Although all types of smoking are not good for optimal health, vaping *could* be the acne-safer choice versus smoking something that is actively burning in your face, forming carcinogens that release free radicals onto your face, eyes, and lungs. Get some topical antioxidants and SPF on your skin to help create a protective barrier against the actual smoke particles that will touch your skin, and do some cardio exercises and deep breathing regularly to counterbalance the lung damage. In TCM, lung and skin health are connected, influenced by, and reflective of each other.

Endnotes

26   *https://www.squattypotty.com/*

27   *https://www.drweil.com/diet-nutrition/food-safety/is-carrageenan-safe/*

28   *https://www.huffpost.com/entry/donald-rumsfeld-and-the-s_b_805581*

29   *https://withandwithin.co/blogs/blog/low-sugar-fruits-glycemic-index*

30   *https://thepaleodiet.com/fruits-and-sugars/*

31   *https://dermnetnz.org/*

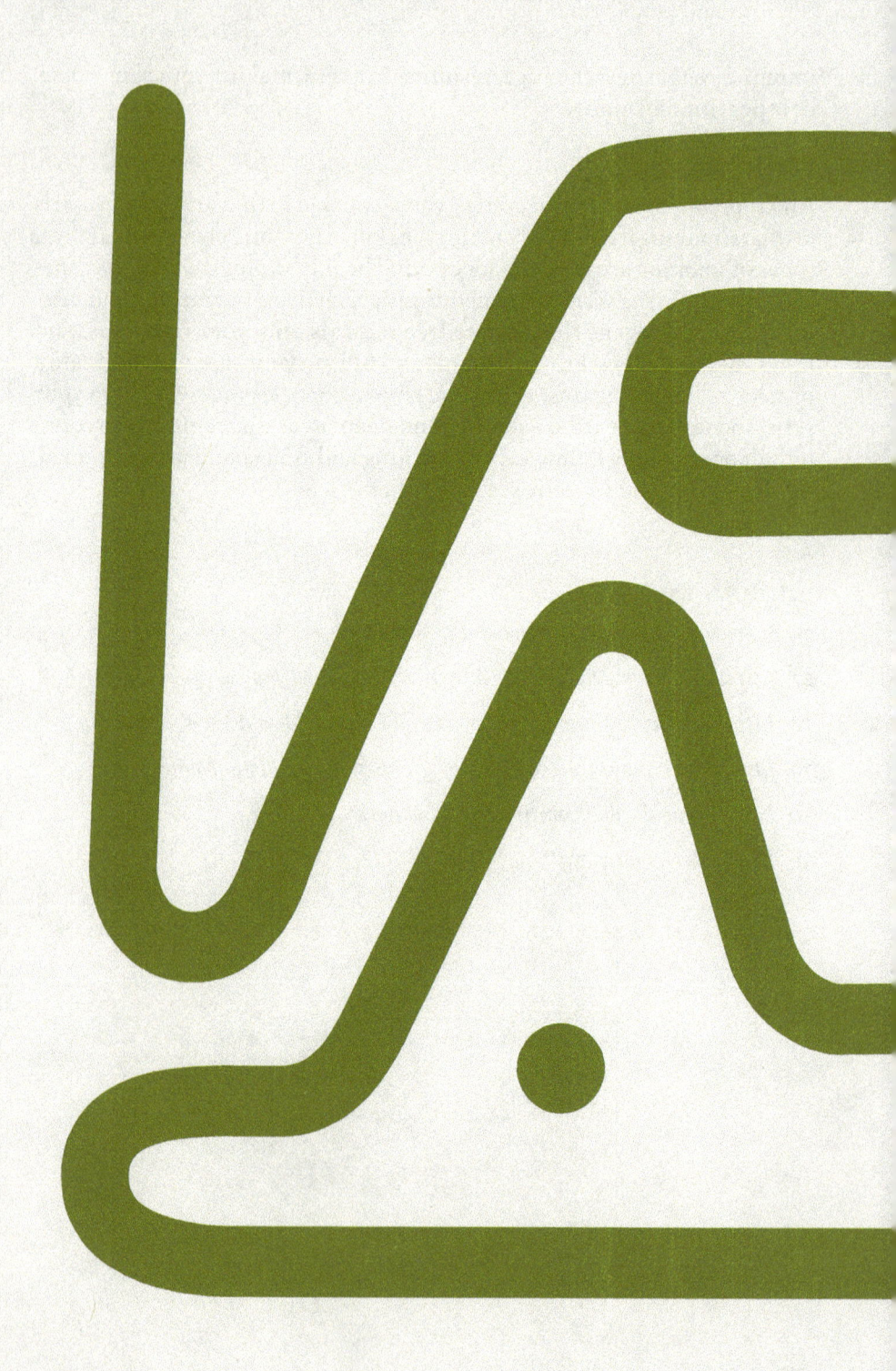

SECTION 6

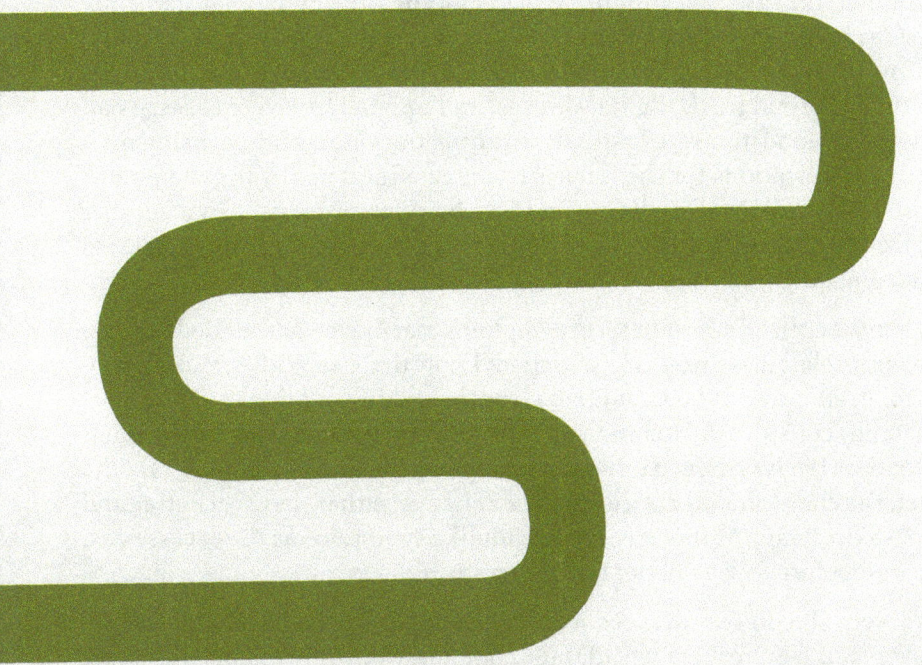

Candida

Though our in-clinic success rate was incredibly high, there were a few that, even with diligent compliance, we weren't able to clear using the With & Within method alone. We found many of these clients had a Candida yeast imbalance, which was holding them back from clear skin.

Even if Candida isn't an issue for you, the knowledge shared in this section is still beneficial if you're looking to strengthen your anti-inflammatory lifestyle. I'll share what we've learned about it and how you can combat it based on our clinical observations.

What is Candida?

Candida albicans is a fungus (yeast is a type of fungus) that naturally resides in the digestive system. When we expose our body to things that throw off its natural balance, this Candida yeast overgrows and colonizes in the intestinal tract, vagina, sinuses, and tongue. In severe cases, it can enter the bloodstream, eventually invading the whole body, causing multiple complications for the intricately intertwined bodily organ systems within. This all involves the gut and liver being compromised by a number of factors (including heavy prescription medication use) and can get real bad, real quick.

When we noticed a certain set of symptoms that looked or sounded fungus- or yeast-related, we would let the client know that the With & Within protocol itself may not be enough to clear their skin, and then we'd suggest that they consult a doctor and/or try the Candida diet to see if it helps their situation. If it was indeed Candida-related, within the first few weeks of the diet, the client should notice a marked change: either they feel better and their skin clears, or they experience flu-like symptoms as the excess yeast dies off before feeling better and clearing up.

We were able to see several clients successfully through the protocol we developed from others we adapted, but a few of these clients didn't get better and had to see functional holistic doctors for a more thorough evaluation, testing, and treatment. In these cases, Candida overgrowth was only a small part of the larger underlying issue.

How is Candida Contracted?

Candida albicans is already present in our body's digestive system. The problem occurs when overgrowth in the body's digestive flora is disrupted, causing the immune system to become vulnerable.

Chronic stress, prescription medications, overprocessed and sugar-containing foods, combined with poor air and water quality all weigh in on lowering our immune systems, making way for Candida yeast overgrowth. These all promote (or are caused in part by) a condition called "leaky gut" that affects the digestive tract and/or an overtaxed liver (where all toxins in the body are processed).

We often see clients with a history of months or years of regular prescription usage, including birth control and antibiotics. Antibiotics work by killing off most of the bacteria in the body – both good and bad – eventually disabling the body's powerhouse, the digestive system. Our guts need good bacteria (probiotics) and enzymes to properly break down food, assimilate nutrients, and dispose of the body's waste. The gut's deficiency in probiotics and enzymes is why it is so common that clients who have been on these drugs for so long eventually end up also suffering from digestive issues.

Antibiotics and other chemicals can also enter the body by way of conventionally raised food-producing farm animals, as 70-80% of antibiotics manufactured annually in the US are sold for use in raising them. Eating a highly processed diet of packaged and fast foods, sugars, and lots of caffeine (especially in coffee, decaf included) combined with a fast-paced or stressful lifestyle can throw off our body's natural, stable, immune-fighting flora.

How Candida Presents

Candida's Physical Symptoms

Commonly associated with Candida overgrowth is general digestive *dis-ease*, including constipation, indigestion, bloating, gas, diarrhea, irregular bowel movements (long and formed every day is ideal), and abdominal pain, to name a few.

Recurring infections are very common with this condition, especially vaginal yeast and urinary tract infections. Dr. Thomas Anstett is a naturopathic doctor I met through the Trinity School of Natural Health who helped me create the With & Within Candida protocol. He reported that in his practice's Candida patients, chronic sinus and upper respiratory issues were way more bothersome than the frequent yeast infections that occur in women. We saw both symptomatic types in the skin clinic, but vaginal and urinary tract infections were more prevalent. A lowered immune system (do you get sick a lot or have intense allergies?) and extreme sensitivity to things like scents and smoke are also symptoms. General bodily discomfort, such as fatigue, muscle aches or weakness, headaches, and pain and swelling in the joints, can also show up. And of course, the body's largest organ, the skin, is also affected.

Stubborn and itchy rashes, eczema, irritation especially within the folds of the skin, general itching, and redness/swelling of the genitals are also common. Oral thrush can pop up: a thick, white coat or lacy-looking spots on red "bases" inside the mouth and throat that are not easily wiped away; not to mention the super stubborn acne that persists, even with super-faithful protocol adherence! We found this acne to occur as stubborn acne that frequently appeared on the forehead, temples, and around the mouth.

Candida yeast thrives on sugar, so anything we eat that turns into sugar, whether sweet to taste like candy or simple carbs like white flour or rice, will feed its growth. It's no wonder that those afflicted with the imbalance tend to have intense sugar, carb, alcohol, and dairy cravings. We may think that we are craving these foods, but it's actually the yeast that wants them.

Candida's Psychological Symptoms

The Candida-inflicted often report brain fog, feeling "spacey" or "unreal," poor memory, an inability to focus, extreme mood swings, irritability, panic attacks, outbursts of anger or crying spells, anxiety, and depression. If you are pretty healthy and take good care of yourself but still feel terrible, there may be an underlying condition that needs to be addressed.

Other Candida Approaches

Conventional Medicine Stance on Candida

Often, Candida is regarded by doctors mostly as a skin condition, and only if there is a white, lacy rash present on the tongue (thrush) or within the folds of the skin (under the breasts, underarms, genitals, between the fingers, middle of the body), irregardless of the plethora of other symptoms mentioned above. The most common approach is to prescribe various topical and oral anti-fungal medications like Fluconazole which often will temporarily improve the condition, but not completely eradicate it, resulting in recurrence.

Ayurveda Stance on Candida

The state of aggravated (or too much) vata in Ayurvedic medicine is caused by insufficient water or fiber, lack of exercise, heavy meat eating, and other factors, says Dr. Vasant Lad. According to the book *Home Doctor, Natural Healing with Herbs, Condiments and Spices* by Dr. P.S. Phadke, constipation may also cause pimples, acne, acidity, ulcers in the mouth, disturbed sleep and heartburn, and in some cases, depression. Taking the digestive cornerstone combination Triphala herbs (Amalaki or Emblica officinalis; Bibhitaki or Terminalia bellirica, and Haritaki or Terminalia chebula), teas made of cardamom, coriander, licorice root, and/or roasted fennel seeds right out of your spice cabinet can help indigestion and flatulence.

TCM Stance on Candida

Traditional Chinese Medicine says that excess heat, insufficient water or fiber, and inefficient functioning of the stomach and spleen disrupt the digestive process, which precludes proper elimination. Warm or hot water throughout the day and nuts and seeds such as almonds, walnuts, pine nuts, pistachios, and black sesame seeds are important to take. Also, the following are not considered Candida-safe in Western protocols, but they are acne-safe in moderation: sweet and moisturizing fruits such as peaches, apricots, pears, and figs.

How to Get it Under Control

With input from Dr. Anstett and by experimenting with different clients over the years, we were able to create a modified acne-safe version of his Candida cleanse program with good results. The cleanse consists of three main parts: 1) Eating a low-glycemic diet, preferably organic and home-cooked with little to no sugars or simple carbs to starve the Candida yeast; 2) Taking herbs to kill off excess yeast and fungus associated with the Candida; and 3) Emphasizing robust elimination (bowel movements) to physically remove the accumulated yeast, fungi, and other toxins from the intestinal tract where they thrive. Taking great care of and resting the body and mind is essential to allow the body to prioritize detoxing and healing during this time.

Support

Although this stricter detox cleansing protocol is temporary, it's always our hope that you'll fold parts of it into your daily "regular" life based on how good you feel when you do these very things. Before you get over the hump, it can be challenging, especially when it seems everyone around you gets to eat what they want without any ill effects (that you can see). Let your community know what you're embarking on, as you may very well find buddies to do the cleanse with. Cheer yourself on and mentally prepare yourself for the weeks ahead, holding fast to your goals of healthier, clearer-skinned living. You will probably slip and that's okay. Just get back up and keep going.

Research the Condition and its Symptoms

Part of the preparation process is to start educating yourself on what Candida is and learning what to expect, along with the dos and don'ts of a successful Candida cleanse. Becoming familiar with what the cleanse entails will help gently ease you into the transition, allowing you to start being conscious of what changes will be needed on your end for a good outcome.

Learning about the common symptoms of Candida yeast overgrowth would be the first step. Write down a list of symptoms you're experiencing, how you hate having to deal with them and how it's impacted your quality of life.

Next, visualize how amazing it will be to be symptom-free: no more yeast or urinary tract infections, lots of energy, the creativity and productivity of a clear mind, and the confidence of going out *sans* makeup with your newly clear skin.

Herbal Supplementation for the Cleanse

While changing your diet will starve the excess Candida yeast, the right herbal supplements will help facilitate their elimination from the body. Doing the cleanse alongside herbs and encouraging robust elimination is necessary for success.

Dr. Thomas Anstett recommends Can-Sol, an herbal tincture, to be taken in conjunction with the diet. The formula contains greasewood, purple loosestrife, and white pond lily, all ingredients known in traditional American herbal medicine that promote healthy digestive flora. We sold it in tincture form because of the inherent potent efficacy of tinctures versus capsules, but it is also available in capsules to make them easier to tote around. He also says there are a lot of Candida cleanse kits on the market and that most of them are ineffective because of their purity, potency, formulation, or dosage. Pure Herbs Ltd., the Michigan-based manufacturer of Can-Sol, is the one he trusts and uses in his own practice. When combined with the rest of the With & Within clearing protocol, our clients generally have had good success so long as they put in the effort, exercised patience, and there were no other underlying imbalances present.

Donna Gates, nutritional consultant and founder of The Body Ecology Diet, says her go-to herbs include turmeric root, oregano leaf, pau d'arco bark, garlic bulbs, peppermint leaf, fennel seed, and echinacea root. She also says that they are much more effective when fermented and sells them as such on her website (along with many other supplements).

I've also heard anecdotal success with taking oregano oil but haven't tested this out to see how well it works. There are plenty of herbal Candida-cleansing supplements on the market, so take some time to research to get a better understanding of the situation. All herbal medicines, though, are usually best used in combination with several others taken several times a day while emphasizing cleansing the body and digestive tract for maximum efficacy.

Hydration for the Cleanse

Detoxing is heavy work on the body, and the more water you drink, the better shape your organs will be to facilitate the cleanup. It'll also help with the purging process, as you'll be flushing out toxins with every trip to the bathroom.

Make it a point to drink fresh filtered drinking water (distilled water was recommended by Dr. Anstett and many other health experts for detoxing and cleansing) and herbal teas. All other beverages are out—yes, even coffee. This will be a difficult adjustment for some, mostly because the yeast has likely been thriving on your consumption of it this whole time. Because of this, you may experience some die-off symptoms (which will be explained shortly).

A trick I love is drinking sparkling water with just one drop of citrus essential oil (it surprisingly tastes a lot like fruit soda) or an herbal tincture (it tastes like a light beer, honestly). It's super refreshing, especially on a hot day or after a rich meal. Do take note of how your body does with the carbonated water; some people with delicate digestive systems may do better with non-carbonated and/or warm, instead.

Detoxing Die-off

At some point during the cleanse (usually within the first week or two) you may experience "die-off" symptoms, or sugar withdrawals. As you starve the yeast, it releases toxic byproducts into your system that can cause symptoms ranging from sweating to headaches to fatigue to a full-on cold or flu-like symptoms. If this happens, don't stop! It simply means that the cleanse is working, and your body is ridding itself of the yeast. Try to take it as easy as possible and be extra gentle with yourself. Carve out extra time to rest and relax, drink lots of water and sweat (Epsom salt baths, steam, sauna) to help facilitate the detox. This phase should pass in a few days.

The Acne-safe Candida Cleanse

Prepare

Food Mindset

The Candida cleanse diet is pretty close to the acne-safe diet, just a bit more refined. The goal of this specific cleanse is to eliminate sugar and foods that turn into sugar, to starve the excess Candida yeast. If you keep an open mind and explore different aisles of your grocery store (or different stores altogether), you'll find there are entire worlds of eating deliciously *and* Candida safely. Many of the ingredients found in traditional and indigenous cooking around the world are actually healing and detoxing for the body, making them naturally perfect for acne- and Candida-safe eating.

Audit your Current Diet

Doing the same auditing, research, and prepping for the Candida cleanse as you did at the beginning of your acne-safe journey will set you up for success. A really important part of the preparation process is to compare your current diet against an acne- and Candida-safe one. Determine what substitutions need to be made, learn what foods *are* safe to eat and find some recipes you'll want to try.

Food journaling your regular diet for a week or two will be helpful so that you can see what your baseline is and then determine what changes need to be made in order to make your diet both acne- and Candida-safe. Reviewing the acne-safe food dos and don'ts will help.

Research Alternatives and Recipes

Let's take coffee for example. If you drink it daily, find beverage alternatives to try while simultaneously weaning yourself off the coffee over the course of a week or two to avoid the cold turkey coffee crash. If you like oatmeal with fruit in the morning, might you experiment with other Candida-safe alternatives like oat bran or cañahua to make a savory bowl instead? If you like a creamy, dairy-laden ranch dressing on your salads, look up recipes on how to make it Candida-safe with coconut milk or choose lemon juice and apple cider vinegar-based vinaigrettes instead.

The cleanse will be much easier if you have a repertoire of go-to recipes, have your kitchen stocked with only acne- and Candida-safe choices, and have an on-the-go food setup that works for you so that you can always have acne- and Candida-safe food with you wherever you go. Or, have your list of restaurants and their Candida-safe meals and proposed modifications for easy ordering.

Purge Your Kitchen

I find it easiest to start any cleanse by purging my pantry and refrigerator of anything that's not "cleanse safe" and getting rid of the no-nos in two different ways: cold turkey or gradually in stages. Either way, it's going to be really helpful to keep your home "safe," so you aren't tempted to cheat! It'll be a lot easier to stick with the plan if all the choices you have in your space are safe to eat.

Ripping off the bandage and going cold turkey would be the fastest way. Everything that's not Candida-safe you can give away, donate to a local food bank, or toss.

The second approach would be to slowly wind down from your regular diet and replace your non-Candida-friendly food staples with "safe" things to ease the transition. This will buy you some time to work into detox mode without the rash abruptness (and possible stress) of the cold turkey method.

However, I don't suggest you wait until you go through your entire five-pound bags of wheat flour and sugar or that monster block of cheese you got on sale before you start this cleanse. The sooner you can get on the cleanse for real, the faster you'll be done with it.

See if you can observe how your body and mind feel after consuming these "no-nos." Doing so may bring to light symptoms you hadn't noticed before, helping you eliminate them more easily.

How to Grocery Shop

For specific foods to emphasize and avoid, check out our extended blog posts in our lifestyle library at withandwithin.co by searching "Candida." TheCandidaDiet.com and The Body Ecology Diet by Donna Gates are also good, long-standing, trusted sources. To keep things acne-safe, abstain from acne-causing foods like animal milk dairy (even if fermented), coconut oil, and sea vegetables (dulse, kelp, seaweeds, algaes), as too much of these may induce acne formation.

Local, Organic and Simple as Much as Possible

The point of the cleanse is to not only rid the excess Candida yeast from the gut, but also to avoid the very toxins like antibiotics, hormones and pesticides found in our food supply that contribute to the overgrowth to begin with. Overly processed foods also are a factor, metabolizing in the body similarly to sugar, while also often containing hidden ingredients. Shop at your local farmer's market and natural food stores as much as you can for the highest quality natural foods in peak season.

Fresh, Frozen or Dried Foods

When stocking your pantry, avoid canned foods and stick with fresh or frozen. Dehydrated food could be okay too, so long as they aren't laden with mysterious seasonings. Reconstitute these foods thoroughly and make sure to drink enough water to compensate.

Meats

Pork is reported to contain retroviruses and parasites that cannot be cooked out. However, I believe this to be true of any conventionally raised animal products, and the chances of consuming healthy meats are much higher when buying local, organic, wild, and/or pastured.

During the cleanse, try to buy only raw and fresh or frozen meat that's unseasoned. The seasonings in pre-made, preserved, pre-marinated, cured, smoked, processed, and seasoned vacuum-sealed meats likely contain ingredients you'll need to avoid for a successful Candida cleanse. Marinating at home can be okay so long as you're making the seasoning yourself from scratch, using Candida cleanse-friendly ingredients. This will be a perfect time to use herbs and spices for their medicinal properties *and* to create your own marinades, sausage spices, sauces, and flavorings to your liking.

Controversial candida and acne-safe foods

Dairy

Some health experts say fermented dairy like yogurt or kefir on the Candida cleanse is okay, but I've seen it still break clients out.

Coconut oil

Coconut oil is highly comedogenic when used topically, and it induces inflamed acne for some of my clients. It is purported to be high in caprylic acid, which is thought to be highly anti-fungal, thus supposedly effective against Candida.

Seaweed and kelp

Sea vegetables may be okay if you don't take enough of them to induce an iodide rash. Iodide reactions have been rare in my practice, but they are still something to watch out for and are relatively easy to spot. If you suspect one, cut out the iodine-rich food or supplement, continue to exfoliate the skin and it should clear up on its own in a few days or weeks.

Meal Prepping

Most Candida cleanse blogs and books will suggest that you cook your food fresh every meal, every day, to avoid the growth of mold and bacteria on your food. This is ideal, but is likely not practical for most. When cooking, make enough to last you two to three meals so that you don't have to cook from scratch every time it's time to eat. Or spend a few hours prepping ingredients that you can quickly cook or assemble for fresh meals each day.

Taking care to use high-quality ingredients, storing them immediately and properly, and eating them within a day or two should be fine—but see how this works for you. We want to avoid being caught starving on the go and then eating whatever food is in sight, which likely will not be the safest choice for your cleanse.

Balanced Meals

Ideally, with each meal, you'll want to eat enough to be satiated and energized but not so much that your digestive system has a hard time processing the food. Remember, we want your body to emphasize detoxing, not digesting. Aim for 25% protein, 25% Candida-cleanse-safe carbs if you need them (seeds, non-glutinous grains or starches) and the remaining 50% veggies. Red meat is okay to have, but you may want to emphasize lighter, easier-to-digest meats like chicken, fish, and eggs to promote the easiest and best elimination possible. Have a fermented veggie with each plate—a bite or two with breakfast and several bites for lunch and dinner. The probiotics will aid in digestion and populate your gut with the healthy bacteria it needs.

TIP: Satisfying soups and stews

Soups and stews are very nourishing and filling and can be a saving grace during the cleanse. They're actually very easy to make, are foolproof as they are very forgiving recipes, and are economical and efficient. Reheating soup makes for a very quick meal; you can pack a hot meal to go by using an insulated thermos with little effort or time.

You basically stir-fry a bunch of aromatics (garlic, onion, maybe ginger), veggies, and the meat of your choice, add water, and then season to taste with herbs or spice blends. If you have some veggie or bone broth, all the better to replace the water with. For stews, you can follow the same recipe, but you'll likely need less water or broth, and to simmer the meat a little longer, depending on what type you go with.

Find your Ideal Meals and Snacks

You'll want to make sure that you're eating enough and eating deliciously so that you feel satisfied after your meals, enabling you to focus on other aspects of your life. Finding your favorite simple meals and snacks you can easily fall back on will be a huge game changer, saving you a lot of time and stress.

Meal Plan Ideas

Cooking at home will be best, but check ingredients to make the best choices when shopping or eating out. Here are some food ideas to start with:

Seasoning blend ideas for all purposes, especially meatballs, meatloaf, stews, omelettes and soups:

- Italian: oregano, basil, garlic, rosemary, thyme, lemon, oil-cured black olives
- Chinese: coconut aminos, ginger, roasted sesame oil, ginger, and green onion, five-spice
- South Asian: tandoori, garam, or biryani masala blends, Ayurvedic recipes
- Southeast Asian: lemongrass, chili, galangal, turmeric, lime, makrut lime leaf, fish sauce, fermented shrimp, and fish pastes
- Ethiopian: *brundo.com* is an Oakland, California based supplier of high quality spices like berbere, abish (fenugreek) and korerima

(black cardamom) imported directly from Ethiopia; find recipe ideas on their site)
- Latin: homemade seasoning blends like sazon (coriander, cumin, achiote, garlic powder, oregano, salt & pepper) and adobo (garlic powder, oregano, salt, pepper, turmeric mixed with lemon juice and oil as a marinade)

Curries and herbs

So many cultures have so many curries, and most of them are rich with health benefits thanks to the potent spice blends' therapeutic effects. Southeast Asian (Malaysia, Singapore, Thailand, Myanmar) and South Asian (India, Sri Lanka) ones are my favorites. Many parts of Vietnam, Laos, Cambodia, and Thailand emphasize eating plenty of fresh herbs and vegetables, eaten with healthy doses of fermented chili, fish, and shrimp pastes. Explore the international section at your market or explore a new grocery store for more ideas.

Soups

- Vietnamese-inspired: simple soup of fish sauce, fish slices (or other protein), black pepper, spinach (or other leafy green), or pho (homemade, to omit sugar traditionally added)
- Malaysian/Singaporean-inspired: laksa (chicken and shrimp stock, curry paste, and coconut milk topped with fried shallots, fresh chili, beansprouts, and cilantro); there are many variations.
- Chinese: egg drop soup, West Lake soup (ground beef with lots of chopped cilantro)
- Filipino: sinigang (tamarind broth soup), bulalo (beef shank in clear broth), tinola (chicken and ginger)
- Thai inspired: tom yum (lemongrass, galangal, ginger & chili broth) or tom ka (same plus coconut milk)
- Simple: chicken, beef, or other bone broth-based soup
- Vegetable soups: cabbage, cauliflower, any leafy green, either chopped or blended
- Candida-safe porridge made from grains like buckwheat, millet, oat bran, quinoa, teff

Salads and lettuce cups

Any protein and fresh vegetables thrown together, in my opinion, counts as a salad. And most any protein can be wrapped in a lettuce leaf for a quick, Candida-safe meal snack or part of a meal.

Dressings

Apple cider vinegar, lemon, or lime and olive oil-based dressings will be the easiest staples, but you can satisfy the creamy cravings by making a Candida-safe mayonnaise as a base, then further customizing:

- Ranch: onion & garlic powder, chopped fresh chives, tarragon, oregano, basil, dill)
- Caesar: anchovies, lemon zest, garlic, mustard seeds, ground and toasted nuts
- Sesame ginger: roasted sesame oil and crushed seeds, coconut aminos, grated ginger, apple cider vinegar
- Citrus Mustard: lemon or lime juice and zest, mustard powder, black pepper
- Avocado Chili: blended avocado, chopped fresh chili, lemon or lime zest, garlic, or other herbs

Sauces

- Salmoriglio, salsa verde, any green pesto
- Cauliflower alfredo
- Pico de gallo
- Guacamole
- Ginger and green onion
- Fish sauce (sugar free) with fresh chili and garlic
- Romesco
- Red chili oil or chili crisp

Snacks

- Almond crackers, celery sticks, radishes, artichokes, asparagus
- Dips: eggplant, hummus (in moderation), garlic toum, homemade ranch, pesto, tapenades
- Naturally fermented foods like sauerkraut, kimchee, pickles made without vinegar
- Dehydrated kale chips
- Roasted garbanzo beans till crisp (in moderation)
- Nuts and seeds; roasted, dehydrated, butters and cracker forms
- Fried chicken or fish skin cracklings

Sweet

Candida-safe sweets are usually based on unsweetened coconut, lime, lemon, seeds, and nuts (not peanuts). Processed foods often contain fake sugars. Avoid them.

- Unsweetened coconut milk- or coconut cream-based drinks and desserts

- A spoonful of 100% nut butter with a sprinkle of salt (brings out the nuts' inherent sweetness)
- Herbal tea blends that are naturally sweet, like kava-kava, cinnamon, rooibos, ginger, licorice, orange and lemon peel, hibiscus
- A bowl of berries topped with coconut cream and toasted seeds, nuts
- Lemon or lime zest, juice
- Stevia may be used in moderation; look for one that's green in color

Eating Out

Eating out during the cleanse may be challenging and frustrating, but is sometimes inevitable and can still be enjoyable. Mediterranean restaurants are generally a good choice because most of their dishes are yeast-free and olive oil is the primary oil used. You can also go to a salad bar to pick your own food, or find a restaurant that serves high-quality ingredients like clean, local grass-fed beef or organic free-range chicken or wild fish.

The simplest approach is likely to ask for your proteins and veggies to be grilled, sautéed, or steamed with only olive oil, salt, pepper, garlic, onions, and fresh herbs. Substitute starchy sides like rice and potatoes with fresh or sautéed greens. I've had Candida-safe dinners at restaurants by requesting these modifications, and they were happy to oblige. At other restaurants, I've had burgers without the bun or condiments, and instead of fries, a side of sautéed green veggies or salad with some lemon wedges and olive oil as my dressing.

Learn how to look at a menu and reverse-engineer it to see what modifications can be made to make it Candida-friendly (cooking at home will help loads with this), or just have a talk with your server so they can help you figure out your options.

> ### TIP: If you don't cook or are vegetarian or vegan
>
> Following the Candida cleanse if you don't cook (most outside meals contain non-safe ingredients) or while vegan can be extremely challenging. Most vegan protein sources are too starchy (beans, hard squashes) or not acne-safe (soy). If you are going to go this route, soups and salads with LOTS of leafy green veggies, soups, and quinoa are going to be your staples.
>
> If you can integrate eggs and bone broth just while you're cleansing, this will help a lot. Beans should only be eaten sparingly (one to two times a week at max, no more than one-third cup each meal), and many of the Candida-safe recipes you'll find online

have garbanzo beans in them. Practice mindfulness and moderation with starchy foods like these.

Elimination – the Whole Point of the Cleanse

VERY IMPORTANT: Do your best and aim for two to three long and formed bowel movements a day to physically rid the excess Candida completely from the gut. You can drink extra water, eat more fiber (marshmallow and parsley teas, flax seed, fibrous veggies like celery, cauliflower, and broccoli), eat more salad and raw veggies (though some may do better with cooked vegetables), and do some digestive-boosting yoga poses to facilitate more successful and complete bowel movements several times a day. Consider colonics and enemas. Eating good food is important, but so is eliminating it effectively. See Section 5 for more information.

What to Do with Your Face

At this point, even while cleansing, you're going to continue breaking out because of the underlying Candida. If Candida yeast overgrowth really is the issue, your skin will clear up in due time. Focus on the cleanse and spend your resources on getting the best quality foods and supplements you can afford while still using acne-safe skin products at home twice a day, as per usual. If you really want something and your skin can tolerate it, you can try adding an additional exfoliant and/or active cleanser to your skin regime, being careful to avoid irritating or sensitizing the skin.

Treatments

If you can afford them, chemical peel treatments would be great, as they'll help your skin more quickly detox, plus you'll get moral support from your esthetician. Your skin may be particularly sensitive, so you might want to avoid extractions, except perhaps for very easy-to-extract or really inflamed ones. Now is not the time to be aggressive with the skin; we want the body to prioritize detoxing instead of healing from treatment or harsh products.

Seeing an esthetician or an integrative therapist like a naturopath can be especially helpful if they are knowledgeable about or experienced in the Candida cleanse. They'd be able to review and troubleshoot any issues you may have while doing it. Estheticians can also help adjust your skincare regimen or make additional product recommendations as needed to strengthen it and assess how much clearer your skin is with each visit, which is motivating.

Itching, Rashes

Icing is going to be the best coping mechanism for itchy rashes. A quick icing session often yields hours of itching relief. If the itching persists, thoroughly air dry the skin and try applying some peppermint and tea tree oil sparingly on the areas, mixing a drop of each with a few drops of aloe vera or hyaluronic acid serum (preferred) or safflower or sunflower oil as needed to dilute them. (Take care as using essential oils neat on the skin can cause burns.) Both the peppermint and tea tree will help to stop the itching, and the tea tree has anti-viral, -bacterial and -fungal properties to support the detox. Itching is a likely sign that the toxins are trying to purge whichever way possible, in this instance, out of the skin.

Extra Resources

There are a plethora of Candida-related resources online. Our own site, *withandwithin.co*, and our Pinterest[32], *TheCandidaDiet.com*, and *The Body Ecology Diet*[33] by Donna Gates are trusted resources for inspiration.

Endnotes

32 *https://nl.pinterest.com/withandwithin/candida-%2B-acne-safe-recipes/*

33 *https://bodyecology.com/*

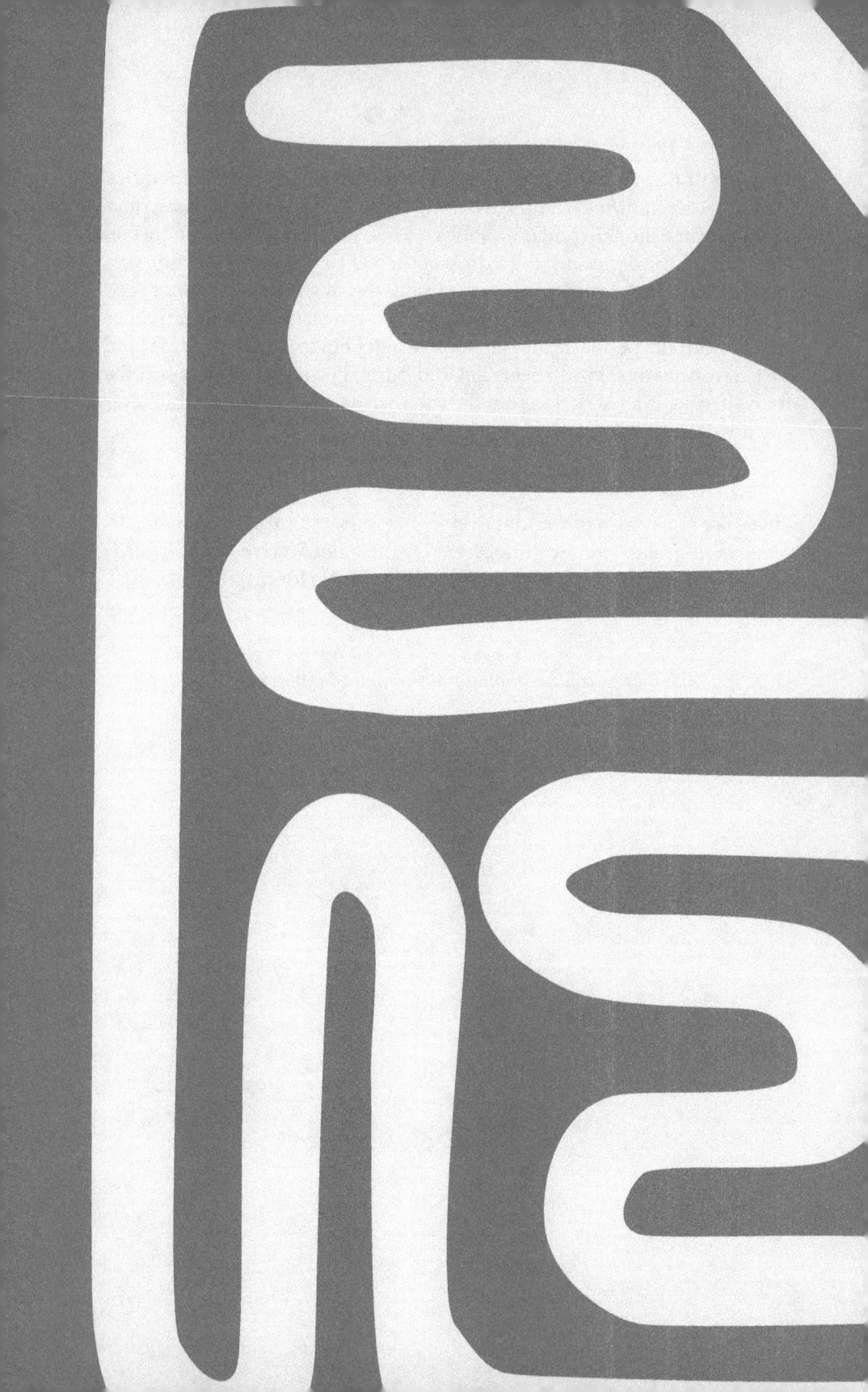

SECTION 7
Working With
a Professional
Esthetician

After having a clinic for over a decade, I realized that with an open mind, some discipline, and consistency, most people were able to clear up on their own (at least significantly, if not completely) so long as they had all the tools needed to do so. However, some clients really benefit from (or need!) actual extractions and treatments, so here are some tips for finding an esthetician near you.

Finding the best and most experienced esthetician to work with will involve research, potentially awkward conversations, trial, error, and hope. You may need to exercise patience and faith; one bad experience at a spa might not mean you should boycott the whole place—the skillset of an individual practitioner isn't necessarily reflective of everyone else working there.

You may find a diamond in the rough, somebody who is excellent with their hands, who would be open to learning new ways of treating skin. Go through the steps of vetting estheticians below, and if you find someone who's professional, is willing to learn and is not defensive with the questions you're asking, and maybe most importantly, has a personality you like, they may be worth a try to work with in clearing your skin. At the very least, they can administer professional chemical peels and LED light treatments before deciding together to venture into extraction territory.

Remember, your main goals are to use the esthetician you find for their extraction skills, LED light treatments, and chemical exfoliation peels, along with encouragement and topical monitoring.

How to Find One

Do an internet search for an esthetician in your area, preferably someone who specializes in (and has lots of professional experience with) acne. Because acne requires more than one treatment, you want to go to a place where regulars go regularly. These local small businesses are more likely to have a regular clientele, while facilities like fancy hotel spas get booked for rarer occasions like bachelorette parties or by out-of-town guests looking to relax.

With this in mind, try searching these terms: acne esthetician, acne clinic, acne facial, acne treatment, facial extractions, medispa acne, acne specialist in your city/state, or if you're in a suburb, perhaps the next city/town over or nearest big city.

Once you get to their websites, here are a few things to look for:

Do they offer acne-specific treatments, and if so, what are they? What product brands do they use for them? (Bonus: using our online comedogenic ingredient search tool, you can audit that brand's acne-specific products to see which ones look acne-safe before using them on your skin.)

Do they offer too many kinds of treatments? The adage "jack of all trades and master of none" may apply here. Be careful if it's a place that does everything under the sun; this could mean that throwing an acne facial on their treatment menu is more a marketing move rather than expertise. They may spend more time perfecting their bikini-waxing or lash-applying skills than on actual facials or acne case studies.

What exactly goes on in their acne treatments and how are they marketed? Do they disclose upfront that more than one treatment will be needed? Do they include skin analysis, recordkeeping, extractions, high frequency, LED, chemical peels, masks, and guidance between appointments?

Do they have case studies with *their own* before and after client photos? Most skincare brands' marketing teams will provide stock before/after photos to estheticians for advertising purposes. By looking at actual case study photos of their own clients, you'll have some proof that your practitioner has actually and personally cleared up clients successfully and that they are not just using promotional marketing photos as their own without actually having gotten positive and consistent results. (Bonus: ask if they have detailed client notes like what and how many treatments were given, products used, what other lifestyle changes were made, etc.)

Can they honestly share case studies of clients who didn't clear up with their program? Hearing how the practitioner handled this and what the client ended up doing can be insightful.

What to Look for & What to Ask

Next, you should interview your short list of therapists by making some phone calls and/or maybe booking some in-person consultations. This phase would be a good way to get a feel for the therapist. Explain that you're following our remote acne management program that's working well, but you need a little extra help, which is where they come in. This helps to set the tone that you are set with the skincare products you are using and are serious about clearing up. As you talk to them, try to see about the following:

- Are they confident in their skills and experience? Do they have specific client case studies they talk about that can be referred to in reference to your type of acne?
- Are they honest? Did they have any clients who just weren't able to clear up, and how do they explain why—other than "client compliance"?
- When sharing their case studies, do they talk about more than just the products they used and the facials they got? Many estheticians might not know all the facets of acne as it is affected by lifestyle like we do; this might not be a deal-breaker for your therapist. However, seeing how honest they are if they don't know about the lifestyle stuff, along with how open they are to learning more, speaks positive volumes.
- Do they seem to be in a very salesy mood? Do they pressure you to sign up for a series of 10 treatments or to buy a whole new set of products right away?
- When you bring up the fact that you want to use them for their extraction skills and chemical peels and only want to use your own skincare products, how do they react? (This is definitely an uncommon request, so there may be some initial defensiveness.)
- Can they describe previous allergic reactions and what they did for that client? Did they implement any new protocols in their practice afterward to prevent the same thing from happening again to other clients?

Products and Tools

Probably the most important thing about your esthetician, aside from getting really great and safe extractions, is the ability to use only acne-safe products during the treatment. Hopefully, your therapist will be on board with using your products (tell them it'll save them some backbar money!). Otherwise, you can point them to our product checker tool and ask that they audit their backbar to see what items in their supply are acne-safe to use on their treatments with you.

Products

In the professional treatment room, the products that are most commonly cloggy/problematic are going to be the creamy moisturizing masks, creams, lotions, sunscreen, and makeup. (Those cold and luscious rubber masks are algae-based, which might be okay because you're only using it once, but with your pores wide open from extractions, it might still be pretty risky.

Section 7 - Working With a Professional Esthetician

Consider icing instead.) Cleansers and toners are generally better but still may contain cloggy ingredients, especially if the cleanser is milky/creamy, oil-based, super foamy or fragranced.

Chemical peels

Chemical peels are, for the most part, acne-safe, as long as they are the liquid versus creamy kinds and are free of seaweed ingredients, so you should be okay receiving these from another professional. The creamy peels are more likely to contain cloggy ingredients, but the resulting exfoliation peeling may outweigh the superficial breakouts you might get from them.

Some professional skincare brands we've used in the past include those listed below. Look for mandelic, lactic, and TCA chemical peels if you can't find the brands below. Salicylic and glycolic acid peels can also be okay but may be more irritating than the previously mentioned ones. In any case, ask your esthetician to consult the manufacturer's training book or contact the manufacturer to get the latest ingredient listings of whatever peel they will use on you to be sure they're acne-safe.

You can try using the company website's professional locator tool to find therapists who use and carry their products. To be listed on the brand site, these therapists should be trained to analyze the skin, perform chemical peels, and recommend skincare regimens. Again, the quality of work from each therapist will widely vary, so use this as a good place to start your search. In any case, use the product checker as much as possible to reduce exposure to any cloggy products.

PCA Skin.[34] Their Sensi Peel, the Ultra Peel I (the 2 is creamy and peels great but is cloggy), the PCA Peel Hydroquinone-free, the PCA Peel with Hydroquinone, the PCA Peel with Hydroquinone and Resorcinol.

Vivant Skincare[35] Both the regular and extra-strength TCA-based ProPeels have garnered successful results in clinic for stubborn acne, hyperpigmentation, and anti-aging.

Skin Script Skincare, Rhonda Allison and Beyond Complexion are other brands we've worked with in the past that also offer professional-grade chemical peels.

Tools

What tools or machines, if any, do they use to help the skin heal or calm inflammation post-treatment? This could be as simple as ice applied directly onto the skin or cooling packs, to more advanced technology machines. Just ensure whatever they use is gentle enough to use when your skin is its most sensitive, post-extractions.

The Treatment

During

Extractions are a very nuanced thing to teach and learn; at With & Within we spent three to six weeks training solely on extractions before allowing estheticians to treat clients on their own without senior esthetician supervision. Here are some tips to help you evaluate how well your esthetician's extractions are going:

The therapist should optimally have short nails, be wearing gloves, and using clean tissue-wrapped fingers to extract! Never bare hands, and absolutely never using their fingernails. If they are using an extractor tool, it should only be used on non-inflamed acne. Using them on inflamed acne can cause serious damage to the skin. No one—including estheticians, nurses, or dermatologists—should ever use metal tools to extract inflamed acne.

Do they extract more than just the sebaceous filaments (often mistaken for and called blackheads) on your nose and chin but completely disregard the non-inflamed acne everywhere else? How do they treat inflamed acne, if at all?

Are you able to take a break from extractions when it gets really intense? The therapist should be looking out for your well-being and initiate breaks if need be. This is a bedside manner thing that you may have to advocate for yourself.

Do they cleanse or tone your skin afterward to help get rid of bacteria and fluids that may have gotten onto the surface of the skin with all the extractions? Ideally, high-frequency and LED are used post-extraction to kill bacteria, reduce inflammation, and speed healing.

Post-treatment Observation

In the days following your treatment, observe your skin's behavior. Do you break out, or does your skin get inflamed? Ideally, post-treatment you'll have little to no inflammation but perhaps have tiny pinprick scabs (from the extractions) and peeling skin (from the chemical peel or enzyme exfoliant).

Section 7 - Working With a Professional Esthetician

If yes, you do get inflamed and the acne doesn't clear, they may not be doing a thorough enough extraction; they may just be draining liquid but not extracting the acne-causing seed. This can be especially true if the acne is recurring in the same exact pores. (Just let the esthetician know next time so they can try to be more thorough.)

If yes, you do get inflamed but the skin clears up, you may be the (rare) type of client who just gets really easily inflamed even after complete extractions.

If yes, you do get inflamed every time you get a treatment AND your skin doesn't seem to be getting *any* better after four treatments in two months, you likely need to find another therapist (and/or check to see if you're holding up your end of the acne-safe lifestyle).

If no, you don't get inflamed, this may be a good indicator that the extractions were complete, but only if they actually did extract acne (and that you're not inflamed because they didn't touch those areas at all).

With the exception of old acne purging, your skin should generally be getting better with each treatment. You may experience some pigmentation left behind by inflamed acne that's healed. This is normal because the pigmentation process started the moment the inflammation set in, not when the esthetician extracted (so long as done properly). It will lift when the pores are clear.

Aftercare

Ideally, post-treatment, you may have tiny pinprick scabs (from the extractions), possibly larger scabs from inflamed acne, and maybe some peeling skin (from the chemical peel or enzyme exfoliant), but little to no inflammation.

Inflamed acne, when properly extracted, should not be as painful (if at all) as before it gets extracted. There may be some soreness from the pressure used, but the general overall pain associated with that one inflamed pimple should be better, or completely gone, afterward.

Stop using your active products (exfoliants, BP, anything that's drying or foaming) after your treatments while your skin heals. This would be the time to use your hydrating and healing skincare products to nurture the skin that's healing from all those extractions and the new skin that's being revealed via peeling from the professional exfoliation treatment. In our clinic, we recommend our clients use their healing regimen for at least a week or until the skin is fully healed—meaning that all the scabs have fallen off, the skin has stopped peeling, and it is back to feeling normal, healthy, and strong. Icing is definitely encouraged during the healing stages, so long as it's done gently and not for too long.

Give It Time

On average, our clinic clients would get to the 90-95% clear mark at around three months, longer if they had particularly tight and difficult-to-extract pores, if they had a difficult time getting their inflammation down, if they weren't compliant with the lifestyle, or if they didn't get the treatments often enough. Aside from a purging period, your skin should improve with each treatment, so long as you're doing your part with all the acne-safe product and lifestyle components.

However, if you're "doing all the things," have ruled out any underlying systemic imbalances, and, at the two- or three-month mark, you still aren't seeing any improvements, it may be time to find a new esthetician, start working with an alternative health practitioner, or check yourself and your compliance to the program.

In Any Case—Remember to Document!

Document your starting point and advancement. Try to have an observant eye on your skin (without scrutinizing or picking at it) so that you can properly track your progress. Some have even gone as far as counting each bump on their skin, but this may not be the best thing for some folks, as it might discourage them motivationally or encourage them to pick. I think getting a feel for how densely packed and how big the bumps feel on your skin, taking notes, and then comparing that to the following week or so is a fair idea.

Learn for Yourself What Clear Skin Really Looks Like

Be mindful of the difference between inflamed and non-inflamed acne and learn to identify them on your face. This is one of the only ways you'll get to know if you're actually clear or not.

Remember, although inflammation will be the first to go away, it's the non-inflamed acne seeds left behind that you need to get rid of in order to get clear. Often, the inflammation goes away and people think they're clear but end up "breaking out again" because the non-inflamed seeds are still on their way up and out of the skin—part of the same purge train coming through and finishing its course. Recall, non-inflamed acne is small and feels like tiny bumps, grains of sand, or Braille. Inflamed acne is when these tiny seeds get lodged inside each tiny pore that's swelling up, causing a larger and often more sensitive or painful bump. Only when the skin is clear of both kinds are you really, truly clear.

Endnotes

34 *https://www.pcaskin.com/*

35 *https://www.vivantskincare.com/*

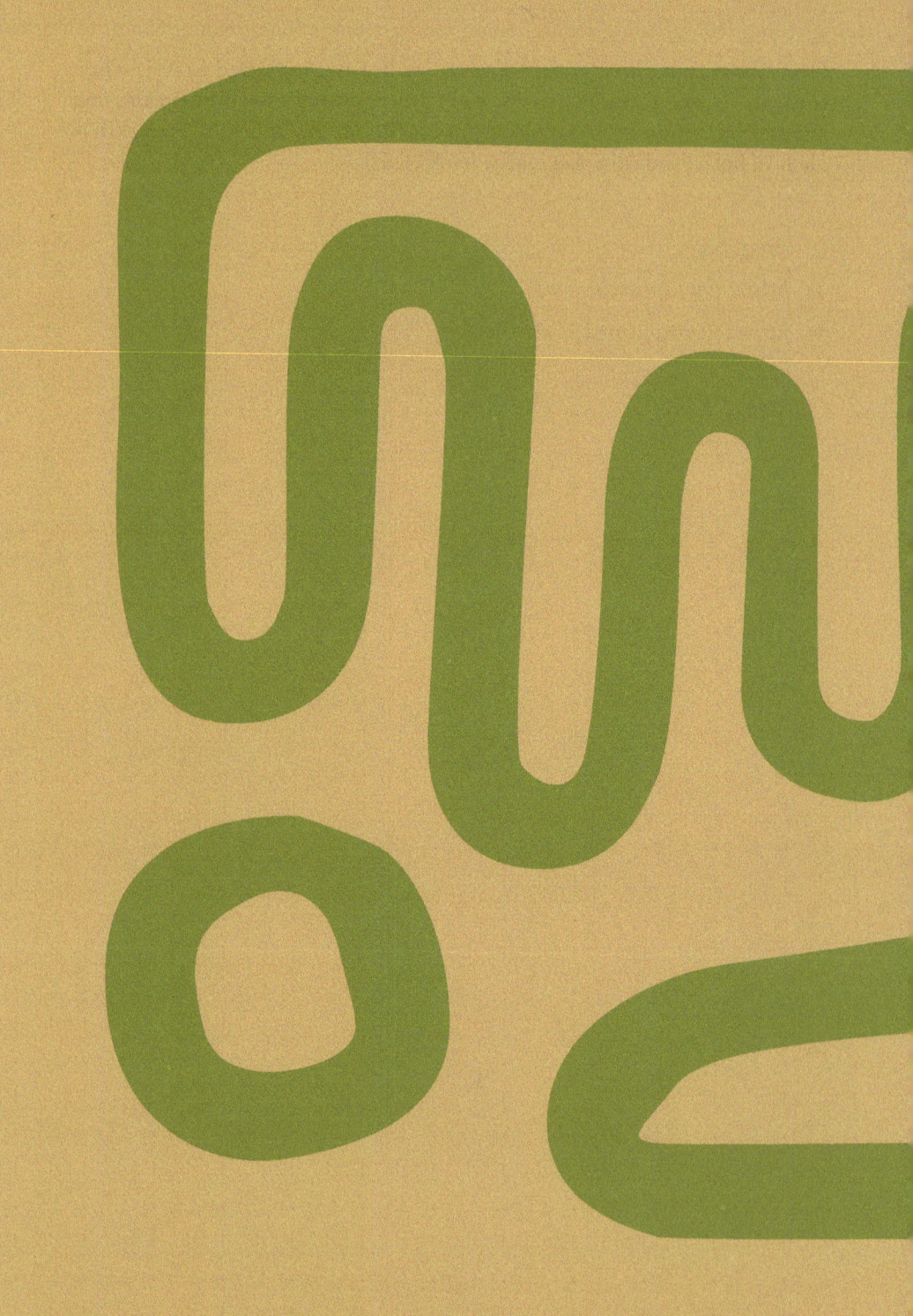

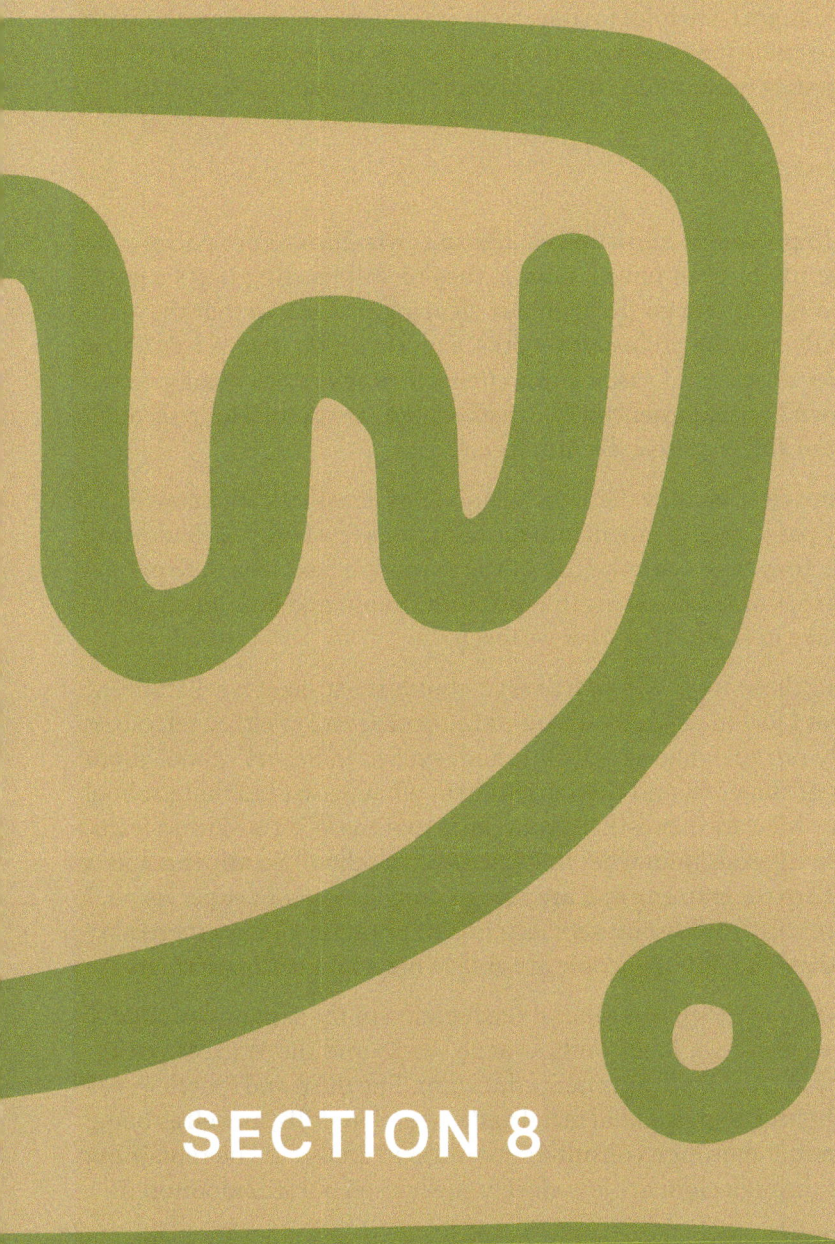

SECTION 8

The With & Within
Standard of Treatment

I thought it might be helpful to share some information about how the With & Within estheticians are trained as well as how we approach our clients when they start treatment and then become more established with us.

Our Therapists

It's really important to me to find estheticians who have experienced acne either recently or even have it now. If they're still battling it, it's a great exercise to have them go through our clearing process so that they can learn exactly how the philosophy works, experience for themselves that it actually does work, and easily guide clients through the clearing process via their own lived experiences. Most estheticians are excited to go through the program and of course, eventually clear up.

At their interview, we quiz the estheticians on basic esthetician knowledge, and if they pass, we bring them into the clinic for a few hours of shadowing to see how they fit in with the rest of the team. We also take note of how coachable they are, how caring they are with clients, and how much initiative they take to learn all of what we teach.

After hiring them, we go through a very rigorous six- to eight-week training. I found that I had to create an entire training program to either refresh or completely retrain what estheticians had learned in beauty school about the basics of skincare, and then teach them what wasn't taught in school about acne. Most former estheticians claim that the With & Within training is more rigorous than what they received in school! So any therapists who complete the training and are able to practice without supervision, I believe, are truly the best estheticians in San Francisco. I have incredibly high standards, and these people are able to meet and maintain them.

The first week, we focus on general reeducation of the skin and products. The second week, we focus on how acne works and the With & Within philosophy of treatment and client education. The third and fourth weeks are spent honing their manual facial and extraction skills, as well as being able to conduct thorough consultations and skin analysis. The remaining weeks five through eight are less closely supervised but still monitored.

For these first four weeks, a senior or training esthetician is by their side the entire time, walking them through both the theory and practical sides of the training. The senior or trainer esthetician will not see any of their own clients during this time unless the trainee is able to sit in to observe or participate during these appointments. Once the trainee is able to perform consultations to our high standard, they will conduct these appointments without supervision and, if needed, will call on the training esthetician if they need assistance.

From the fifth week onward, as the trainee grows more proficient with the work, the trainees will perform their appointments on clients with less supervision but have a senior or training esthetician come in to sign off on the completion of extractions and review of client homework emails. In these client homework emails, we:

- Sum up any areas of concern or extra attention that was gone over during the appointment.
- Give clear written instructions on how the client should take care of their skin while it's healing.
- Communicate what product regimen changes to make once their skin heals up from treatment. This is especially important if a new way of using an existing product is needed or if a new product is being introduced to their regimen.
- Give ideas of any lifestyle suggestions that the esthetician thinks could be beneficial in strengthening their clear skin lifestyle regimen going forward until their next appointment.

Our Acne Treatments

Generally, we see new clients for treatments every two weeks to help facilitate the purging process, spreading out the visit frequency as the client clears up. Around the two-month mark, we're able to stretch the visits out to every three or four weeks until they get to the maintenance mode stage, coming in at least once a season. For some clients that have particularly inflamed or active acne, we'll have them come in once a week during the purging stage until the skin and acne are in a manageable state: inflammation and sensitivity under control, pores less densely packed and able to tolerate exfoliants. The more intense the acne is, the better these more frequent visits help the client gain more immediate control of their skin while, most importantly, alleviating the painful soreness associated with severely inflamed skin.

Along with all the lifestyle stuff, we also monitor how the client's product usage is going. If we find they're going through their products too quickly, we let them know so that they don't fry their skin or waste their money. I purposely did not offer employee commission on product sales in my business because I did not want to promote pushy sales practices to our clients or cause any friction between team members in regards to sales goals and clientele conflicts.

The Initial Consultation Appointment

We emphasize the lifestyle educational aspect of our program because, without this, many clients would probably continue to break out even after switching up all their products, falsely believing they need to rely on treatments to stay clear. The goal of With & Within is always to empower clients by teaching them how to gain self-awareness about their body and skin, learn what their triggers are so that they can "self-diagnose" and course-correct to prevent new breakouts and maintain clarity after the series of treatments they get with us.

During our time together, we educate them in real-time with acne-safe lifestyle "homework" assignments and hold them accountable to making these changes when they come back for their follow-up appointments. After about three months of treatments (clearing out the old existing acne) and education plus lifestyle integration (preventing new acne from forming), they'll be clear, and we'll send them on their way to maintain their clarity with all the tools they learned from working with us. And if they happen to break out or need some help down the line, we're always there, ready and willing to help.

No full treatments during the consult

This initial appointment does NOT include a full treatment. On a topical level, there are several reasons for not jumping right into a full extraction session at the first meeting.

The first reason is the most common: the skin is simply not ready for the incredibly thorough extractions. At the time of the consult, clients' skin is most often imbalanced, compromised, and/or sensitive from products and/or medications that they've used prior to coming to With and Within.

Second, the skin needs to be prepped with a properly balanced and active skincare regimen for at least two weeks for a successful extraction session, much like an athlete needs to train prior to a victorious marathon win. At the consult, we put together a skincare regimen bespoke to the client's complexion, which offers the correct exfoliation and moisture levels the skin needs for an effective follow-up treatment. Also, inflammation is often at its highest, so employing the regimen and anti-inflammatory lifestyle for a couple of weeks prior to treatment will help bring it down, making for more effective extractions and faster healing.

Third, because we have never worked on the client's skin before (and given the nature of our extraction-heavy signature treatments), we want to rule out possible allergic reactions. By giving the client's skin a couple of weeks to get to a healthy baseline and acclimate to the skincare regime, we can negate any possible adverse reactions associated with the basic skincare products of the program.

Potential Clients Call to Inquire

Potential new clients call us to find out about booking an appointment. Partly due to our small team and number of calls (and the time needed to answer every question each caller has), I created an FAQ and require all new/prospective clients to read this before booking their consultation. This helps conserve the energy of my small team to prioritize caring for the clients we have in-house and give the prospective clients a taste of the self-initiative and commitment they need to work with us. I instruct my front desk team that if a prospective client exhibits any hint of doubt at the time of booking, they should encourage them to call back when they're 100% ready. My therapists love their work so much, and it's deflating to exert so much energy toward a person who is not committed to the work, especially when there are so many others more motivated who could instead be taking our coveted after-work evening appointment slots.

Potential Clients Book Their Consultation

Once they do their homework of thoroughly reading our website and are ready to commit, we book them for a consultation and have them fill out their intake forms that cover the wide variety of acne contributors outlined in this book. We also point these clients toward our blog and social media outlets so that they can explore resources we provide outside of our treatments and to get a jump-start on their clear skin journey. Many of them also purchase and start to use our products to prepare their skin for treatment.

Intake Form Review

On the day of the appointment, the esthetician reviews the intake forms to familiarize themselves with the new client's case. During the appointment, they explain everything in detail to uncover that person's individual acne-causing habits and imbalances, teaching them how to correct these habits and bring things back into an acne-safe, clear-skinned balance.

Skin Analysis

Next is the in-depth skin analysis. We cleanse the skin, take confidential photos at different angles, and analyze the skin for clarity and degree of inflammation. We also do a few test extractions and test out some active homecare products to find which are the best fit for that person's skin.

The skin analysis helps the therapist get an idea of what condition the overall skin is in and what steps are needed to clear it up safely. Many clients come in with skin that is way too oily from using oil-based cleansers, way too dry and sensitive from using products that are too harsh or being used incorrectly, or some are super inflamed because of their unsuccessful attempts at trying to self-extract. Some even experience allergic reactions and don't even know it!

Another goal of the skin analysis is to figure out the right skin regimen for that client. The regimen's role in the first couple of weeks is to stabilize the skin so that it can be as dry or oily as it *naturally* wants to be—and not because of outside topical factors. From there, one can truly see the skin as it naturally exists and then further refine the products to help balance any natural dryness or oiliness for optimal anti-acne action.

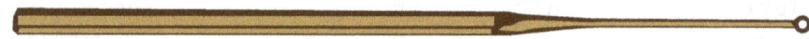

The With & Within extraction tool of choice: the buck ear curette. It's full circle shape free of sharp edges give perfect leverage around the pore for extracting non-inflamed seeds without harming the surrounding skin.

Test Extractions

These test extractions help the therapist determine the condition of the client's pores and gives the client a sense of what the full extraction treatments will be like, as well as how the skin will heal in the days following. We give the client a mirror to show them what types of acne are on their skin, the tools we use to extract them and how they actually work.

Disinfecting and Healing the Skin

Post-extractions, we employ two technologies to clean and promote healing of the skin using the high frequency and light emitting diodes (LED) machines. As effective as they are, they still don't make acne seeds jump out of the pores, so no matter their marketing claims, extractions are still very much needed.

Widely considered old-fashioned in lieu of today's more modern, expensive and sometimes more invasive beauty contraptions, we find the high frequency machine incredibly effective in helping to reduce inflammation. This time-tested device uses radio frequency emitted through a glass wand that's gently rubbed over the skin covered in loose knit surgical gauze. The space between the wand and the skin helps to create ozone, a natural and safe gas that, when used in this way, is known to kill bacteria, reduce inflammation and speed healing of the skin. (For electrical safety reasons, omit if pregnant).

Light Emitting Diodes (LEDs) are another excellent tool we employ. First developed by NASA to conduct plant growth experiments and eventually pain reduction and wound healing for astronauts in space, LED is a safe and painless skin treatment that uses varying wavelengths of light to treat the skin and body for a variety of conditions and concerns.

Post-extractions, we use LED with excellent results, speeding healing by several days. There are LEDs for different purposes—some more acne-focused (with blue light bulbs) than others, like anti-aging or pain-focused (with red light bulbs). We had both in the clinic, and to be honest, we couldn't really tell which one of the two worked better but saw that clients consistently did their best with any LED than without.

Product and Chemical Peel Patch Testing

The product testing portion helps the therapist teach the client about the active product sensation scale of 1-10 (1 feels like water, 10 feels like fire) used to describe how exfoliants and chemical peels feel on the skin. From here, a bespoke skincare regimen is created for the client to use at home in between their clinic visits.

We also patch-test chemical peels on the client's skin during this appointment to learn of any possible allergic reactions prior to applying it all over their face. The chances of allergic reactions are low, but I want to take extra precautions for our clients' safety. We repeat this patch test on the neck, jawline, or inner arm anytime we think a client may need to use a new chemical peel prior to applying it all over their face on their return visit.

Finishing the Treatment

Finally, we tone, apply any spot treatments or serums as needed, then sunscreen to conclude the hands-on portion of the appointment.

Product Audit

Time permitting, an audit of the products a client uses will be included. Most clients opt to go the most efficient route by getting rid of everything they're currently using and starting anew with With & Within products. Some are on a budget or have emotional ties to products they use, so the auditing process will help give them an idea of what might be safe to continue using. When these products run out, they will be replaced by With & Within products. The product audit is an important part of the consult because it helps show the client the very likely triggers in their cases of acne, along with the marketing tricks the multi-billion-dollar beauty industry employs in search of sales.

Treatment Plan and Homework Email

Finally, the esthetician will review with the client their treatment plan, explain how to take care of their skin post-treatment, how to use their new clearing regimen products, and reiterate the biggest "homework" assignments to focus on until they come back for their follow-up treatment.

The main focus is pretty much always around lowering the skin and body's inflammation (allowing for a more comfortable purge), product usage guidance to loosen impactions (allowing for more productive extractions during the next visit), and preventing new acne from forming (to start the clear skin lifestyle prevention phase).

Follow-up Treatments

Our corrective treatments are very thorough and therefore, extraction-heavy. Depending on what the client's skin needs are that particular day, we might include some sort of exfoliation (either with steam and enzyme or a dermatological-grade chemical peel) and/or a moisturizing, healing treatment. We'll use the high-frequency machine and may also suggest adding on an LED-light treatment to help reduce inflammation and encourage faster healing time.

The homecare regimen is adjusted as the skin progresses, and we continue to coach clients on acne-safe lifestyle changes to stay on the path to self-sustainably clear skin. There are many bits and pieces that can drastically

Detailed Treatment Notes

Our estheticians take great care in very careful treatment note-taking, documenting exactly what products are used in treatment, the client's clarity percentage, and any other relevant information to helping them get their clearest. We also copy and paste their homework email in their chart so we can keep track of any skin regimen changes to make, if any, and any lifestyle shifts we'd discussed during the appointment. The client can easily refer to this during their time away from the clinic, and with our careful note-taking, the therapist can hold clients accountable for their clear skin efforts.

Post-treatment—What to Expect

We tell the client to expect to leave the consultation treatment just a bit red and bumpy. After the regular follow-up clinic treatments with extractions, we tell them to expect a lot more redness and bumpiness, along with scabbing, peeling, inflammation, redness, and/or hyperpigmentation of the skin as it heals. These post-treatment effects are temporary and take anywhere from overnight to a full week before their skin normalizes. And as long as they follow a proper skin-healing regimen, gently ice, and refrain from picking, their skin should heal beautifully.

The client begins to get clearer and clearer with each treatment until they are completely and self-sustainably clear! Eventually, the treatments become about maintenance and prevention rather than correction, and they can continue to use their clearing regimen of skincare products and employ their acne-safe lifestyle to prevent new acne from forming.

"Popzits"

In between full treatments, we offer short five- to ten-minute appointments to emergency extract inflamed pimples (called "popzits") that creep up before a client's next full treatment to discourage them from picking it themselves. The client gets one of these appointments for free between each scheduled full treatment, with subsequent popzits costing $20, which goes straight to the esthetician as a tip as they often have to rush a bit or skip a meal/rest break in between clients to fit these in.

Bad extractions aren't good for anyone, risking infection, scarring, and prolonged anxiety. Having the client come in for these popzit appointments also allows the esthetician to make any adjustments or suggestions to further their program along (and the client can pick up any products they might need).

Consistency, Clarity, and Maintenance

The client experience after the treatments is similar to those doing the work remotely, as discussed earlier in the book. There is an acclimation stage for the skin to get used to the new regimen. The skin will purge, but the acne-safe lifestyle, products, and treatments help this process along quickly. As clients clear up and understand how to maintain their clarity an acne-safe lifestyle and a balanced skin regimen, the time between treatments stretches.

Remember: consistency is the real key to getting and staying clear. Once your skin clears, it's wise to stick to the acne-safe lifestyle! If you start using cloggy products and eating acne-causing foods, you will most likely break out again. The regimen and lifestyle might be difficult to get used to at first, but with some patience and determination, your skin will begin to clear, and your routine will become second nature.

It's important to remember that for many with the gene, there is no final "be-all, end-all cure" for acne—it is a chronic genetic disorder of the pores—so even though you will clear up, you must continue the acne-safe lifestyle to stay clear.

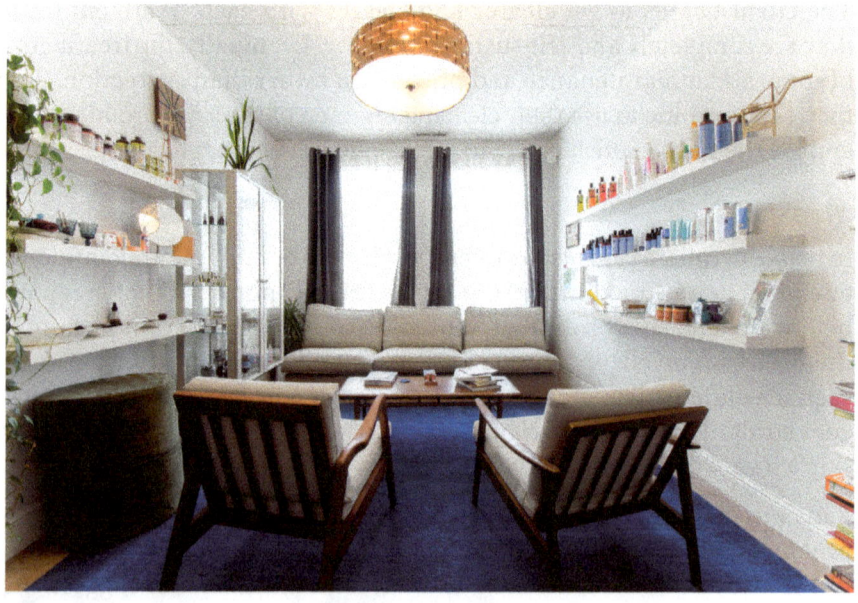

Section 8 - The With & Within Standard of Treatment

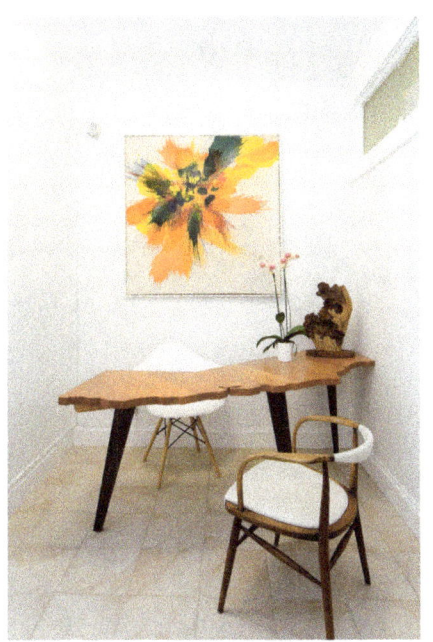

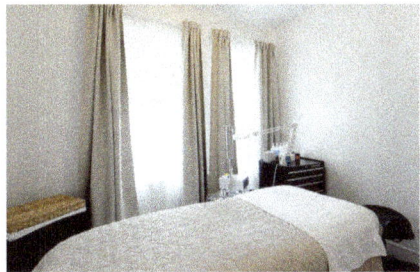

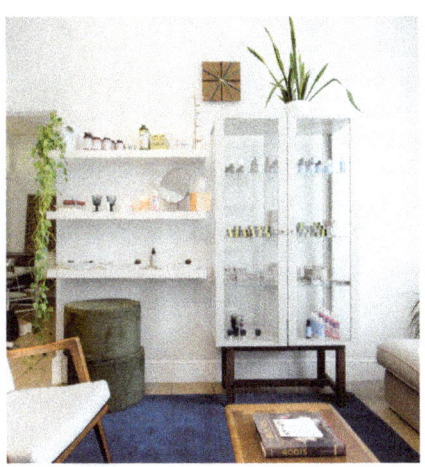

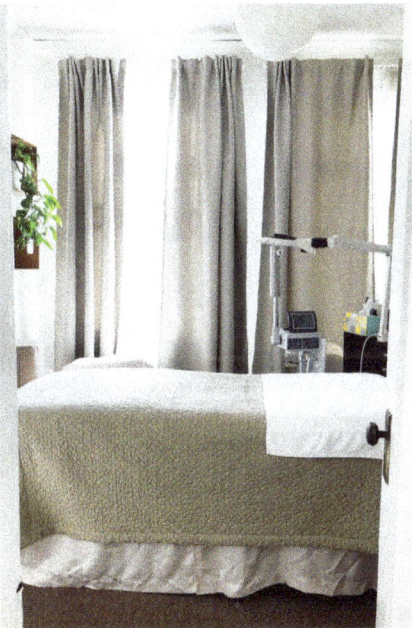

Our 2489 Mission Street, San Francisco, California location in 2015 - 2019.

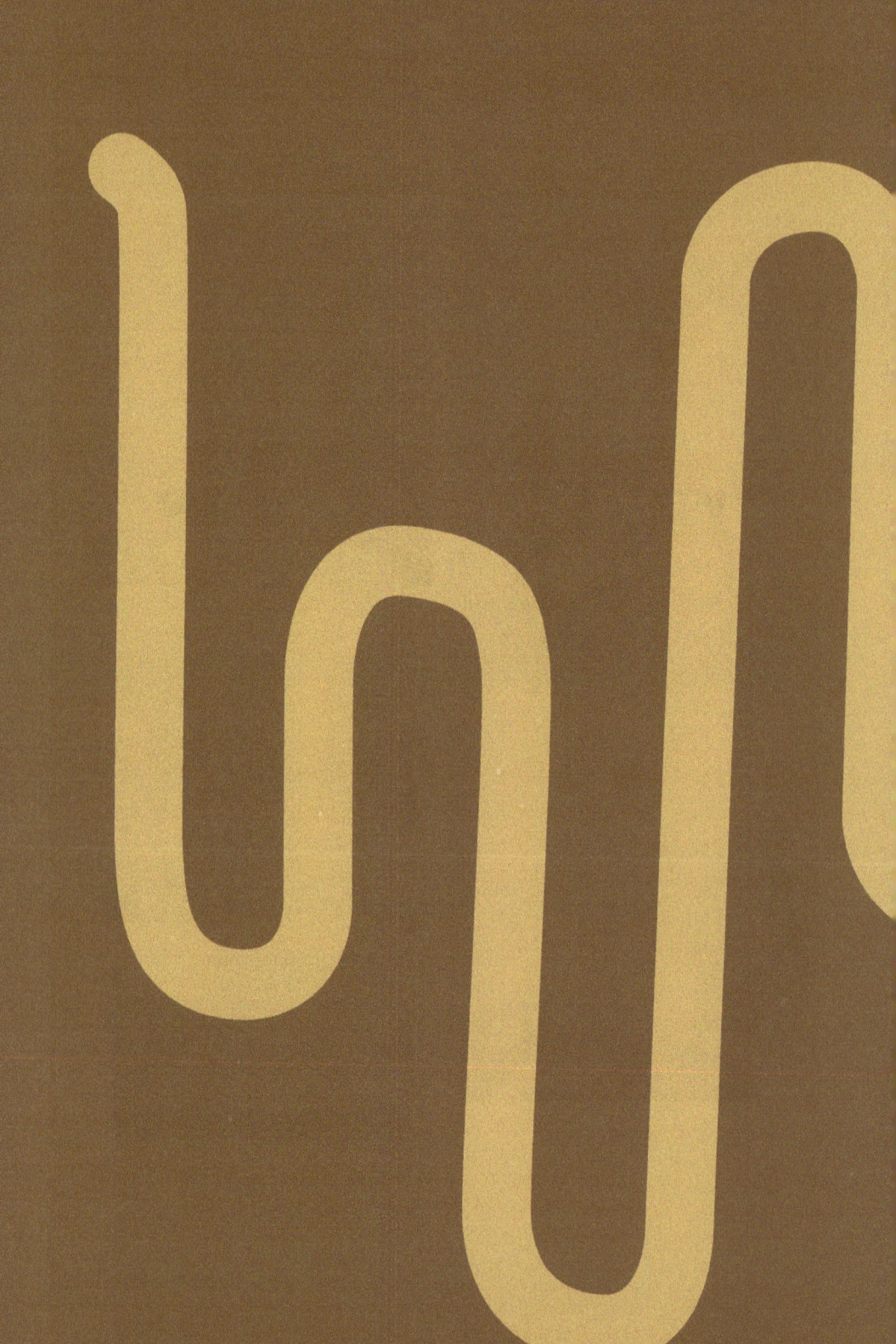

SECTION 9

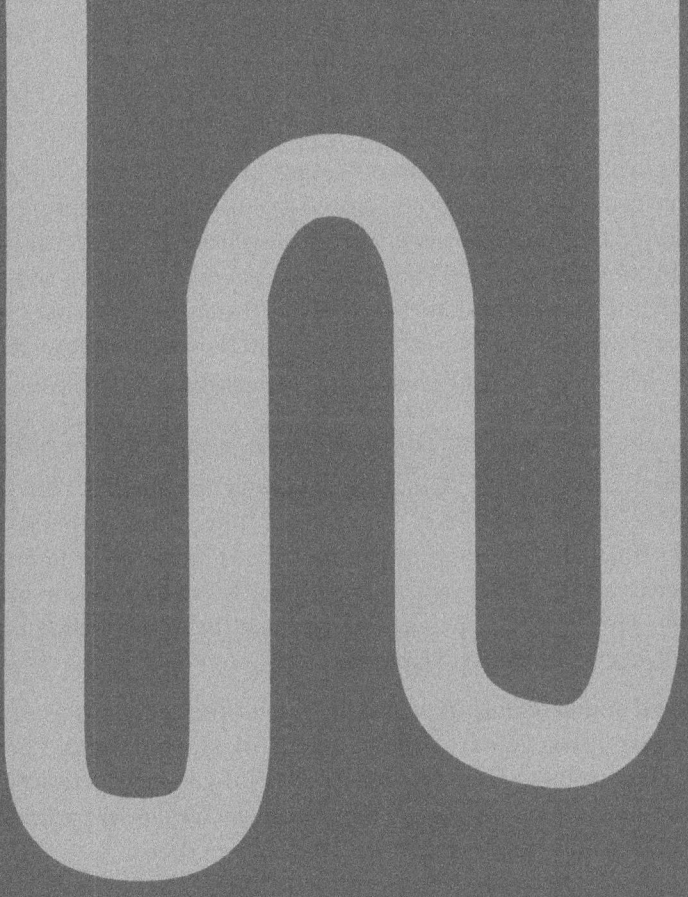

Feeling Stuck?
Let's Reassess

Let's Check-in

Mindset Check

So maybe you've hit a block in your clear skin journey and need some encouragement. Let's do an honest mindset check to make sure we have all our bases covered. Remember, topical products will only do so much, and lifestyle changes may be needed to really clear you up.

Are Your Expectations Reasonable?

Achieving 100% clear skin 100% of the time is not a realistic goal. This is a game of management, not complete elimination or perfection. Just like the seasons of nature and our moods, things change, and our bodies adapt to those changes. Give your body some grace for being the ever-fluctuating biological miracle it is. Also, social media has warped our sense of reality. Don't be swayed or discouraged by it!

Have You Given the Program Enough Time to Actually Work?

In today's fast-paced world of instant gratification, we forget that things of nature—like the human body—need time to integrate changes and produce the outcomes you want to see from them. With both in-clinic and remote clients, clearing up happens on average at the three-month mark and sometimes takes longer for more stubborn cases (like hard-to-control inflammation, very oily skin, really tiny and tight pores that *need* extractions, non-compliance, or other factors).

Are You Really Doing All the Things, and Doing Them Correctly?

Do an honest audit of all aspects of your acne-safe lifestyle. Are you cheating with dairy "sometimes"? Or having coffee "only with friends?" Are you still using that favorite (cloggy) makeup or hair care product of yours just "once in a while?" Or still working yourself to exhaustion and your sleep habits aren't consistent or great? All these little cheats add up and can definitely keep you from clearing up.

Record and take note of your daily habits and food intake and write down whether or not you are doing your FULL skincare regimen plus icing at least two times a day (and an extra time if you are exercising or sweating in between). This way, you can honestly see if there are any loopholes your clear skin may be sinking into—and correct them.

Are You Using Enough Product?

Sometimes, clients want to stretch out the life of their products, but you need to use enough of them for them to actually work. Find the balance of using just enough product for them to do their job; not so much that you're over-exfoliated, dried-out or over-moisturized, or not using enough, resulting in an ineffective result.

Stress

Stress management is HUGE. Though difficult to identify and control at first, it is a must. Stress can affect all areas of your life, much like a domino effect. If left unmanaged, this can override all the "acne-safe" things you are doing. Day-to-day care is very important, but bigger self-care adjustments may be necessary, like seeing a therapist, consulting a doctor about anxiety management or more significant lifestyle choices, like moving or changing jobs.

Diet

If you are struggling with particularly stubborn or aggressive inflamed acne, try refining your diet further with the suggestions given in Section 5, Acne-causing foods/Secondary triggers. Our past clients with these types of acne had success following those guidelines, combined with improving their lifestyle and getting frequent professional skin treatments.

Picking

Picking can severely hold back the clearing process for all folks, especially those who experience picking as a means of body-focused repetitive behaviors (BFRBs). If icing your face and the program isn't helping, you may need more support. There are many communities and resources available online and in real life for those with BFRBs.

The underlying condition under picking is usually anxiety, so finding approaches that help to alleviate this—including seeking therapy—may be key to getting this under control.

Is There a Larger Systemic Condition at Play?

For some, acne will persist (or temporarily get better and then come back with a vengeance or plateau) because of an underlying systemic imbalance. The most common underlying condition holding our clients back from fully clearing up was a Candida yeast imbalance. Other things to consider were prescription drugs that had acne as a side effect or birth control pills, usually when they weren't taken on a regular schedule. A few clients had persistent acne on their chin until a visit to their OB-GYN revealed they had cysts that needed to be monitored and treated. One had a particularly aggressive cyst that, when removed, finally allowed her chin acne to clear.

Chronic stress was the other big systemic issue (besides Candida yeast overgrowth, see below) that overrode any acne management protocol!

If these points resonate, I recommend consulting with an alternative health functional doctor who can utilize both conventional and holistic medicinal approaches in evaluating your condition, diagnosing it, and coming up with an effective action plan to get it under control. Many of our clients opted to do their own elimination diet and follow the With & Within Candida cleanse protocol to see if it would help alleviate (or entirely eradicate) their symptoms, including the extra persistent acne.

Compliance + Lifestyle Tracking

Keeping track of and journaling about what you've been doing is one of the best ways to figure out exactly what is or isn't working for you. There are many moving parts when adjusting to and maintaining an acne-safe lifestyle. Being honest and accountable for the role you play is a major factor in getting clear. You can track your sleep (when you sleep and wake and how you feel upon rising), stress levels, diet, how often you did your skin routine, how inflamed your skin is day to day, etc.

Strengthen Your Program

Your Regimen Needs Some Tweaks

If you're still breaking out and you're "doing all the things" perhaps your products are not strong enough and you need to up your exfoliation. If you are using an introductory-level exfoliant and your skin has grown accustomed to it, you may need to add an additional method of exfoliation (like an exfoliating acid cleanser or serum if you're already using an exfoliating toner) in your regimen to really get that dead-skin-cell-sloughing, acne-purging action going.

If you are still inflamed you may need to ice more, incorporate benzoyl peroxide gel, or get a bit stricter on your diet/stress management to try to get inflammation down even further. Cutting down nightshade vegetables or grains and adding some anti-inflammatory supplements can also be worth trying.

If you are too dry or flaky perhaps your regimen needs more moisture added to it and/or your exfoliants are too strong. The exfoliant itself might be too strong or may need to be used differently/less often. In either case, stop using the active product until your skin is back to normal. Then, work the active product back into your regimen one to three times a week, slowly increasing as your skin needs it and as you can tolerate it.

If you're too oily the extra sebum may be creating a barrier, preventing your active products from penetrating into the skin, so making some adjustments to slightly dry the skin may be in order.

Regimen Adjustment Ideas for Stubborn Acne

If You're Doing the Basic Regimen Twice a Day and Are Still Purging But Feeling a Bit Dry:

Are you dry only in certain places?
- You're probably over-exfoliating. Are you rubbing extra hard or applying extra exfoliant in certain places, making those areas peel? Stop exfoliating there altogether. Let your skin heal, then carefully and slowly try working the exfoliant back in; this almost always takes care of the area-specific over-exfoliation.

Or are you dry all over?
- Your skin is probably dehydrated and lacking water or lipid dry and lacking in oils. Are you waiting in between regimen steps when washing your face? This is a very common culprit that's easy to fix. Don't wait between steps. If you find the need to wait for products to dry before moving on to the next step, you're probably using too much product to begin with. Wash your face, ice, pat dry, tone, serum (if using), then moisturize as soon as possible.

You may need to give your skin a break from active products. If you are using both an exfoliating toner and exfoliating serum, as long as the dryness or peeling isn't severe, you can keep using the toner but should temporarily stop using the serum. As your skin acclimates without irritation, slowly work the serum back into your regime, applying it only on areas that need it or slowly working it into your regular routine, applying it all over the face as needed and tolerated. If you're visibly peeling or the skin is very irritated, stop all exfoliants and slowly reintroduce your primary exfoliant before integrating the second one if it's still needed.

You might need to go slow if you are very sensitive and may only tolerate toning once a day (or even once every other day) versus twice. However, if you're still purging acne, this isn't the best approach because you need more regular exfoliation to facilitate the flushing of acne from the pores; reducing your exfoliation slows this process. Exceptions can be made if your skin is truly sensitive, hopefully building up usage over time. Don't try to use a product that's just too strong or use it too quickly. Slowly try to acclimate your skin to the active products you have, or find another product that your skin can tolerate twice a day instead.

You might just need to moisturize, period. Always moisturize after washing or getting your face wet, even if it's just a quick rinse at the gym before working out or running home, where you'll do your entire regimen. Your face can and will dry out in the meanwhile, dehydrating and sensitizing your skin over time. This is true even for clients on their way to the clinic for treatment; some would wash but not moisturize their faces before leaving the house, and by the time they got to the treatment room, we couldn't apply a chemical peel because they were too dried out and sensitized for it.

You might need to switch to more moisturizing products: either a non-foaming moisturizing face wash or switch to a more hydrating moisturizer or sunscreen, or layer extra moisture under your moisturizer/SPF. This way, you can continue using the same active products that are keeping your skin clear (or the purging going).

If you're doing the basic regimen twice a day, are still purging but feeling a bit oily:
- If you aren't already, switch to a foaming or more active cleanser (like a mandelic acid or BP cleanser). Foam it up, leave it on the skin for a few minutes to work like a mask, then rinse off.
- Try switching to a lighter-textured, less- (or non-) moisturizing SPF.
- If you're oily only in certain areas, skip moisturizing these areas (but still apply SPF for protection).
- You can try using a powder mineral SPF on top of your moisturizer to protect from the sun but also to soak up excess oil.
- Look at your food consumption; are you eating greasy, oily foods or foods that increase cortisol/oil production, like coffee or peanuts?
- Are you particularly stressed? People with elevated cortisol levels and lots of stress often report feeling oilier than usual.

If you're already doing the basic regimen twice a day and have inflammation under control but are still purging acne, try:
- Bumping up your exfoliation action by adding an exfoliating serum to your regimen. Start off using it once every other night, working

up to every night, then every night plus every other morning, eventually twice a day. Allow at least a week or two at each stage increase before strengthening the regimen to avoid sensitizing and over-exfoliating the skin.
- You *might* be able to use a facial scrub but ONLY if you aren't inflamed. Try mixing some baking soda with your face wash and using this once or twice a day. Sometimes, skin isn't inflamed but becomes so after scrubbing is introduced, so please proceed with caution.
- Audit your acne-safe lifestyle and diet and make sure you aren't doing or using anything that could be causing more seeds to form! This especially includes makeup.
- See a professional for a chemical peel to help flush the impacted pores faster than homecare.

If you're already doing the basic regimen twice a day but inflammation is still a problem, try:
- Increasing your icing time twice a day, up to 30 minutes each time. You can ice additional times per day, watching for irritation and dryness (making sure to moisturize after each time your face gets wet).
- Adding benzoyl peroxide gel to your regimen. See *Section 1, Understand Products, Using BP for Acne and Rosacea.*
- Consider integrating LED light treatments either at home with the handheld units or in the professional setting with the professional hands-free panels.
- Consider taking anti-inflammatory supplements like Zyflamend or Optizinc. Omega fish oils rich in Omega-3s and turmeric combined with black pepper are all good choices.
- Consider eating a very low-glycemic diet if you aren't already. You can also try omitting nightshades and grains to see if that helps with systemic inflammation.
- Evaluate your low-inflammatory lifestyle. Are you stressed? Sleeping okay? Eating more sugar or high-glycemic foods than usual? Retaining water? Hormones, PMS? Experiencing pain or soreness from an injury or...?

Finally, if you've gone through this entire section and are still breaking out, seeking out a skin professional in your area may just be what you need. Some clients will need extractions from a skin therapist if their skin is purging too much or too quickly, especially if they have a hard time controlling the inflammation. Others may need the help of an integrative practitioner who can help identify the root cause. Candida overgrowth may be a factor, as was the case for many of our standard protocol-resistant clients.

Professional Help: an Esthetician

You may need the help of a licensed skincare therapist in your area. Chemical peels alone can help get those seeds up to the surface (and eventually out of the skin) much faster than not—but if you can find an esthetician who can also do thorough extractions, that would be ideal. Check out *Section 7, Working With a Professional Esthetician* for more information.

"You will quickly recognize Kim is committed to getting results and arming you with the knowledge to maintain clear skin. I would highly recommend With &Within to anyone who is committed to changing their life and getting radiant skin!"

- KH

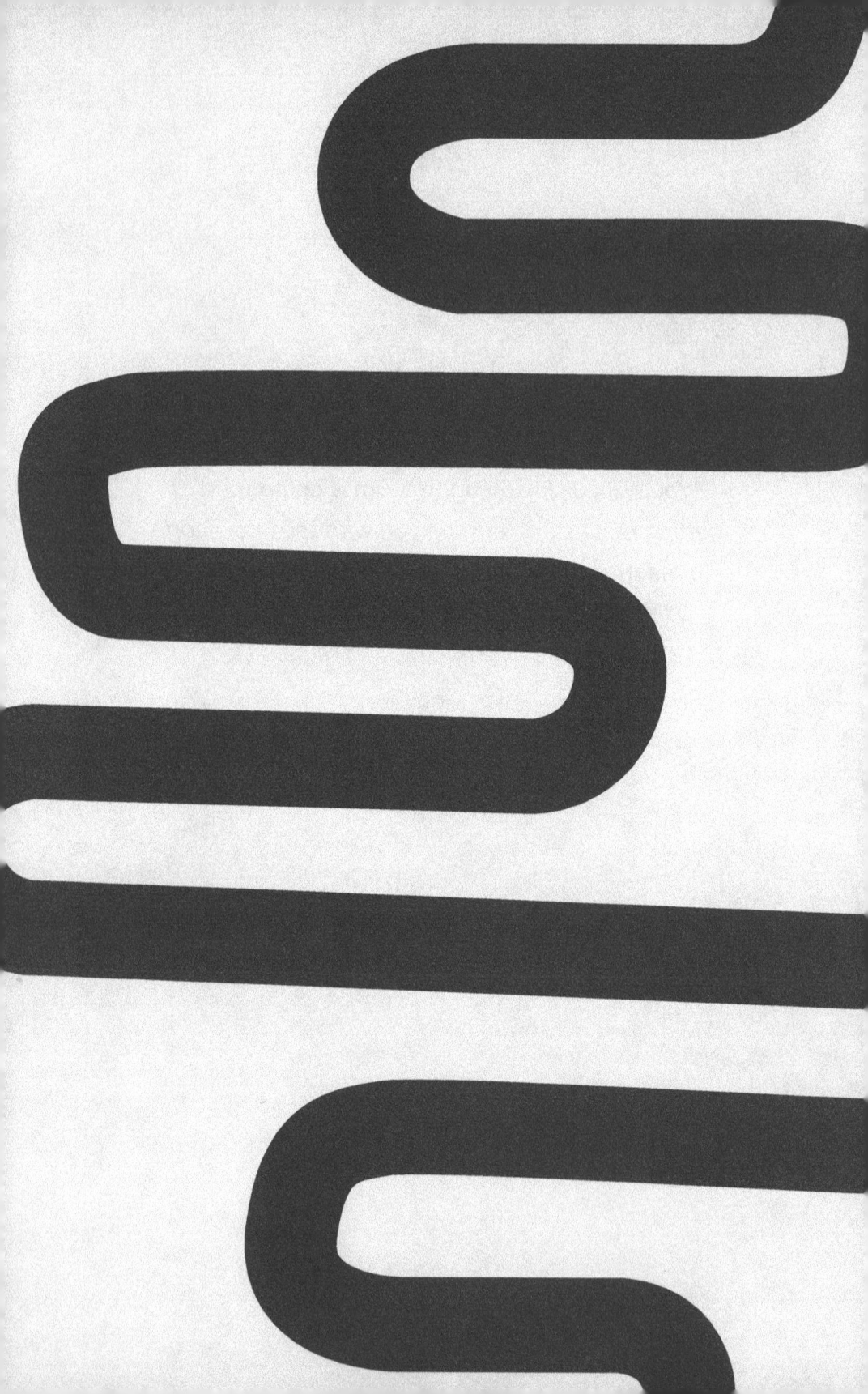

SECTION 10

Maintaining Your Clear Skin

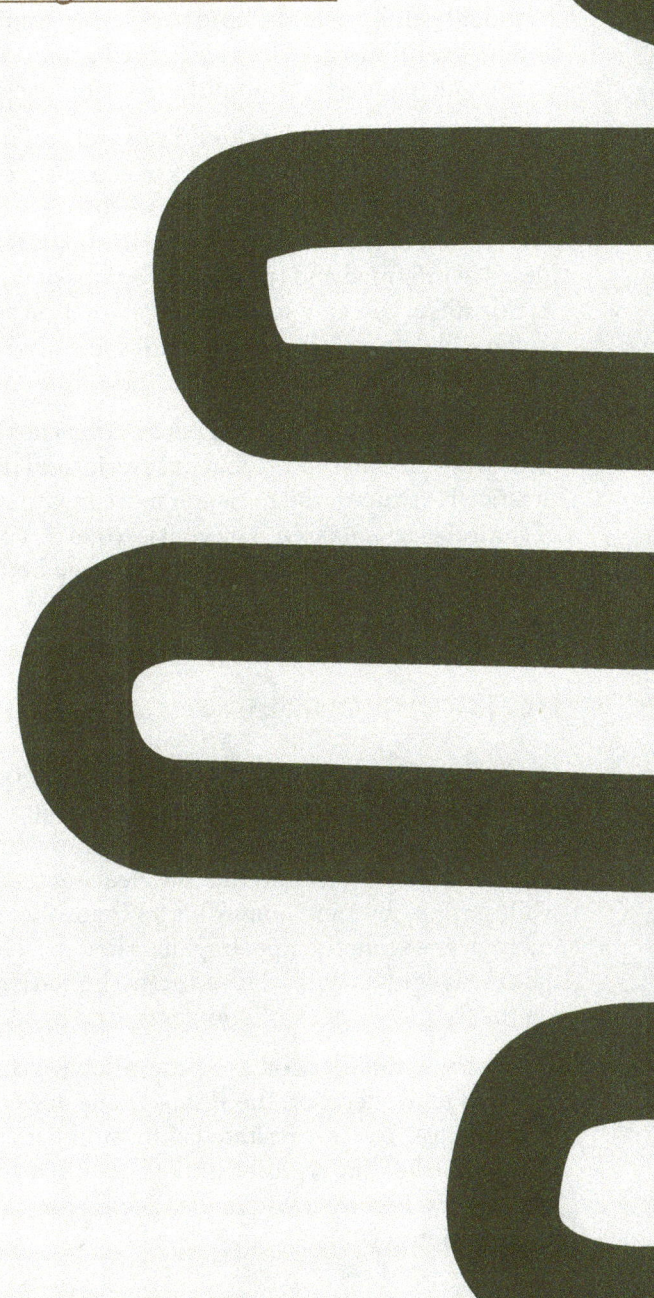

By taking your before, progress, and after photos, you'll be able to have a clear visual record of where you started and where your skin is now. You'll also want to go back to the goals you set forth for yourself when you started this clear skin journey. Was it to drastically reduce the time for getting ready in the morning or skip wearing makeup altogether? To feel more confident going out and facing people? Or simply to reduce physical pain and messy pillowcases from inflamed acne? Whatever these goals were, circle back to see how you would answer these now.

On the topical level, you should see and feel more flat areas on the skin and less of the bumps and lumps of active acne. Pain from inflamed acne has abated; perhaps your pillowcases are no longer soiled in the morning. The texture of the skin is smoother in all kinds of light, as both the larger lumps of inflamed and the smaller bumps of non-inflamed acne are gone. At this stage, you may see some pigmentation spots where acne once was, which will naturally fade over time (especially with the help of brightening products or treatments).

Realize that 100% clarity and perfection is not the goal, nor is it realistic. Acne will still come and go, but its severity and frequency should have been drastically reduced; you're clearer most days than not, and you have a sense of control over your skin. The goal is to get to a place of knowing when you do break out, why, and how to fix it (or even better, prevent).

What Does My Maintenance Regimen Look Like?

Once clients reach clarity, their regimens may or may not change, depending on a few factors. Some skin needs the same amount of exfoliation to keep those acne seeds from forming, so they can stick to the same regimen for years. Others may find that the clearing regimen their skin thrived on while purging becomes too strong for them once their skin clears up, resulting in over-exfoliation: peeling, irritated, or flaky skin. For these folks, a modified regimen with reduced active ingredients will do, perhaps reducing the frequency of exfoliation or switching to another type altogether.

Try just one modification at a time, allowing at least one month for each to see its true effects on the skin, as acne does take some time to form (if it's going to). To reset irritated skin, stop using all your active products and use the healing regimen until your skin has returned to a healthy and healed state before slowly reintroducing any active products or regimen modifications.

Pay attention to your skin, and it will let you know what it needs. Reevaluate your regimen every so often, even if only every season as the weather changes, but more so when you notice changes in your skin (i.e., products start to sting or burn, or you get oilier/drier than usual). Also, make sure to take into account the seasonal outdoor and indoor climates that you're in, as those can be big factors in what your skin needs and can tolerate at any given time.

Regimen Adjustment Ideas

If you're doing the basic regimen twice a day, are clear, and in maintenance mode (no longer purging) but feeling a bit dry:

- Are you rubbing extra hard or applying extra exfoliant in certain places, making those areas peel? Stop and let your skin heal, then try working it back in not as aggressively; this may take care of the area-specific over-exfoliation.
- Are you using enough product? Sometimes, clients want to stretch out the life of their products, but you need to use enough of them for them to actually work. Try using just a little bit more Hydrating Cleanser on dry skin while washing and Hydrating Cream when moisturizing.
- Up your moisturizing game. Switch to a non-foaming, more moisturizing face wash while keeping the rest of your active products the same. Or switch to a more hydrating moisturizer or sunscreen or layer extra moisture under your moisturizer/SPF.
- If you're using a more drying exfoliating toner (like With & Within Mandelic Toner), try alternating with something more moisturizing (like With & Within Hydrating Toner).
- If you are using an exfoliating toner AND exfoliating serum, keep up with one, but stop using the other (but you can continue using serum as a spot treatment if tolerated).
- If you aren't using an exfoliating serum, try toning with your active product just once a day versus two.
- You can also look into incorporating a moisturizing face mask like the Skin Script brand Goji Berry and Yogurt Mask. Wash, ice, tone, and mask for 15 to 30 minutes, then rinse and moisturize.
- Incorporating Omega-3 fish oils into your diet may also be beneficial for skin moisture; allow several weeks to see the effects.
- Try integrating the holistic hydration practices as outlined in Section 5, The Digestive System, Diet and Acne, Eliminate.

- Consider colonic cleansing; it's thought that impacted material is lining the colon, preventing water absorption through the colon, which is responsible for a large portion of the body's hydration. Doing a cleanse will help eradicate this impacted layer, allowing water to absorb more freely into the colon.

If you're doing the basic regimen twice a day, are clear, and in maintenance mode (no longer purging) but feeling a bit oily:
- Switch to a foaming cleanser (if you aren't using one already).
- Try switching to a lighter-textured, less- (or non-) moisturizing SPF.
- If you're oily only in certain areas, skip moisturizing these areas (but still apply SPF for protection).
- You can try using a powder mineral SPF on top of your moisturizer.
- Perhaps integrate an exfoliating or slightly drying cleanser, like a mandelic face wash.

Benzoyl Peroxide users

If you were using BP gel, are now clear, and inflammation has been completely under control for at least two to three months, you may be able to cut down or stop using it altogether.

Start this slowly by gradually reducing your BP usage in half. If and when you fully wean off of BP, icing along with the lifestyle changes should be enough to keep you clear and keep your inflammation under control. If you find yourself breaking out again, reevaluate your acne-safe lifestyle, or else you may have to incorporate the BP gel a bit longer till your acne isn't as active (usually in your 30s).

Anti-aging

A lot of the products you're already using to control acne also happen to be anti-aging! This is especially true if you are using With & Within products because I've built antioxidants into most of the products we formulate. As long as you have good active products to stimulate exfoliation, strengthen with antioxidants, and protect with a good quality sunscreen, your topical line of defense against acne, sun damage and "aging" skin is ready to go.

Remember that aging largely has to do with things that are *not* topical: diet, overall health, sense of happiness and fulfillment, and the most influential, genes. Stress management, a strong and mobile body, peaceful mind, balanced diet, and robust digestion are the keys to long-term health. Collagen taken internally via supplements or hearty bone broth can also help plump the skin. These, along with topical approaches, work to preserve the genetic physical makeup we have been given.

- Regular chemical exfoliation, such as with multi-functional mandelic acid or retinol (topical vitamin A), which to date is the only ingredient proven to directly boost collagen production. Try using this one of these at night under your moisturizer.
- An antioxidant serum will help strengthen and prevent breakdown of the skin. A Natural Difference's Rejuvenation Concentrate (with powerful antioxidant Spin Trap) is a With & Within favorite that also moisturizes. Vitamin C serums can help brighten and protect the skin at the same time (but like silicones, they can break out a small percentage of folks, so be careful).
- Protect the skin from the #1 aging source, the sun, with a good sunscreen applied generously and regularly along with physical protection like wide brim hats, large sunglasses, long sleeves and pants, and seeking shade.

If your skin starts to become a bit dry, incorporate extra moisture into your skin and body, both topically and internally.

You can look into facial acupuncture, facial yoga, or skin treatments at medical skin spas like intense pulse light (IPL) or laser therapy.

Incorporate gentle facial massage techniques when applying products to encourage blood circulation, lymph drainage, and muscle relaxation. This is especially great to soothe headaches, soreness, and teeth grinding/jaw clenching. Always stroke upward and outward against gravity, and think positive thoughts.

Reintroducing Questionable Variables

If you want to reintroduce old (and cloggy) favorites or new questionable products, do so one at a time, preferably for three months each (unless you break out, you can stop sooner than that) so you can clearly tell if your new breakouts are due to the recently introduced variable.

Should you break out, go back to the basic twice-a-day clearing skincare regimen as a baseline to clear up:

- Cleanse (foaming if you're not dry, non-foaming if you are dry)
- Ice (a swipe or two all over as a preventative is great, even if you are clear but ice for longer if your acne is inflamed or purging)
- Tone (preferably an exfoliating one, like our Mandelic Toner)
- Exfoliating and/or antioxidant serum (if using)

- Moisturizer and/or SPF (or benzoyl peroxide gel, for those with inflamed acne using it at night)

When Do I Need Treatments?

Treatments can be done for maintenance, corrective (acne purging, brightening) or preventative (acne, anti-aging) reasons. Make sure that the products used are acne-safe, and research the ingredients if possible to avoid post-treatment breakouts. If you are correctively treating the skin for active acne, treatment frequency can range from every week to every three weeks, depending on how long it takes your skin to heal from extractions and exfoliation. If you are treating the skin preventatively for acne or aging, every one to three months should work for most (it can range) for best results.

Importance of Maintaining an Acne-safe Lifestyle and Diet

Maintaining this way of acne-safe living is ideal to keep you clear and your body its healthiest. However, when some clients are cleared up, they choose to reintroduce certain foods or products to see if they are reactive to them and, if so, how. Starting from a baseline with clear skin will enable you to more clearly and quickly see what triggers remain for you to continue being mindful of.

Remember the delayed effects—that products can take days to months, and diet can take about a month to show up on your skin as acne. Intentionally introducing a new variable and keeping a record of it will be helpful for reference purposes.

If you do experience breaking out, you know what to do: stop the now-confirmed acne-causing variable, go back to the acne-clearing lifestyle, use your active skin regimen, and you'll clear back up soon enough.

Scarring

There are two types of physical marks left behind after the skin heals from trauma like acne: textural and hyperpigmentation (which shows up as colored dark, brownish spots and/or redness). However, the most challenging scars to deal with are the potentially lingering psychological effects.

Textural

Textural scarring is when the surface of the skin looks rough or dimpled; ice pick, "craters," or pockmarks are terms often used to describe these kinds. This is actual structural damage to the tissues deeper in the basal membrane layers of the skin and not simply an issue of color, like the surface-level pigment scarring as described below.

Textural scarring is best treated with modalities performed as soon as the skin is healed and clear, either at a dermatologist or medical aesthetics practice via puncturing (such as micro-needling with a micro-pen, with or without platelet-rich plasma; or TCA cross), machine treatments (IPL, lasers, ultrasound), injectables, and more. Seek a practitioner who has extensive experience working with skin tones like yours. Darker skins need extra care with these technologies and can get burned by too-hot laser machines more easily than lighter tones.

Regular professional extractions with precise acne treatments while you are purging will drastically reduce the chances of new textural and pigmentation scarring and speed the healing of any scarring that has started to develop. Get your acne and inflammation under control before beginning any scar treatments for the best results.

Hyperpigmentation

Also known as pigment "scarring," it looks like red, brown, or darker-colored spots left over from old, inflamed acne that's since healed.

Brown and darker-colored pigmentation (aka post-inflammatory hyperpigmentation, or PIH) is treated quite successfully with in-clinic chemical peels and at-home brightening products. This pigmentation is the result of melanocytes—the pigment-forming parts of the cell located in the upper epidermis layers of the skin—reacting to the trauma of inflammation and acne. Products, chemical peels, and skin treatments targeted towards pigmentation brightening, supported by adequate topical hydration will speed up the brightening of these spots, evening out the skin tone.

Red pigmentation (aka vascular pigmentation) generally takes its own time to heal without any extra skincare products. This pigmentation is the result of blood vessels healing from the trauma of inflamed acne that will eventually reabsorb back into the body. However, I have seen IPL face treatments fade this pigmentation up quite quickly, and it may be worth the investment. Be wary of products marketed with anti-redness properties, as they often contain cloggy seaweed-derived ingredients.

Hyperpigmentation

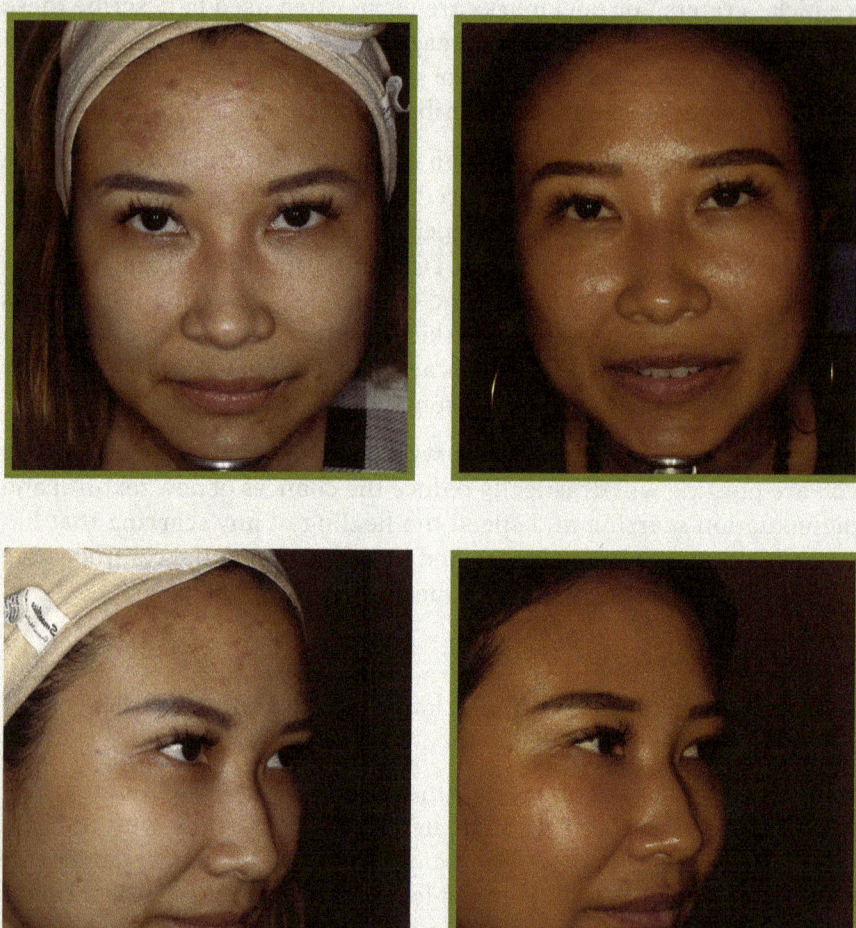

This tanned-skin client had inflamed acne that she picked, that left PIH (brown) scarring. After getting the acne under control and integrating skin picking alternatives, both her acne and pigment scarring completely cleared up.

Section 10 - Maintaining your Clear Skin

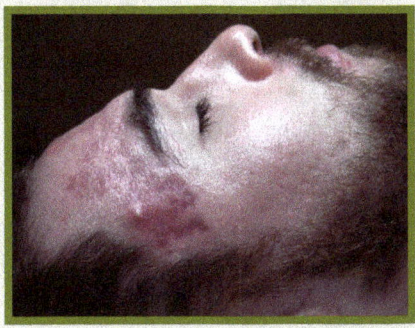 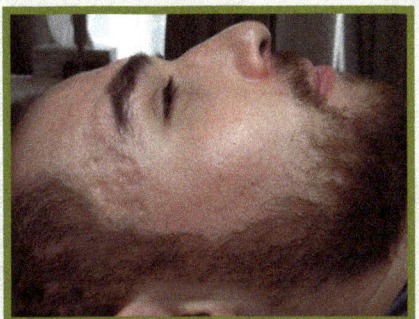

This light-skinned client had severely inflamed acne that left deep vascular (red) pigmentation scarring. Just one LED treatment at a medispa dramatically cleared it up in just a few weeks' time.

Some stubborn pigmentation of either color may remain because a full extraction of the acne seed still hiding inside the pore needs to take place. If a pore is still clogged with the acne seed stuck inside, the pigmentation will remain because the pore is never able to fully heal with it in the way. Expert corrective acne treatments with safe and thorough extractions will take care of this.

Psychological and Emotional

Create and stick to a lifestyle that focuses on self-care, fulfilling work and relationships, rest and relaxation with a low-glycemic diet, reasonable and regular exercise, enough quality sleep, and effective stress management. Taking care of the body sets a good foundation for a peaceful and rested mind.

Seek out ways to understand and exercise compassion for yourself, build up your self-esteem, and appreciate yourself for how far you've come. Explore talk therapy, journaling, take frequent five-minute breaks throughout your day, focus on one thing at a time, optimize your time and energy toward things that are worth your time, learn to accept and be easy with yourself and others, and find creative outlets and relaxation techniques.

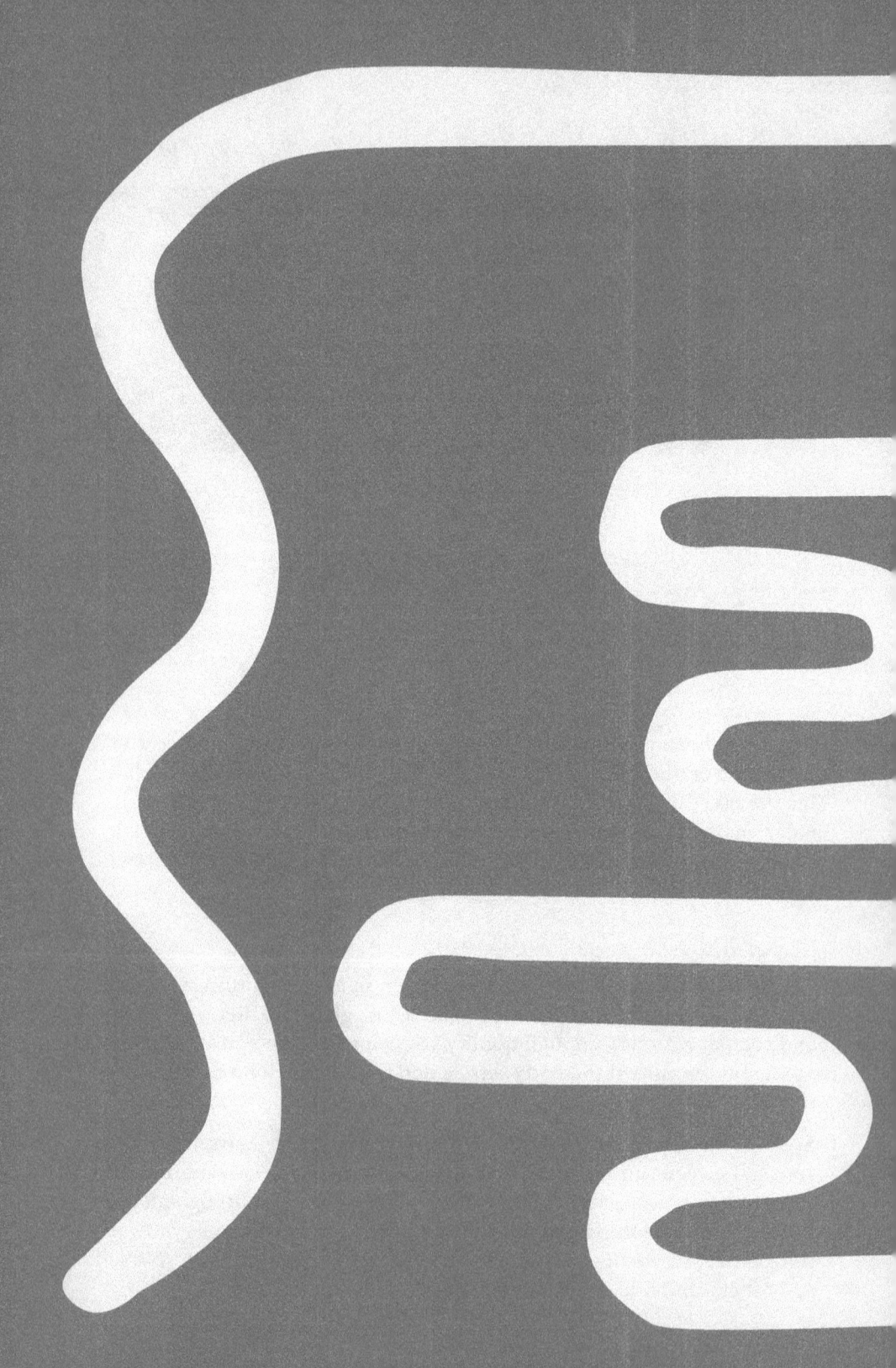

SECTION 11

Additional Resources

Clear Skin for Everyone

With & Within Lifestyle Library Blog

For more in-depth explanations and study updates, read our Lifestyle Library Blog posts, follow us on our social media, and sign up for our newsletter. We are constantly researching, testing, and sharing our work, and these are the first places we share our discoveries.[36]

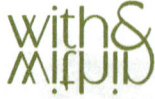

START HERE   DIY TOOLS ⌄   SHOP   SUPPORT ⌄   LOG IN   🔍   🛒 0

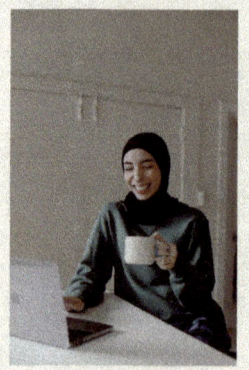

Welcome to our clear skin lifestyle library

Herein is the bread and butter of the acne-safe lifestyle, that will accelerate and prolong your results. Switching up your skin products is a big part of the battle, but implementing what you learn here will help you not only maintain your clear complexion, but also promote a healthier life in the long term.

All
body
candida
digestion
food
hair
holistic health
hormones
kim
lifestyle
makeup
products

Candida safe noodles

As we all know, an important part of doing the candida cleanse properly is to avoid

Read more...

Malassezia folliculitis, aka "fungal acne"

"Fungal" acne is a popular (and incorrect) term used to describe a skin condition that looks like acne, but actually isn't...

Read more...

Soy and acne: why we avoid this food for clear skin

Here at with & within, we encourage our clients to adopt several healthy dietary changes, one of the most important being the...

Read more...

Hidden offenders that are keeping you from clearing up

Using your active and acne-safe skin regimen and eating acne-safe, but still breaking out? here are a few sneaky culprits you...

Read more...

Sensitive peely face? could be overexfoliation. or... who you're making out with!

often times we get clients complaining of sensitivity and peeling around the mouth, and lower half of the face. we find that...

Read more...

Mask-ne part 2: masks i've tried and my faves

Ok so maskne is still a thing and since my last really long post about it, i've done some research...

Read more...

Books on Skin

ACNE RX by Dr. James E. Fulton
The With & Within philosophy and treatment protocol are based largely on this book, which is full of in-depth information about the science, biology, and history behind acne. Dr. Fulton also chronicles his personal journey; having suffered from severe cystic acne since birth, he spent decades looking to solve his acne problems before he eventually became a dermatologist and biochemist specializing in the research and treatment of acne. Through his work and the work of Drs. Gerd Plewig and Albert Kligman, vitamin A (which eventually got bought out by American pharmaceutical company Johnson and Johnson, which reformulated it into a comedogenic base and rebranded it as Retin-A) and BP were stabilized specifically for the treatment of acne.

Radiant Skin from the Inside Out: The Holistic Dermatologist's Guide to Healing Your Skin Naturally by Alan M. Dattner
Dr. Dattner's philosophy on acne as described in this book is the one that most closely aligns with what we've seen in clinic.

Clearing Concepts: A Guide to Acne Treatment by Dr. Mark Lees, PhD and LE
Dr. Lees has been in the professional skin circuit for decades, and his philosophy is very similar to Dr. Fulton's, with some variances. Like Dr. Fulton, he did his own comedogenic ingredient research, and it was through Dr. Lees' work that we were able to confirm avocado oil's comedogenicity.

Comedogenic Ingredients

We've listed the most common comedogenic ingredients in *Section 1, Product Shopping Tips*. You can access the complete list for free on our website's Product Checker.[37]

The world famous With & Within product checker

https://withandwithin.co/pages/product-checker

With diligent researching, compiling and updating of our comedogenic ingredient database, anyone anywhere can copy and paste questionable product ingredient listings into our free and easy to use machine to quickly see if it is safe for acne-prone skin to try using. Largely based on the published ingredient research work of Dr. Fulton and Dr. Lees, we also continue to add our own clinical research findings to help our clients shop smart.

With & Within Products and Shop

Our shop is carefully curated with products that we've sourced, tested in clinic and, in most cases, formulated ourselves to be truly acne-safe. Here is some basic information about our products, the very same ones that have cleared and maintained thousands of complexions over the years in our San Francisco clinic. Visit our site for more information and instructional videos: *withandwithin.co*

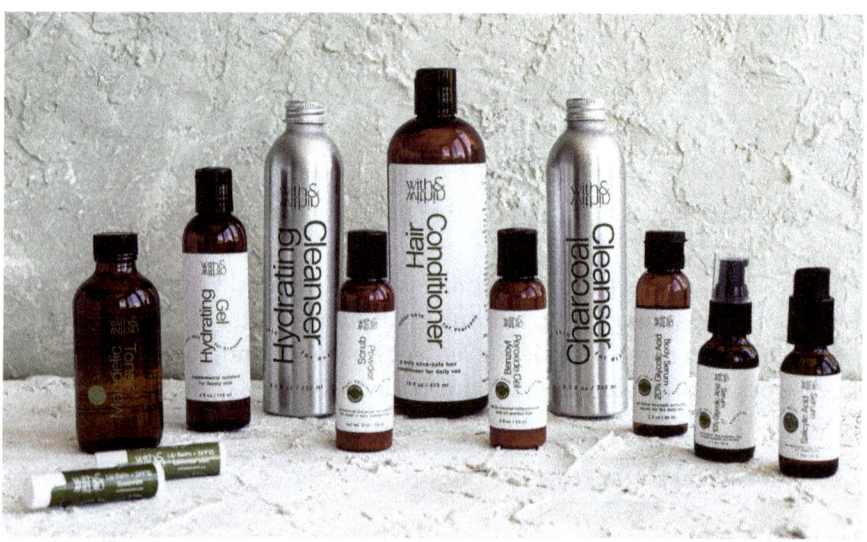

Cleansers

We have two basic cleansers: Charcoal Cleanser for normal to oily/combination skin types and Hydrating Cleanser for normal to dry/dry skin types. They are meant to gently yet effectively cleanse the skin, preparing it for active treatment products.

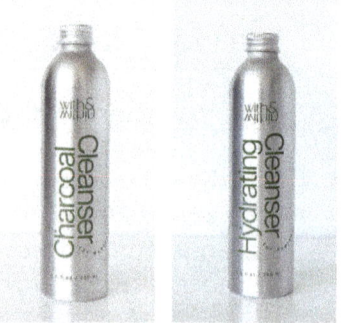

Section 11 - Additional Resources

For a thorough cleansing of face makeup, waterproof eye makeup, SPF, and general dirt and grime, try our cleansing washcloths. Use your cleanser as normal and before rinsing, and use a wet wrung-out washcloth to gently wipe off your cleanser and debris. Finish off with several splashes of warm water to remove any residual cleanser before proceeding with your regimen.

Active Exfoliating Products

We have five active products in our line. Four of them are exfoliants: Mandelic Toner, 2% Salicylic and Glycolic Serums (10% for the face and 20% for the body). The fifth is our Benzoyl Peroxide Gel (BP Gel).

Mandelic Toner is our signature multi-functional active product that purges acne, brightens pigmentation, and encourages strong, clear skin. This active product alone is enough for most to achieve and maintain a clear complexion, but for those who need extra support, we also have Salicylic and Glycolic Acid Serums to further exfoliate the skin. Salicylic acid is particularly exceptional for purging acne, while Glycolic brightens while exfoliating (but can be irritating for sensitive skin). We recommend acclimating to using the toner twice a day for several weeks before integrating an exfoliating serum.

When used correctly, our Benzoyl Peroxide gel reliably helps to control inflamed acne and some forms of rosacea. For best results, use it with Hydrating Gel alongside an exfoliant as tolerated.

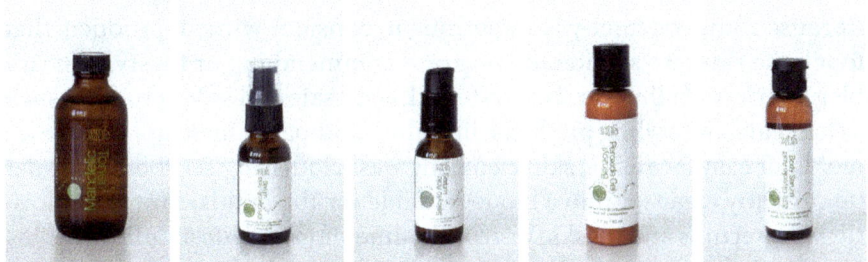

Moisturizers

We offer two moisturizers: our Hydrating Cream and Hydrating Gel.

Hydrating Cream is good for most skin types, offering moisturizing, soothing, and strengthening antioxidant support, designed to be used at night or in the daytime under your SPF. Hydrating Gel is designed to be used with

BP Gel or layered under Hydrating Cream, but for the oiliest of skins, this may be enough to use on its own.

We also offer Hydrating Toner, which can be used to add even more moisture to one's regimen.

Sunscreens

We offer three different sunscreens, each offering different amounts of moisture.

Safeguard SPF 40 is our most moisturizing formula, good for normal to dry and dry skin, and it can be used on both the face and body. It's also water resistant and stays in place. I like to apply this thoroughly in the morning and reapply throughout the day using one of the following sunscreens:

Clear Choice Sport Shield SPF 45 offers light moisture and is suitable for normal to oily or combination skin. It's very easy to apply and is great for the body.

Tizo SPF 40 is a formula that is not at all moisturizing, so it's ideal for oily skin or those who like a matte finish. It comes tinted and untinted and can be used as a makeup primer.

We also carry Illuminare liquid foundation makeup, and though it does contain SPF 20, for best sun protection, we recommend first applying sunscreen prior to applying this or any makeup.

Extra Products

Because comedogenicity is something to consider with all products that touch the skin, we sell in our shop or recommend in our lifestyle library blog a variety of clinic- and client-tested, acne-safe accessory products such as hair care and styling products, lip balm, toothpaste, makeup, silicone ice molds for easy face icing, skin cleansing washcloths, dry scrubbing powder (to turn any cleanser into a biodegradable scrub), antioxidant, and moisturizing serums and masks. Visit our online shop and lifestyle library blog for more information, including how-to videos and additional resources.

Body-Focused Repetitive Behaviors (BFRB)

In addition to the common urges to pick at pimples, we also find that picking can be the physical manifestation of other stressors that may be better addressed with the additional support of a mental health professional. Picking becomes more serious of an issue when it persists, even without the bumps of acne present. Here are some tips from Kristin Southwick, a marriage and family therapist who specializes in BFRBs:[38]

Honestly and Compassionately Assess

Being truthful and assessing what your answers to these questions are may reveal some ideas of how serious your picking problem is and maybe will raise self-awareness or inspire different approaches when the urge arises.

- On a scale of 1-10, how difficult is it for you *not* to pick your skin?
- How do you feel about your skin, and yourself, in general?
- How do you feel about your skin, and yourself, after you're done picking? (Defeated, out of control, and devastated are common answers.)
- Have you ever felt out of control with your picking, stress or other activities and emotions?

Other things to think about: How and when did the picking begin? Do major life changes or incidents intensify these behaviors? Do you enter a state of trance-like deep thought while picking? With compassionate and truthful answers, you will likely find the real underlying motivating force underneath the picking—perhaps it's conflict within a relationship, struggles in life, or maybe even a genetic disposition.

Brain Activity and Picking

Picking usually happens when the person's basic needs are out of balance—they're either hungry, tired, or maybe just need to use the bathroom. They are usually also anxious, needing to do something with their idle hands. Being able to raise self-awareness when you want to start picking and taking a moment to evaluate what's happening (or what basic needs are not being met) are the first steps to managing compulsive picking.

If you catch yourself picking—stop and ask yourself what else is going on. Are you tired and perhaps just need to get ready to rest? Are you hungry, which is making you feel cranky, and need to eat something? Are you angry and need to calm yourself down with some fresh air and a quiet walk around the neighborhood?

Picking Alternatives

Once your mindset check-in is complete and basic needs are identified, try fulfilling those needs to see if that helps to calm your nerves, taking the itch out of your fingers to pick. Having an alternative plan of action for when you feel compelled to touch your face is helpful so you have something to keep your hands busy at the ready. These can include:

- Lotion — Applying body lotion to your hands or body, giving yourself a nice massage.
- Fidget toys — These are great to keep your hands busy and off your face. There are many you can get online, like squeeze balls, playdough, Rubik's cubes, fidget spinners, etc.
- Oral distraction — Chewing gum or eating something crunchy like carrots can offer a satisfying sensation.
- Meditation apps and guided relaxation videos —Simple Habit, Calm, and Insight Timer are a few apps I love. Search YouTube for quick 1- or 2-minute meditations.
- Physical distraction — Grabbing some ice from the freezer and rubbing that on your face is a great tool to get inflammation down and get you to focus on the cold sensation while doing good for your acne, too.
- Physical movement — Jumping around, screaming into a pillow, or going outside for a quick walk around the block can help offer some quick and easy relief for the nervous system.
- Deep breathing — Using this simple technique instantly helps to calm the nervous system and oxygenates the brain for a calmer state of mind.

Tools to Help Curb Picking

- No skin-extracting tools! Toss them or freeze them in a large ice block and keep them in the freezer. In the time it takes for that ice block to defrost, the craving to pick may go away.
- Use a removable matte-finish dulling spray (available at hardware or craft stores) on mirrors you'll pass by or use to lessen visibility and discourage picking.
- Positive affirmations—they really work! To keep it simple, think of one word that helps to invoke a positive feeling. Peace, calm, or even a small picture reminder could help.
- Getting your nails done could be a good motivator to keep them in good shape by not picking your skin. If your nails are long, perhaps they'd be too long to pick your skin with.
- Set an alarm to go off a few times a day for a self check-in. Where am I? How am I feeling? Am I picking my skin?

Further BFRB Resources

Websites such as The TLC Foundation for Body-Focused Repetitive Behaviors[39], Stop Picking[40] and Skin Pick[41] are great online resources for community, professional referrals, tools, and even apps to help manage picking (as well as other BFRBs).

Identifying and contacting a Cognitive Behavioral Therapist who specializes in BFRBs can be a lifesaver. They can offer personalized support and get to the root of the BFRB with talk therapy. Kristen Southwick is an LMFT who specializes in BFRBs and has provided many of the tips and tricks mentioned in this section. She's available for professional training and personal therapy sessions via videoconferencing and can be contacted by email[42]

The book *Skin Picking: The Freedom to Finally Stop*, by Annette Pasternak, PhD, seems to be a highly recommended resource for the dermatillomania community.

Food

The Omnivore's Dilemma by Michael Pollan

It was this book that changed my life and view of how to eat for the better of the world. Though quite dry and wordy in the first few chapters, this book informs the reader about the food supply systems of our country by tracing the origins of four different meals from plate to farm: conventional industrial (McDonald's), organic industrial (an Amy's Organic brand frozen dinner), organic closed loop farm (Polyface Farm), and strictly locally sourced (where he grows, barters, and forages his own meal). His extended research thoroughly explains the inner workings of the food industries in America and the environmental and nutritional impacts they have.

Food Rules by Michael Pollan

Michael Pollan's short and sweet book, *Food Rules*, is the best quick and easy-to-digest resource on how to eat for the health of self and the world. He concisely explains why whole, nutrient-dense foods and supporting your local ecosystem are so important, and it will help you create a mentality to eating that is skin-safe, nutritious, delicious, and more sustainable.

Eating on the Wild Side by Jo Robinson

So we know to eat healthy—but when you're in the grocery store buying salad greens, which types of lettuce are the most nutritious? What exact variety of apples has the highest antioxidants? And once you've picked out your fruits or veggies, how do you prepare them to coax the most nutritional value out of them? This book guides the consumer to the most flavorful and nutritious foods at the market and divulges tips on how to best prepare them.

With & Within Lifestyle Library and Pinterest pages

Find more resources for recipe ideas, food substitutions for cheese[43], cooking oils[44], and coffee[45] and other dietary guidelines. We've also got several relevant lifestyle and food idea boards on Pinterest.[46]

www.pinterest.com/withandwithin

General Wellness

Prescription for Natural Cures (Third Edition): A Self-Care Guide for Treating Health Problems with Natural Remedies Including Diet, Nutrition, Supplements, and Other Holistic Methods by James F. Balch, MD, Mark Stengler, NMD, et al.

This book is a bible that we constantly refer to when clients complain of another systemic issue that is not within our scope to diagnose or treat. It includes both allopathic and naturopathic diagnosis descriptions and treatment descriptions, and it discusses most body ailments from Candida imbalance and recurring nosebleeds to constipation and ear ringing.

The New Chinese Medicine Handbook: An Innovative Guide to Integrating Eastern Wisdom with Western Practice for Modern Healing by Misha Ruth Cohen

A longtime San Francisco wellness community pioneer and veteran of Jewish descent, Dr. Misha was one of the first to use TCM to treat the first HIV and AIDS patients in San Francisco. I was fortunate enough to be one of her patients when she helped me a lot with hormonal balancing issues.

The Complete Book of Ayurvedic Home Remedies: Based on the Timeless Wisdom of India's 5,000-Year-Old Medical System by Vasant Lad

I found this at an Ayurveda retreat in Sri Lanka. I liked that it was easy to understand and offered many practical insights and tips to try while back at home after leaving the retreat.

Nourishing Traditions: The Cookbook that Challenges Politically Correct Nutrition and Diet Dictocrats by Sally Fallon, Mary G. Enig et al., Jan 1, 2001

I haven't read this cover to cover, but I've attended the conference and agree with most of the research that was presented. However, they emphasize the use of fermented dairy, which I recommend acne-prone folks to avoid.

Communication and Relational Skills

Seemingly out of place in direct relation to clearing one's acne, I've personally found these actionable resources too valuable to omit.

Communication and relationships are perhaps the most scary and challenging yet essential and rewarding parts of our lives. Learning the skills to improve how we show up for ourselves through self-awareness and in more conscious relationship with others helps to reduce daily overall stress and anxiety, lowering cortisol production and systemic inflammation.

Difficult Conversations: How to Discuss What Matters Most by Bruce Patton, Douglas Stone, and Sheila Heen

This book walks through several relatable scenarios to help you understand how to break down and engage in challenging conversations in a very easy-to-follow, actionable text.

Authentic Relating and *Non-Violent Communication*[47]

Authentic Relating offers fun, interactive practices to learn and deepen relational, emotional, and communication skills. *Non-Violent Communication* offers a simple framework and language guides to remain emotionally aware and connected during tough conversations.

Nedra Glover Tawwab, MSW, LCSW

Nedra is a licensed therapist, relationship expert and NY Times best selling author who teaches people how to create healthy relationships by teaching them how to implement boundaries. Her philosophy is that a lack of boundaries and assertiveness underlie most relationship issues, which can be alleviated by creating healthy relationships with self and others.[48]

Dr. Nicole LePera

Also known as "The Holistic Psychologist," Dr. LePera blends her background of traditional psychotherapy with holistic lifestyle practices, in her book "How to Do the Work." Informed by multiple philosophical approaches and filled with actionable steps, readers can learn how to cultivate self-awareness, compassion and understanding of self, to be in better community with others for a more vibrant, authentic and joyful life.[49]

Ahran Lee[50]

Ahran is a Korean-American multidisciplinary artist, coach, facilitator and speaker in the San Francisco Bay Area. She facilitates experiential workshops that help folks—especially BIPOC's—learn and integrate relational, communication and community building skills through play, art and fun.

Self-care and Meditation

Here are just a few of the writers and teachers whose work I love, follow, and have gotten so much solace and many lessons from.

Diego Perez is an Ecuadorian American poet, philosopher, and author who writes under the pen name Yung Pueblo. Grounded by his longtime Vipassana silent meditation practice, his writing focuses on the power of self-healing, creating healthy relationships, and the wisdom that comes when we truly work on knowing ourselves. I highly recommend his books *Inward, Clarity & Connection* and the latest release, *Lighter*.

Lalah Delia is a Black American spiritual writer, certified spiritual practitioner, wellness educator, and the founder of Vibrate Higher Daily, a vibrational-based living online community and mentoring program, as well as the author of the beautifully published book with the same name. I find her work very grounding in a strong feminine way that reminds me to stay regal and honor my highest self.

Manoj Dias is a Sri Lankan Australian meditation teacher born and raised in the Theraveda Buddhist tradition, a speaker and the author of *Still Together*, a gorgeous book that makes starting to meditate simple, approachable, and leads with learning how to cultivate self-awareness and meaningful relationships through the core teachings of mindfulness and Buddhist meditation. I love using his app *Open* for meditation, learning series, breathing, and physical exercise.[51]

Rupi Kaur is a Punjab Indian Canadian poet, illustrator, photographer, and author of several best-selling poetry books. Her messages are raw and empowering, accompanied by her own illustrations, and about womanhood, abuse, inequality, violence, growth, and most importantly: peace. At the core of her work is human dignity.

Simple Habit is my favorite meditation app, with hundreds of 1-5 minute guided audio tracks perfectly suited for any scenario (before a big meeting, going for a run or rest breaks, for example), designed to make meditation easy to integrate for even the busiest folks. They even have tracks for kids.[52]

Endnotes

36 *https://withandwithin.co/blogs/blog*

37 *https://withandwithin.co/pages/product-checker*

38 *https://www.bfrb.org/*

39 *https://www.bfrb.org/*

40 *https://stoppicking.com/*

41 *http://skinpick.com/*

42 She can be contacted at kristinsouthwick@gmail.com.

43 *https://withandwithin.co/blogs/blog/acne-safe-cheeses-galore*

44 *https://withandwithin.co/blogs/blog/cooking-oils*

45 *https://withandwithin.co/blogs/blog/kicking-the-coffee-habit-for-clear-skin*

46 *https://www.pinterest.com/withandwithin*

47 authenticrelating.co and cnvc.org

48 *https://www.nedratawwab.com/* and *https://www.instagram.com/nedratawwab/*

49 *https://theholisticpsychologist.com/* and *https://www.instagram.com/the.holistic.psychologist/*

50 *https://ahranleecoaching.com/* and *https://www.instagram.com/ahranmakes/*

51 *https://o-p-e-n.com/referral/1VL7IHovTkXFss3ChLBxUrZHptv2*

52 *https://simplehabit.app.link/DDUD1GtQzDb*

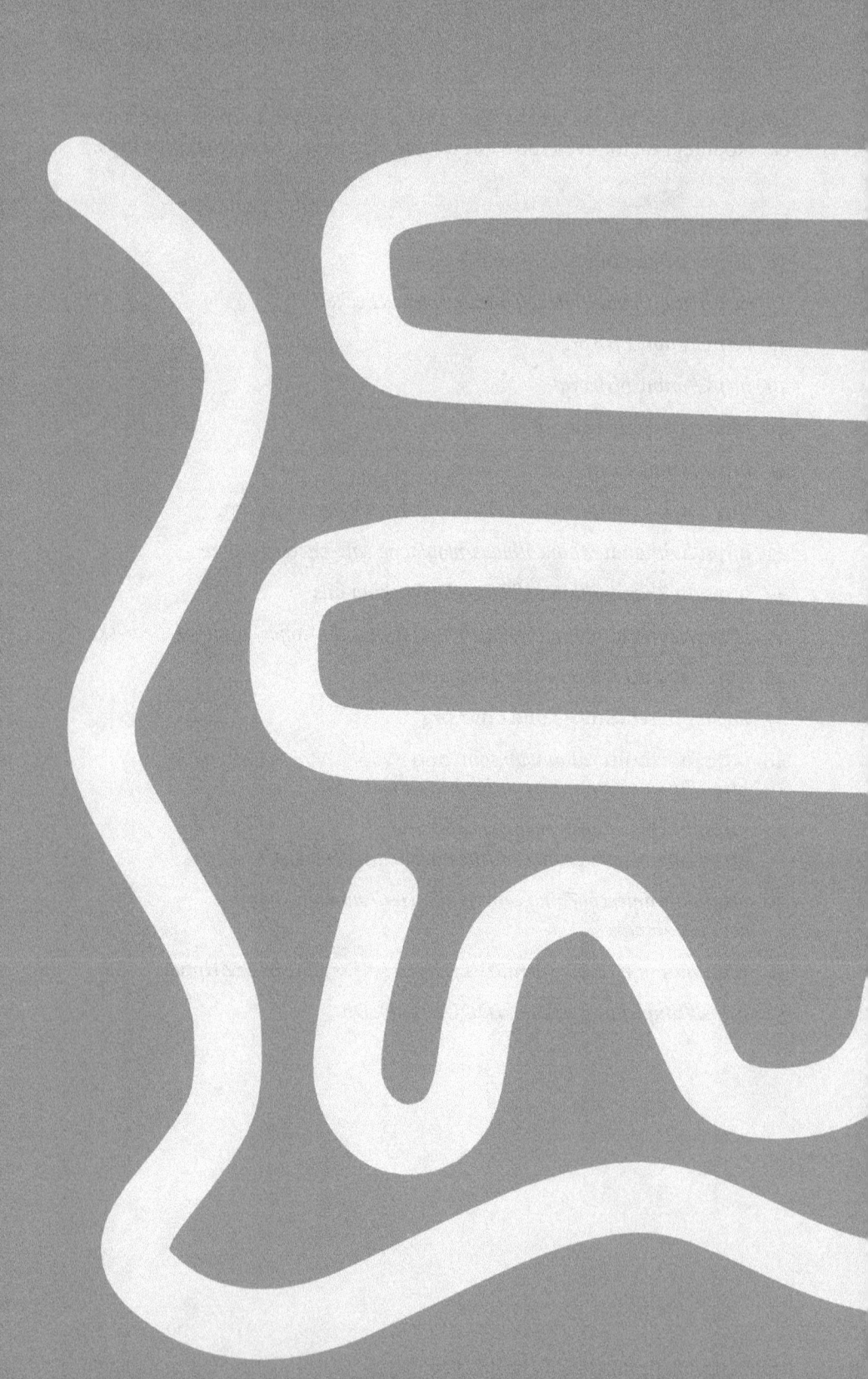

SECTION 12
Finale

Finale

After you've finally cleared your skin and have it under control, aside from the maintenance and reduction in physical scars, it's important to acknowledge and continue to nurture any emotional scars that may be left behind from the effects of acne. The most rewarding part of this work has been seeing our clients' personalities change from quiet and shy to confident, happy, and making eye contact again, with their true personalities finally allowed to shine through.

Take care to pat yourself on the back for the hard work you put into getting here. Be aware of when depression and/or low self-esteem try to make their way into your life and learn how to combat it. Some ideas: seek out a therapist to learn skills to better manage difficult emotions, create and live by positive affirmations and reminders, learn to believe and accept compliments and how to be assertive, build positive relationships, recognize what you're good at, and continue to hone those skills. Give yourself compassion for rough days, move your physical body, get plenty of fresh air and water, eat well, and take really good care of yourself. Hopefully, throughout this self-care journey, you've realized that you are more than the skin on your face and are more empowered to take control of your own health and life.

That's all I've got! Every single thing I know and can think of in regard to acne and what I've learned and seen over the years is here in this book. I hope that you feel more empowered and able to take agency over the health of your skin to clear up for good and contribute what you will to the world with your newfound confidence and self-actualization! I look forward to hearing about your journey and hope that you get in touch with us on our website at withandwithin.co to share your story. Thank you for reading along and allowing us to assist and inspire you on the journey of liberation for all, through wellness with & within.

Gratitude

I acknowledge and offer my gratitude to the Indigenous Ramaytush, Ohlone, Mukwema and Confederated Villages of Lisjan peoples, on which their land (San Francisco and Oakland, California) I was born, raised and occupy, creating this work herein.

To my mom, Julie Yap, who taught me self-care, independence, freedom, responsibility, and unconditional love. She is the embodiment of the American dream, having overcome so many obstacles and sacrifices to single-handedly and selflessly provide the very best for me and our family as a Chinese immigrant from the Philippines. She gave me the trust, freedom, wisdom, and unconditional love to explore my very unconventional path in life, ultimately leading me to this work. To my birth father, whose character has influenced me deeply despite the distance of time and space. To my ancestors, who, over the centuries, made sacrifices in new lands and cultures for future generations they would never get to know, along with other loved ones that have passed on, I love, honor, and feel you guiding me toward my highest self and hope to make you proud.

To my mentors, specifically acne pioneers Laura Cooksey and Dr. James E. Fulton, whose work and research paved the way for me to create With & Within. Fellow estheticians Shilpa Makhija, Julie Pruitt, and colleague Corey Chan, who were my biggest supporters when I contemplated starting this business: thank you for being the push I needed to reach beyond my comfort zone and humble beginnings.

To my clients who have trusted and believed in me and my ability to help them live healthier, clear-skinned lives, especially the ones who supported me emotionally as friends and professionally as clients, including those who flew in from out of state just to visit our clinic, got us published and featured in the media and those who gave me pep talks when I needed them most.

To all my teachers, leaders, mentors, and teammates through the years—personal and professional—who helped contribute to the evolution of myself and my business that's changed so many lives for the better. Special thanks to Kerry Watson for all of her help, partnership as an employee turned clinic licensee, and loyalty all these years, especially for her help in compiling our comedogenic ingredients list and testing products on her very sensitive skin. An additional heartfelt thanks to Masha Chepovetsky for all of her support.

To everyone that I've ever been in community with; from my chosen family, my soul siblings, food friends, clients-, fellow healers- and entrepreneurs-turned-close friends, coaches and confidantes, mentors, every single person that worked with or for me. Everyone I've ever crossed paths with has influenced who I am today. I acknowledge, honor, and am grateful for all the shared moments of joy, grief, learnings, laughs, adventures, and everything in between. Special thanks to the amazing women who helped this book come to life; Tara Majuta, Debbie Burke and Hester Van Toorenburg. Duizend maal dank to Hester for her pregnant patience and persistence with this perfectionist newbie, bringing my work to incredible life.

And to everyone fighting the good fight towards true liberation for all (especially my first social justice teachers: Dr. Connie Wun (imreadymovement.org), Dr. Kiona (reroottravel.com), Bianca Mabute-Louie (biancaml.com), Michelle MiJung Kim (michellemijungkim.com), Terisa Siagatonu (terisasiagatonu.com), Favianna Rodriguez (favianna.com), Ericka Hart M.Ed. (ihartericka.com), Amanda Seales (amandaseales.com) and Angela Davis): Thank you for bravely, consistently and lovingly putting the work in to keep us on the path towards collective wellness, reclamation and healing. It is my hope that my work instills some of the self-care and self-preservation needed for us all to better ourselves and by extension, our world.

About Kim and With & Within's Story

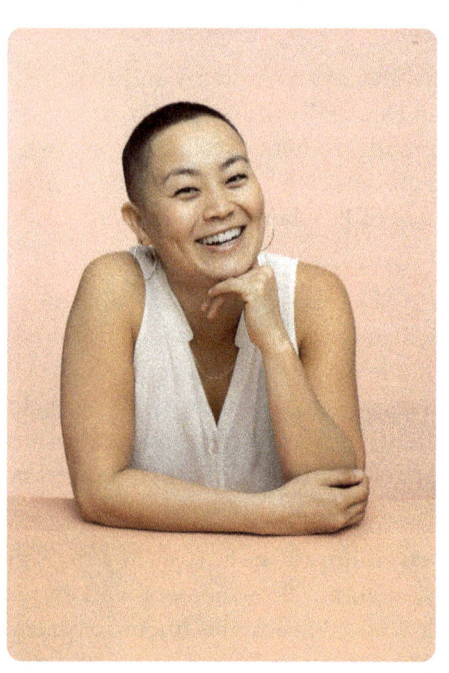

Born as a first-generation Filipino Chinese American raised in San Francisco by a single mother and her maternal grandparents, I was a high-achieving but unconventional learner who unexpectedly dropped out of high school in junior year and received my California High School Proficiency Exam certificate. (Shout out to my high school counselor Lowell Denny III, who taught me that I could thrive outside of the conventional educational construct, and shared with me his love of Celia Cruz and passion for politics, among many other things.) With my newfound freedom, I focused on working in fashion retail full-time before eventually finding a spa reception job at the iconic Spa Radiance in San Francisco's Marina District. At the front desk and trapped behind the cash register, there wasn't much opportunity to build real relationships with clients, let alone make a meaningful impact on others. So I quit, went to work for a credit union to save up some money, and then applied to beauty school.

Section 12 - Finale

The San Francisco Institute of Esthetics and Cosmetology was the newest beauty school in town, and I was in one of their very first graduating esthetician classes in 2004. After that, I worked everywhere I could. Starting out at the neighborhood hair and nail salons, I gradually expanded my experience and learned about Ayurveda, where I became fascinated by holistic medicine and intrigued by the similarities Ayurveda has with the Traditional Chinese Medicine I grew up with.

After that, I learned about luxury levels of service and microdermabrasion, helping to open San Francisco's first five-star resort spa, Remede Spa, at the St. Regis Hotel. From there, I tried my hand at the medical skincare industry at a laser hair removal clinic, which gave me an opportunity to learn about what it takes to start a new business from scratch. I was responsible for building out and opening a brand-new office, generating and closing new sales leads, recruiting, hiring, and training a brand-new staff of nurses and selling and managing inventory, all while working ten-hour days, six days a week. Here, I experienced my first round of burnout.

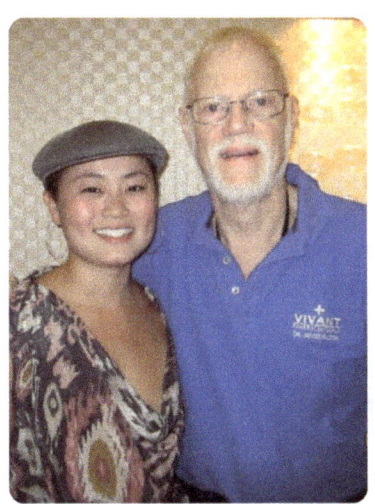

With Dr. James E. Fulton, at his 2011 Advanced Aesthetics training conference.

I then went on to work alongside Laura Cooksey, co-owner and lead esthetician of Face Reality Skincare in San Leandro, CA. It was really satisfying to witness the transformational life changes they experienced (and to perform extractions). I learned that Laura had her own acne cleared up by Oakland-based esthetician Kat Leverette of Clinically Clear Skin Rehab Center of Oakland, CA. Both Laura and Kat had read a very impactful book called *Acne RX* by Dr. James E. Fulton III, and Laura based her practice on his techniques. If there was anyone who knew anything about acne's ins and outs, it was Dr. Fulton, and I was fortunate enough to study with him in person over the years before his death in 2013. Yet, as much as I appreciated my time at Laura's clinic, our treatment and business philosophies started to diverge. And since she had no plans to open a location in San Francisco, I decided to take the leap and open the first holistic acne clinic there.

I started With & Within (then called SkinSALVATION) in Unit #503, a 150-square-foot room within the Activspace building in San Francisco's Mission District overlooking Twin Peaks. It was a great and fun time, as so many brand-new business owners were opening up shops and offices in this brand-new building. The networking with fellow entrepreneurs was off the chain and inspiration wildly contagious. I worked alone seven days a week, and within a few short months, had a year-long, 100+ person wait list. A few clients of mine, inspired by their experience and results from working with me, even went on to beauty school to become estheticians and employees of With & Within. Several of them have gone on to open their own acne clinics. Over time, we grew into a beautiful 1500-square-foot clinic with four treatment rooms in the heart of the Mission District.

The clinic and I were professionally successful, but the years of surviving as a small business (even though we were growing) in a city like San Francisco were tough. Eventually, my mental and physical health started to deteriorate. In 2017, I got really sick as a result of years of stress. I was depressed, cranky all the time, and lethargic, no matter how many hours of sleep I got or how well I ate. Though my conventional medical test results all came back normal, my naturopathic and allopathic integrative doctors confirmed specialized test results that showed particular estrogen hormones directly linked to breast cancer in my system were alarmingly elevated. My cortisol hormone levels were off the charts, and my blood sugar was dangerously high. As a wellness expert already doing all the "healthy lifestyle things," stress was the only other variable I had left to tackle. I had to make a change and practice what I preached to my clients for so many years: to practice self-care and to create and honor boundaries that would preserve my health and happiness, and ultimately, my life.

Running a brick-and-mortar while managing the never-ending operational aspects was literally killing me. How could I keep this work alive, continuing to help folks who really needed it, while preserving my personal quality of life and sanity? It would have been silly and selfish to shut it all down and walk away when so many people could be helped with the exact solution I held in my head and hands. I had to get out of the treatment room, the brick-and-mortar, and start observing it from a bird's-eye view. I had to see the forest through the trees, so to speak.

After observing how several remote clients were able to maintain their skin clarity, I started to see that ongoing treatment, although beneficial, was not necessarily essential for most clients. After all, these people were able to keep their clarity by self-diagnosing and course-correcting by using the lifestyle lessons we taught them in the clinic without relying on the actual facial treatments. Creating and sharing resources that folks could access remotely was also more efficient because we were able to help so many more people in the same time frame with the same effort. In the treatment room, we could only help one person per hour versus using that same hour to write a blog post that hundreds of folks could access, implement, and share. In other words, people didn't need to be saved; they just needed access to the tools to become empowered to save themselves. And maybe, from time to time, be reminded they had these powers within.

Although *skin* was always the focus, the "magic" we were performing in the clinic was really just teaching our clients how to build and maintain a low-inflammatory acne-safe lifestyle, while supporting and holding them accountable to it. The research I did, which was backed by the advice my integrative doctors gave me to manage my stress, hormone, and bloodwork imbalances, was in alignment with all the things we taught our clients for years. It turned out that pretty much everything we told our clients in the treatment room to clear their skin was the same holistic practices integrative practitioners would have their clients use to lower systemic inflammation, calm the nervous system, and rebalance hormones.

In 2023, we changed our name to With & Within to expand our focus around skincare to include all these huge lifestyle components that could be beneficial for everyone, everywhere, not just for, but especially for, those with acne: eating natural, delicious foods with culturally diverse ingredients and flavor profiles. Simple rituals and practices for daily use to help ease the everyday grind of life. Travel to explore new worlds, ways of living, thinking, and being.

This practice and book have been many years in the making, and I am so grateful that you are here to use it. I hope that what you've learned from this changes your life for the better, rippling out to the community and world around you. Thank you for allowing me the chance to help you rediscover the intuition that lies within you to heal and live well. ☺

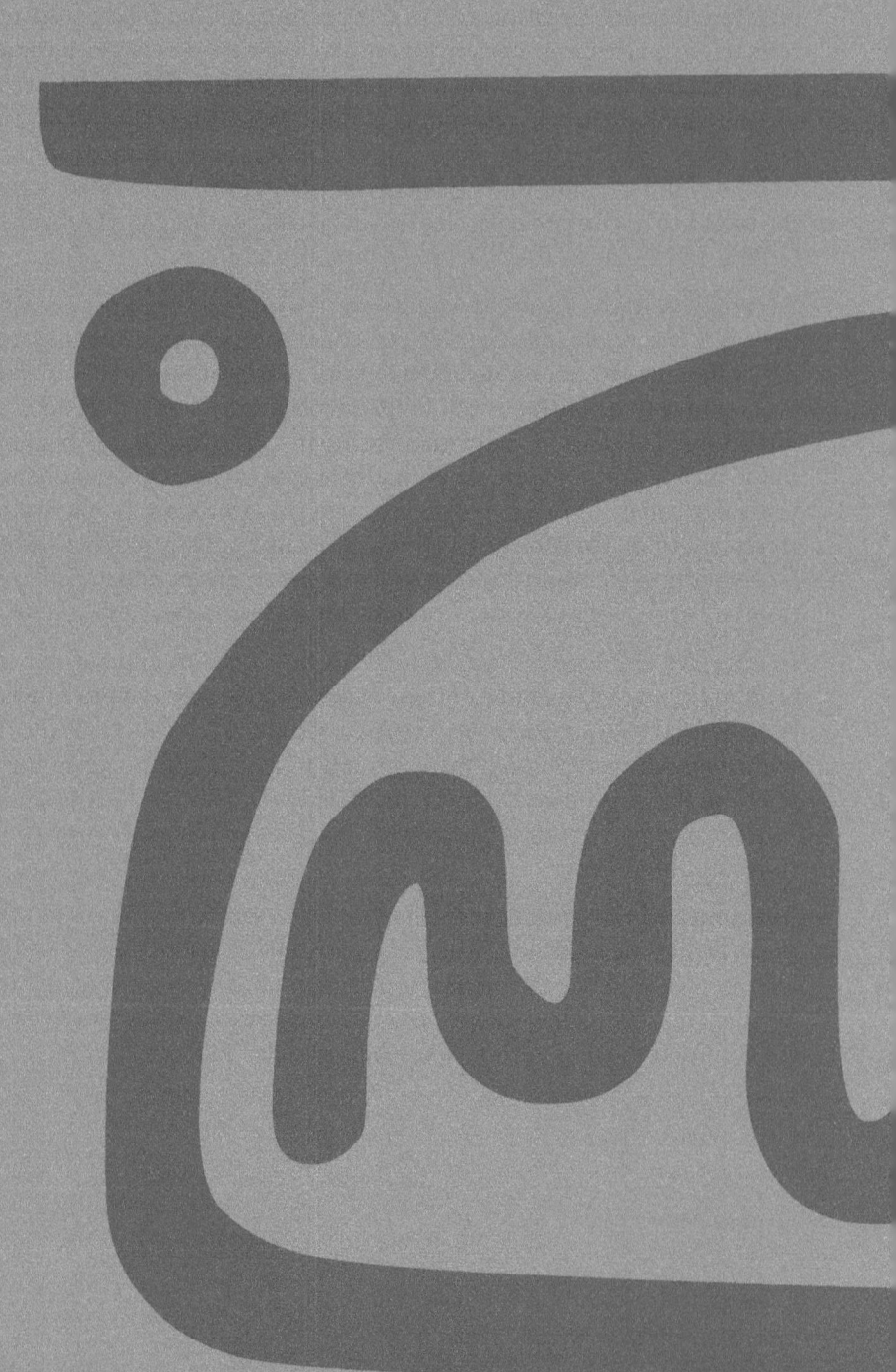

SECTION 13

Glossary

Glossary

Acne "seeds" or Impaction (the root of every Blemish, Breakout, Eruption, Lesion, Pimple, Zit): The accumulation of dead skin cells, oils, comedogenic ingredients, and sometimes hair that clumps together within the base of a pore, causing an obstruction of the pore's natural detoxing function, resulting in what is commonly known as acne. This must be extracted thoroughly in order for the pore to completely clear.

Benzoyl Peroxide: An over-the-counter topical skin ingredient (also commonly found in topical prescription medications, usually combined with antibiotics) used to control acne, and some cases, rosacea. It reduces inflammation and acne formation by drying up the skin's excess oils, releases oxygen into the pore to kill acne-causing bacteria, and exfoliates the cellular walls within to purge acne seeds.

Blackhead: See Sebaceous Filament and Comedone.

Candida Albicans: A type of yeast that is a natural part of a healthy digestive system's bacterial flora. Systemic imbalances such as chronic stress, frequent prescription drug use, or excessive processed food/sugar consumption cause it to overgrow, causing multiple health-related issues, particularly acne management protocol resistance. If left untreated, it can become serious and fatal. Conventional and natural methods of treatment are available.

Comedone: A blocked pore containing an acne seed. Can be open or closed; both are forms of non-inflamed acne. An open comedone, aka blackhead, is a black-capped acne seed or plug that stretches the pore opening wide and appears black at the surface because the oils have oxidized from the air. A closed comedone, aka whitehead, is the same acne seed or plug inside a pore whose opening is shut and not exposed to the air, thus flesh-colored, hiding under the skin's surface.

Dermis: The middle and thickest layers of the skin where blood circulation is rampant, lying just underneath the epidermis and on top of the subcutaneous skin layers. The dermis is where hair follicles, pores, sweat glands, and nerve endings live. If physical damage on the skin reaches this layer of the skin, permanent textural and pigmentation scarring can occur.

Dry Skin: Skin that is naturally lipid/sebum dry all over the face (even the T-zone area), even at the end of the day. Dry skin requires some extra external and internal care to replenish moisture in order to keep the skin flexible, waterproof, and healthy. Skin that is too dry can create cracks in the skin where bacteria, viruses, and other foreign bodies may enter.

Epidermis: The uppermost layers of the skin we can see and touch. This layer is actually made up of dead skin cells that are getting ready to slough off on their own but is also where pigmentation is produced. This layer serves to protect the deeper, blood-filled layers of the skin underneath. You can liken the epidermis to the top crust of a pie, the fruit being the dermis and the bottom crust being the subcutaneous layers.

Exfoliation: The act of removing dead skin cells from the outermost layers of the skin to reveal new skin underneath. This usually results in finer lines and wrinkles, brightened hyperpigmentation, and purging of acne seeds. There are physical, chemical, and enzymatic ways of doing this.

Extractions: Manual removal of acne seeds from the pores, usually and preferably by a licensed esthetician by way of fingers or extraction tools. These must be done carefully to avoid scarring or infection. Depending how deep the pores are, the extraction can be shallow or deep. Complete extractions are a must to ensure the pimple does not recur in the same pore.

Follicle/Pores: The root of every hair has a bulb called the follicle, and the cavity or sac that surrounds it all is called the pore. One of the primary functions of hair is to wick dead skin cells, sebum, and other toxins created at the base of the pore out of it.

Hyperpigmentation: There are two types: vascular (red in color) and post-inflammatory hyperpigmentation (brown in color, aka PIH). Vascular pigmentation happens when blood vessels appear as a trauma response and often (eventually) get reabsorbed by the body. PIH happens when melanocytes create darker pigmentation as a trauma response. As long as there is no acne seed or other debris stuck inside the pore, these marks often naturally fade away on their own. This natural fading may take years or require additional products or treatments to lift.

Icing: Dubbed "the poor man's antibiotic" by Dr. Fulton, this process involves gently applying ice directly onto the skin to calm, prevent inflammation, speed up healing, and drive active products applied afterward to go deeper into the pore—where the acne starts. Often written off as not important, when done consistently, it is an incredible game-changer for the treatment of acne.

Inflamed Acne: A type of acne that presents as red, swollen, and often sore bumps that can be both soft (cystic) or hard (nodular). Once inflammation is down, access to the acne seed is easier, allowing that pore to clear. If left untreated, inflamed acne can grow in size and severity and may eventually leave permanent textural scarring. See Nodules and Cysts.

Keratin: Fibrous structural proteins that make up the skin, hair, and nails of the human body.

LED (light-emitting diode): First developed by NASA to conduct plant growth experiments and eventually pain reduction and wound healing for astronauts in space, LED is a safe and painless skin treatment that uses varying wavelengths of light to treat the skin and body for a variety of conditions and concerns. Blue lights are used for acne-prone skin by killing bacteria and slowing down oil production. Red lights are used to relieve inflammation and boost collagen production for anti-aging purposes, smoothing fine lines and wrinkles. Red lights can also relieve pain and bruising, speed up the skin's healing process, and help with hair loss and psoriasis. Green lights can help with skin cancers, and amber/yellow lights can help relieve redness.

Mallorca Acne: Also known as sun acne, summer acne or *acne aestivalis*, a condition where the skin exhibits allergy-like reactions to the sun's UV rays and fats (in sebum or creams, SPF's). Small 1mm weeping bumps form around hair follicles, often on the body but not usually on the face or neck. It affects about 20% of the population, is prevented by avoiding sun exposure and thick oily creams, and is treated with BP gel or adapalene along with sunburn remedies such as applying cold packs or soothing ingredients like witch hazel or chamomile extract. Also see Section 4, The Acne-Safe Lifestyle, Polymorphous Light Eruption (or Heat Rash).

Melanocytes: Cells that are primarily responsible for the color of our skin, located in the deepest layers of the epidermis. They are also responsible for emitting excess pigment in response to trauma, injury, or inflammation, such as in the case of post-inflammatory pigmentation after a cut or inflamed pimple heals.

Nodules and Cysts (also see Inflamed Acne): Both are more advanced types of inflamed acne. Nodules are inflamed acne lesions that measure 1 cm and below, are hard to the touch, and may be painful. Cysts are inflamed acne lesions that measure larger than 1cm, are are soft and sometimes hot to the touch, are filled with pus or other semi-liquid/solid, are usually painful, and can be purple or blue due to blood collecting under the surface.

Non-inflamed Acne: A type of acne that presents as small, often densely packed, usually painless, skin-colored bumps, not to be confused with sebaceous filaments. See Comedone and Sebaceous Filament.

Normal/Combination Skin: The most common skin type where the skin is neither oily nor dry after washing, but in the afternoon, the T-zone area is often (but not necessarily) oilier than the cheeks. The differences between the two aren't necessarily extreme but can be affected by the season, environment, diet, and stress.

Oily Skin: Oily skin is greasy to the touch all over the face, including on the cheeks, within an hour or so after washing. This is usually part of one's natural genetic makeup, but overproduction of sebum can be exacerbated by lifestyle, diet, internal and external factors, and using products that are too moisturizing for the skin.

Over-Exfoliation: This happens when active products (with exfoliating ingredients) are overused so much that visible superficial wrinkling and flaky peeling skin is a result. Often this can be accompanied by a tight and shiny appearance, dehydration, redness, general irritation, and sensitivity.

Pus: A white, yellow or even green liquid containing white blood cells that the body creates as a defense mechanism against bacteria. Left untreated, pus can digest living skin tissue, resulting in textural scarring.

Retention Hyperkeratosis: Retention means keeping. "Hyper" means too quickly or too much. Keratosis is the overgrowth of skin cells. Coined by 1970s' acne researcher Dr. Albert Kligman in relation to acne, this term means too many dead skin cells are shed and get stuck in the pore. When they clump together, they create an acne impaction, or acne seed.

Sebaceous Filament: Commonly and erroneously called "blackheads," these are plugs made of sebum in the pores, are typically the same size, and are usually found on the nose, chin, and sometimes upper cheeks near the nose. These behave differently than acne in that they do not get inflamed or turn into pimples and will always come back no matter how much you try to remove them. They plug up the pores to prevent bacteria from entering the body and help facilitate moisturizing sebum to come up to the surface of the skin. For the real blackhead, see Comedone.

Sebaceous Hyperplasia: Most common in oily skin types, these are overactive pores whose skin cells proliferate, almost erupting onto the surface of the skin. These pores look like tiny volcanoes with the pore opening acting as a tiny crater for the oil to come out of. Some are treatable with TCA peels or cauterization but usually come back, thus requiring maintenance treatments.

Sebum/Oil/Lipids: Made up of a combination of fats, cholesterols, and fatty acids, this is what the skin naturally creates in order to stay lubricated, flexible, and waterproof. It's part of the skin's natural barrier function against bacteria and debris from entering the body.

Seeds: See Acne Seeds.

Sensitive/Sensitized Skin: Skin that is prone to unpleasant reactions (burning, stinging, pain, redness, inflammation, general discomfort) from stimuli that's normally well tolerated by the general public. There are two types that are commonly confused with each other: sensitive and sensitized. Truly sensitive skin is a long-term condition from genetics or as a result of trauma, disease, or major allergic reaction that cannot tolerate much stimulation or products, active or not. Sensitized skin is a short-term acute condition as a response to an external factor; the skin eventually heals, and with careful reintroduction, can reacclimate to using the active product again safely.

Sloughing: When your skin sheds, revealing newer layers of skin underneath. See Exfoliation.

Under-exfoliated: This happens when active products (with exfoliating ingredients) are so underused that there are little to no visible results. Often, this can be accompanied by a dull, lackluster complexion due to the buildup of dead skin cells.

"Choose good habits, choose good products, choose honest experts and there is no doubt that With & Within will improve your life!"

- LT

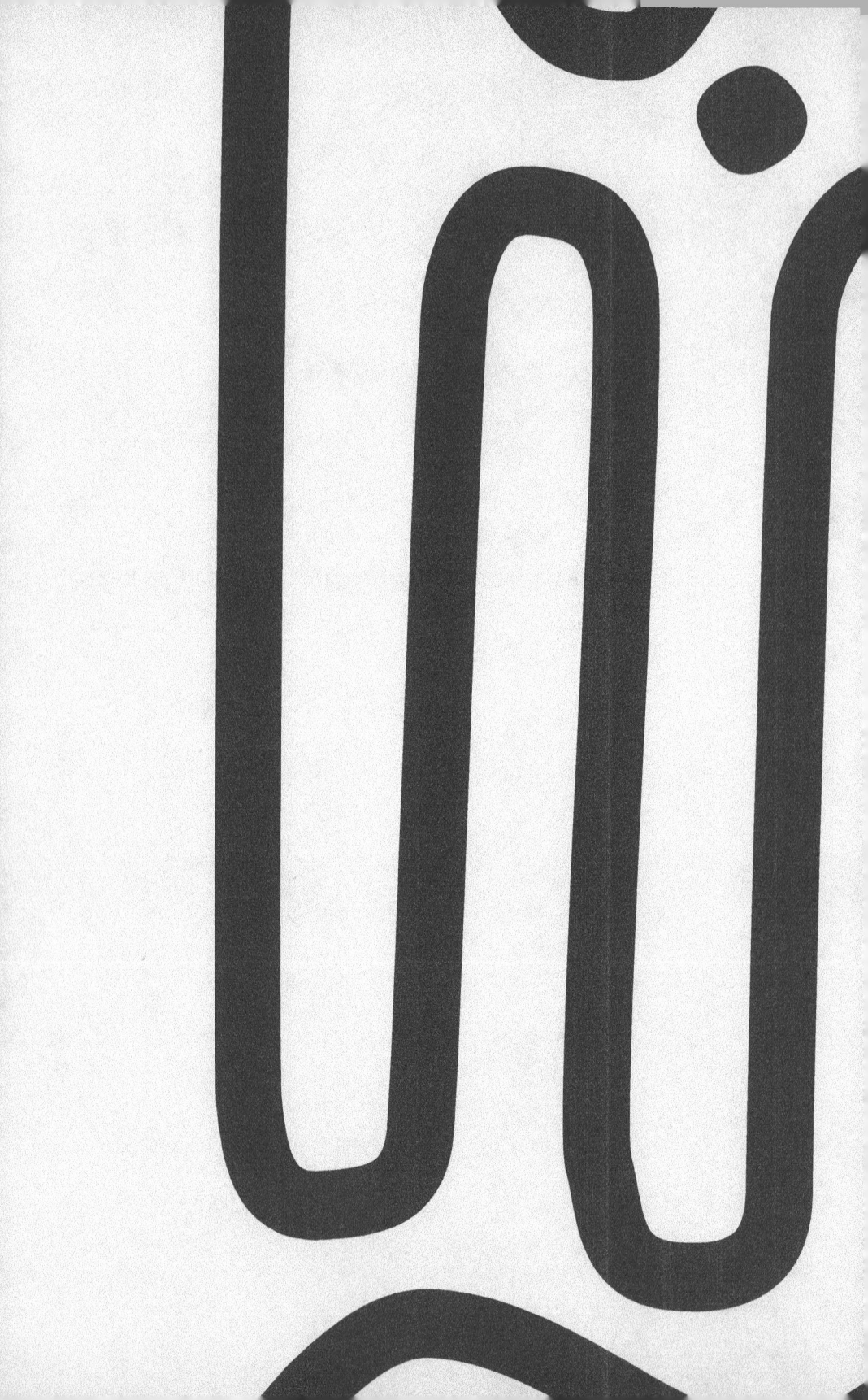

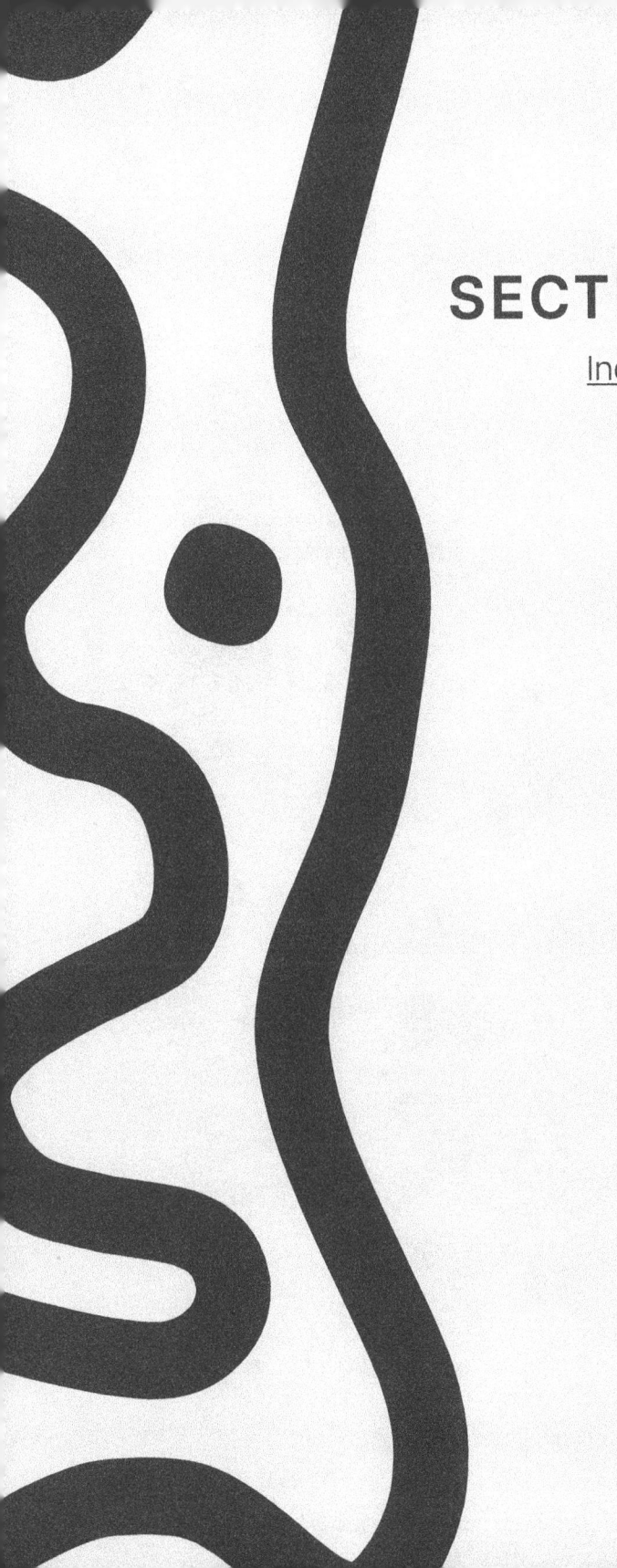

SECTION 14
Index

Index

A

Accutane, 130, 140
    See also isotretinoin
acne
    about, 26
    acne aestivalis, 322
    acne cosmetica, 119, 162
    acne mechanica, 119
    acne seeds, 26, 112–113, 115–116, 118, 320
    acneiform drug eruptions, 130–131, 231–233
    bacteria and, 118
    blackheads, 115–116
    body acne, 119–120
    comedones, 115–116, 320
    dietary acne, 122
    face map, 197–199
    genetics and, 112, 162, 274
    inflamed acne, 117–118, 133–137, 260, 261, 262–263, 321–322
    inflamed vs. non-inflamed, 262–263
    Mallorca acne, 120–121, 322
    non-inflamed acne, 115–116, 132–133, 322
    picking, 102–107, 119, 279, 302–305
    recurring, 120
    stress and, 151
    types of, 119–125
acneiforms, 124, 125–131

Acne Rx (Fulton), 299, 315
adrenaline, 151
affirmations, 19
allergy medicines, 233
Alpha Hydroxy Acids (AHAs), 43–44
androgen-rich foods, 89, 158, 199, 227
Anstett, Thomas, 239, 242, 243
anti-aging tips, 290–291
antibiotics, 53, 117, 118, 125, 139, 239
antidepressants, 232–233
artificial sweeteners, 225
Ayurveda
    about, 144–145
    on acne, 145–146
    on Candida, 240–241
    on dairy, 219
    eating alone, 206
    heating foods, 196
    oil pulling, 56
    on rosacea, 126
    warm beverages, 207

B

bacteria, 118
bacterial folliculitis, 129–130
barber shops, 165
beard burn, 184
beauty salons, 165
belly massage, 208

Section 14 - Index

benzoyl peroxide (BP), 45–50, 84–85, 119–120, 290, 301, 320
Beta Hydroxy Acid (BHA), 43
birth control, 121, 124, 158, 185, 231–232
blackheads, 115–116
blood sugar, 154, 207
blue lights, 322
body acne, 119–120
The Body Ecology Diet (Gates), 245
body-focused repetitive behaviors (BFRB), 102, 279, 302–305
body lotions, 182
body scrubs, 91–92
bowel movements. *See* elimination
bromides, 124, 228
bug sprays, 194–195
bulletproof drinks, 223

C

caffeine, 121, 124, 126, 239
camping, 192–195
Candida yeast imbalance
    anti-fungal medications, 240
    cause of, 238–239
    cleanse program, 241–253
    described, 18, 124–125, 238, 320
    die-off symptoms, 243
    herbal remedies for, 242–243
    physical symptoms, 239–240
    psychological symptoms, 240
Can-Sol, 242
carminatives, 207
carrageenan, 219, 228
Charcoal Cleanser, 29, 60, 98, 300
chemical peels, 141, 252, 259
chocolate, 230
chronic pain, 155

cigarettes, 235
cleansers, 60, 73–74, 300–301
clearing process
    about, 50–52
    purging, 20–21, 66–68
    what to expect, 20–21, 65–69
    See also products
coconut oil, 246
coffee, 123, 124, 156, 158, 222–223, 239
cold medicines, 233
colonic cleansing, 165, 290
combination skin, 27, 30–32, 323
comedogenicity, 34–35
comedones, 115–116, 320
constipation, 187, 208, 210, 211, 213–214
Cooksey, Laura, 12, 17, 313, 315
cortisol, 151, 153, 159, 176, 222
cosmetic tattoos, 165
cystic acne, 117, 118
    See also inflamed acne
cysts, 117, 322

D

dairy, 218–221, 246
dating, 183–185
Davis, Leola, 159
deep breathing, 19
dehydration, 33, 187, 188
deodorant, 182–183
dermaplaning, 169
dermis, 320
diet
    an acne-safe diet, 216–218
    for Candida cleanse, 246–251
    coffee, 123, 124, 156, 158, 222–223, 239

dairy, 218–221, 246
fermented foods, 207, 212, 247
food cravings, 152
grains, 217, 225, 227
healthy fats, 213
high-androgen foods, 89, 158, 199, 227
nightshades, 217, 225, 227
peanuts, 90, 123, 158, 227
restaurants, 230–231
soy products, 123, 156, 158, 220, 221, 233–234
sugars, 18, 224–226
sweets, 229–230
vegetarian diet, 216
water-rich foods, 214–215
while traveling, 186, 189–190
young adult men and, 156–157
dietary acne, 122
digestion
brain-gut connection, 205
carminatives, 207
chewing and, 204–205
constipation, 187, 208, 210, 211, 213–214
elimination, 213–216
fiber, 211
herbal teas, 207, 210–211
hydrochloric acid (HCl), 212–213
mindful eating, 206
probiotics, 207, 211, 212
soft foods, 205
stress and, 152–154
travel and, 188, 191, 193
yoga poses for, 208–209
dimethicones, 38, 39, 57, 100
dinner parties, 190
drug-induced folliculitis. *See* acneiform drug eruptions
drugstore products, 140

dry cleaning, 178
dry skin, 27, 28–29, 88, 89, 320–321

E

electrolysis, 168
electrolytes, 187, 188, 214, 215–216
elimination, 213–216, 252
See also constipation
enzymes, 212, 239
epidermis, 321
estheticians
chemical peels, 259
finding, 256–258
products and, 258–259
tools and, 259–260, 270–271
treatments and, 260–262
estrogen, 156, 157, 159
exercise
cold weather sports, 176
high-intensity, 154–155, 175, 176–177
as self-care, 163
skincare and, 171–175
swimming, 176
weightlifting, 175, 176
exfoliation, 33, 42–45, 114, 141, 166, 173, 321
extractions, 103–107, 114, 141, 260, 261, 270, 321
eyeglasses, 178–180

F

face maps, 144, 197–199
face washing, 70–74, 88
facials, 163
females with acne, 156, 157–158

fermented foods, 207, 212, 247
fertility treatments, 158
fiber, 211
fight-or-flight response, 151
fish oil supplements, 213
follicles, 321
food cravings, 152
foods. See diet
foundation, 96–97, 302
friction-induced acne, 119
fruit, 225–226
Fulton, James E.
    about, 12, 17, 299
    acne protocol, 139
    Acne Rx, 299, 315
    on benzoyl peroxide, 12, 45
    on dimethicones, 57
    on icing, 76
    on iodides, 219
    on oils, 56, 61, 71
    on pyoderma faciale, 131
    on retinols, 43
    on stubborn body acne, 120
    on teenage acne, 156

G

Gates, Donna, 242, 245
gender-affirming therapy, 124, 158–159
Gershon, Michael D., 152
ginger, 210, 222
glycolic acid, 43
golden milk, 223
grains, 217, 225, 227
Gua Sha, 183

H

hair
    hair products, 92–93, 100–101
    hair salons, 165
    heat styling, 101
    textured hair, 59
hair removal
    dermaplaning, 169
    ingrown hairs, 166–167, 168, 169–171
    laser hair removal, 168
    metal spring tool, 169
    shaving, 166–168
    threading, 168–169
    waxing, 168
haldi doodh, 223
halogen drugs, 130, 131
hand cream, 182
hats, 180–181
heat rash, 196–197
helmets, 180–181
herbal remedies, 210, 242–243
herbal teas, 207, 210–211, 222–223
herpes simplex, 126–127
high-androgen foods, 89, 158, 199, 227
high frequency machines, 270–271
high glycemic foods, 122, 224–226
hirsutism, 171
hormones
    about, 123–124, 150–151
    adrenaline, 151
    cortisol, 151, 153, 159, 176, 222
    estrogen, 156, 157, 159
    reproductive hormones, 90, 121, 123, 155–159
    serotonin, 152, 153
    testosterone, 156, 157, 159

hormone shots, 121, 232
hot springs, 164–165
hot tubs, 165, 176, 228
hyaluronic acid, 43, 83
Hydrating Cleanser, 28, 30, 60, 289, 300
Hydrating Cream, 28, 29, 30, 60, 289, 301–302
Hydrating Gel, 28, 47, 48, 60, 196, 301–302
Hydrating Toner, 289, 302
hydrochloric acid (HCl), 212–213
hyperpigmentation, 44, 120, 292, 293–295, 321

I

icing, 25, 74–77, 166, 167, 188, 191, 321
Illuminare foundation, 96-97, 302
improvement
    not seeing, 278–284
    speed of, 15, 20, 112, 262
inflamed acne, 117–118, 133–137, 260, 261, 262–263, 321–322
inflammation, 118, 188–189, 222, 224, 227
infrared saunas, 164
ingrown hairs, 166, 167, 168, 169–171
insoluble fiber, 211
intersex, 157
iodide acne, 130–131, 137
iodides, 124, 130–131, 228, 233
isotretinoin, 129, 130, 131, 140, 159
IUDs, 124, 232

J

jade rolling, 183

jet lag, 188

K

keratin, 322
keratosis pilarsis, 127

L

lactic acid, 43
laser hair removal, 168
laundry, 70, 177–178, 184, 191
laundry detergent, 119, 178, 191
leaky gut, 239
LED treatments, 68, 270–271, 322
Lester, Tiffany, 152, 165
Leverette, Kat, 108, 315
lifestyle changes, 162

M

magnesium, 211, 214, 216
makeup
    brushes and sponges, 98–99
    dyes in, 95-96
    ingredient lists, 94–95
    mineral makeup, 64, 96–97
    removing, 71–72
malassezia folliculitis, 128–129
males with acne, 156–157
malic acid, 43
Mallorca acne, 120–121, 322
mandelic acid, 43, 44
Mandelic Toner, 44, 289, 291, 301
massage oils, acne-safe, 163–164
massages, 163–164
McBride, Kami, 207

meats, 89, 158, 227, 246, 247
medications. See prescription medications
meditation, 19
melanocytes, 322
melatonin, 159, 188
menopause, 156
menstruation, 123, 157
milia, 116
moisturizers, 60–63, 85, 182, 301–302
mosquito bites, 194–195

N

nightshades, 217, 225, 227
nodular acne, 117, 118
    See also inflamed acne
nodules, 117, 322
non-inflamed acne, 115–116, 132–133, 322
normal skin. See combination skin
nut milk, 220
nutrition. *See* diet

O

oil pulling, 56
oily skin, 27, 29–30, 46, 89–90, 323
The Omnivore's Dilemma (Pollan), 218, 305
OptiZinc, 77, 189, 283
oral contraceptives, 124, 232
over-exfoliation, 33, 81, 87, 323

P

pain, 155
paleo diet, 218
papules, 117
papulopustular eruptions. *See* acneiform drug eruptions
PCOS (Polycystic Ovarian Syndrome), 121, 154, 157, 158
peanuts, 90, 123, 158, 227
perioral dermatitis, 127–128
Perricone, Nicholas, 158
pets, 185
picaridin, 195
picking, 102–107, 119, 279, 302–305
pillowcases, 177, 184, 191
pimples. See cysts; nodules
Plan B pill, 185
pockmarks. See scarring
Pollan, Michael, 218, 305
polymorphous light eruption (PMLE). See heat rash
pores, 321
post-inflammatory hyperpigmentation (PIH), 293, 321
PPE masks, 181
pregnancy, 121, 123, 157–158
prescription medications, 121, 124, 131, 231–233
Price, Weston A., 218
probiotics, 207, 211, 212, 239
product checker, 299–300
products
    about, 34–36
    auditing, 52–55
    cleansers, 60, 73–74, 300–301
    comedogenicity, 34–35, 57–59
    demographic brands, 58–59
    drugstore products, 140

fragrance, 56–57
low pH, 36
moisturizers, 60, 85, 301–302
oils, 56, 58, 61
order of layering, 78
packing, 186
serums, 81–84, 291
sunscreen, 28, 36–41, 63–64, 139, 193–194, 291, 302
toner, 79–81
underusing, 87–88, 279
vitamin E, 55, 58
With & Within, 300–302
protein powders, 228–229
psyllium husk, 211
puberty, 123, 156
purging, 20–21, 66–68
pus, 117, 118, 323
pustules, 117
pyoderma faciale, 131

R

red lights, 322
regimen. See skincare regimen
reproductive hormones, 90, 121, 123, 155–159
restaurant dining, 230–231
retention hyperkeratosis, 112, 323
retinols, 43
rosacea, 77, 125–126, 131

S

Safeguard SPF 40, 39, 63, 176, 302
salicylic acid, 43
saunas, 164
scarring, 118, 293

sebaceous filaments, 116, 260, 323
sebaceous hyperplasia, 323–324
seeds. See acne seeds
self-care, 12, 163
self-compassion, 20
self-tanners, 182
Selye, Hans, 150
sensitive skin, 32, 324
sensitized skin, 32, 324
serotonin, 152, 153
serums, 81–84, 291, 301
shaving, 166–168
shea butter, 29, 31, 32, 56
shower tips, 90–94
shrimp, 130, 137
silicones, 38, 39, 57, 100
Simple Habit meditation app, 19
skincare regimen
    adjusting, 85–89, 281–284, 289–291
    applying products, 78–85
    face washing, 70–74, 88
    icing, 74–77
    for maintenance, 288–292
    shower tips, 90–94
skin types, 27–32
sleep, 152, 159, 184, 188
sloughing, 324
smoking, 235
soluble fiber, 211
soybean oil, 55, 124, 233–234
soy products, 123, 156, 158, 220, 221, 233–234
SPF (Sun Protection Factor), 36, 40–41
See also sunscreen
spironolactone, 140
steroid acne, 130
steroids, 126, 130, 131, 234
stress

about, 123–124, 150
chronic stress, 153
fight-or-flight response, 151
See also hormones
sugaring, 168
sugars, 18, 224–226
summer acne, 322
sun acne, 322
sunburn remedies, 322
sunscreen, 28, 36–41, 63–64, 139, 193–194, 291, 302
supplements, 189, 233–234
sweets, 229–230
swimming, 176

T

teenagers, 156
teeth brushing, 72
testosterone, 156, 157, 159
textual scarring, 118, 293
threading, 168–169
thyroid issues, 158, 233
tocopherol, 55
toner, 79–81
Traditional Chinese Medicine (TCM)
    about, 142–143
    on acne, 142–144
    on Candida, 241
    on dairy, 219
    face maps and, 144
    heating foods, 196
    on rosacea, 126
    warm beverages, 207
transgender, 157, 158–159
travel
    camping, 192–195
    climate considerations, 187
    diet and, 186, 189–190

jet lag, 188
packing skincare products, 186
turmeric lattes, 223

U

under-exfoliated skin, 324

V

vitamins, 233–234

W

water, drinking, 207, 214–216, 222, 243
waxing, 168
Weil, Andrew, 219–220
whitehead. *See* comedones
With & Within
    acne face map 197-199
    chemical peel patch testing, 271
    esthetician training, 266–267
    initial consultation, 268–272
    popzits, 273–274
    product audit, 272
    products, 300–302
    skin analysis, 270
    treatments, 267–268
Wu Wei, 16–17

Z

Zyflamend, 77, 189, 283

Photo credits

Shutterstock
Mariana M: Blackhead, page 115

Yurakrasil: Whitehead, page 115

Marina Demeshko: Sebaceous filament, page 116, top image

ThamKC: Sebaceous filament, page 116, bottom image

Vchal: Milia, page 116, left milia image

Nau Nau: Milia, page 116, right image

Zay Nyi Nyi: Papule, page 117

Ukki Studio: Pustule, page 117

Gnepphoto: Cyst, page 117

Science Photo Library
Dr. P. Marazzi: Nodule, page 117

skinSALVATION inc. and skinSALVATION skincare inc.
Before & After Photos

Clinic Photos

Photo with Dr. James Fulton

Rezel Apacionado
rezelkealoha.com

Product photos

Lauren Tabak
laurentabak.com

Author Photo

www.ingramcontent.com/pod-product-compliance
Lightning Source LLC
Chambersburg PA
CBHW070802040426
42333CB00061B/1794